Brain-Robbers

Brain-Robbers

How Alcohol, Cocaine, Nicotine, and Opiates Have Changed Human History

Frances R. Frankenburg, MD

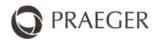 PRAEGER

AN IMPRINT OF ABC-CLIO, LLC
Santa Barbara, California • Denver, Colorado • Oxford, England

Library of Congress Cataloging-in-Publication Data

Frankenburg, Frances Rachel, author.
   Brain-robbers : how alcohol, cocaine, nicotine, and opiates have changed human history / Frances R. Frankenburg.
     p. ; cm.
   Includes bibliographical references and index.
   ISBN 978–1–4408–2931–4 (alk. paper) — ISBN 978–1–4408–2932–1 (eISBN) I. Title.
[DNLM: 1. Substance-Related Disorders—history. 2. Behavior, Addictive—history.
3. Brain—drug effects. WM 11.1]
RC564 .F73 20H
362.29—dc23   2013040015

ISBN: 978–1–4408–2931–4
EISBN: 978–1–4408–2932–1

18 17 16 15   3 4 5

This book is also available on the World Wide Web as an eBook.
Visit www.abc-clio.com for details.

Praeger
An Imprint of ABC-CLIO, LLC

ABC-CLIO, LLC
130 Cremona Drive, P.O. Box 1911
Santa Barbara, California 93116-1911

This book is printed on acid-free paper ∞

Manufactured in the United States of America

The letter from Freud to Fleiss is reprinted by permission of the publisher from *The Complete Letters of Sigmund Freud to Wilhelm Fleiss, 1887–1904*, translated and edited by Jeffrey Moussaieff Masson, pp. 116–117, Cambridge, MA: Belknap Press of Harvard University Press, Freud Correspondence, Copyright © 1985 and under the Bern Convention by Sigmund Freud Copyrights. Copyright © 1985 J. M. Masson for translation and editorial matter. By permission of the Marsh Agency Ltd on behalf of Sigmund Freud Copyrights.

Contents

Acknowledgments

I am grateful to the following: Ross Baldessarini, Ruth Becker, Sandy Becker, Greg Binus, Isis Burgos-Chapman, Debbie Carvalko, Gary Cole, Lucy Cole, Lindsey Conkey, Andrea Cordani, Nitigna Desai, Charles Drebing, Marguerite Foley, Charles Frankenburg, Robert Frankenburg, Susi Frankenburg, Fran Grace, Ela Grynberg, Larry Herz, Megan Kelly, Bill Lebovich, Shannon LeMaster, Alan Mandell, Joan Margeson, Jennifer O'Leary, Mark Oldham, Doreen Perry, Ania Terajewicz, Joan Tycko, and Mary Zanarini.

Introduction

Friends and family linger over a meal with a bottle of wine. A young man chews some coca leaf before descending into a mine in Bolivia. An anxious and bored soldier lights a cigarette. A nurse relieves a patient's pain by administering a morphine injection. Alcohol, cocaine, nicotine, and opiates are four plant-derived molecules that please our senses, energize and distract us, lessen our pain, and generally improve our lives. When used to excess, a different picture emerges.

History can be viewed through the lens of these four valued substances. Even though politics, personalities, and the horrors of war usually take center stage in history, the story of humanity is played out on a wider stage. What people choose to drink, snort, smoke, or inject is influenced by thousands of years of agriculture, civilization, and exploration, and, in turn, these choices have changed the world.

At the time of the American Revolution, rum and tobacco satisfied the hunger of people for mind and mood-altering substances. People were willing to pay good prices for these two products, even though neither was essential for physical health or prosperity. This successful commerce, founded on the backs of slaves in the southern states and the Caribbean, fueled the economic foundation of the United States. The chapters about alcohol and nicotine will put these enterprises into a greater context.

Another example has to do with a little-known trade triangle between England, India, and China. Opium was illegal in China, but England sold Indian-grown opium to the Chinese anyway, waving the flag of "free trade." England wanted Chinese tea and porcelain, and to get these goods she traded cloth and machinery to India and then opium from India to

China. This drug trafficking infuriated the Chinese and precipitated the Opium Wars that began the "century of humiliation" for China. Mao Zedong eventually rid China of opium, but nicotine addiction now plagues that country. A separate chapter in this book describes the Opium Wars in some detail.

Some people become dependent on these substances. Dependent people are steady customers, and this means that selling drugs is good business. The notion of taxing this business is irresistible. Taxes on molasses (distilled to make rum) were one of the irritants that sparked the American Revolution. A few years after the Revolution, George Washington, now responsible for paying for a government himself, used military force against Americans who were protesting tax on whiskey. Governments become addicted to the revenue from these substances. However, sometimes, concerned about harm, legislators ban the substance, as happened in the United States with Prohibition. When governments step in to prohibit, criminals rush in to smuggle. Societies are often unsure of whether to ban, regulate, tax, or prohibit some substances.

People get so much pleasure from these substances that they do not need much persuasion to use them. The exception is nicotine. Some of the advertising of the tobacco companies is described in the chapter about nicotine and also in the chapter about women and cigarettes.

These small molecules have such intriguing, helpful, and damaging effects that they have fascinated scientists and have been part of many academic discoveries. For example, a debate raged among nineteenth-century scientists about the nature of fermentation, the seemingly miraculous process by which ordinary sugar is changed to alcohol. In a similar way, scientists have wondered how it is that opiates, coming from the simple poppy, a flower that blooms and dies in a few months, can lead to such powerful effects on us. Scientists investigating these puzzles have made advances that have changed our understanding of how our bodies work. These substances loom large in the history of medicine.

Although a theme of this book is the global importance of these four substances in the stories of empires, commerce, and biochemistry, we will also examine the effect of these substances on the lives of some individuals and families. Some of these people changed the ways in which these four substances were used.

The politically powerful Adams family of the United States was touched by alcohol in many ways—some good, some bad. Lydia Pinkham, a Quaker teacher from Massachusetts, created best-selling patent medicines that were sold in bottles identified by a label with her face.

She and her family profited from her kindly visage and her alcohol-filled potions. Carry Nation was another well-known American woman of the nineteenth century who preached fervently against alcohol and tobacco. She vandalized saloons and stirred the pot of temperance that bubbled over to lead to Prohibition.

William Stewart Halsted, one of the most creative American physicians, invented a form of cocaine anesthesia and yet throughout most of his distinguished medical career, he was addicted to cocaine and morphine. Sigmund Freud started his career by writing excited papers about cocaine and ended his life with a morphine overdose because of tobacco-caused cancer.

The body organ most affected by substance abuse is, of course, the brain. Each of these four substances leads to pleasure through the aptly named "reward pathway" in the brain. These four molecules slip into the brain and interfere with the working of the brain's *own* molecules—the neurotransmitters. The reward pathway is slippery. Some people can use these substances for pleasure or relief of anxiety, but others are unable to be moderate in their use, and this leads to addiction, which is the ongoing use of substances despite the harm that they cause. Why would someone persist in such an activity? The various theories about addiction are described in a separate chapter.

The history of the use of substances goes back to the beginnings of civilization. Technology plays a role. Distillation, known to the Babylonians and perfected by the Celts, leads to stronger alcoholic beverages than does simple fermentation. The invention of the syringe made it easier to use drugs—both for good and for bad; the creation of the cigarette on the other hand has only benefited tobacco companies. Chemical advances, such as the isolation of cocaine and morphine, the active ingredients of the coca leaf and opium, have made it possible to use these substances in pure forms. The addition of acetyl groups to morphine resulted in heroin, a substance more addictive than opium or morphine. A disconcerting theme of this book is that these advances have made addiction easier.

1

Alcohol

Introduction

Alcohol, or ethanol, is a simple molecule with complicated effects. It consists of only nine atoms (two carbons, six hydrogens, and one oxygen) and is produced by yeast, a modest single-celled fungus. Alcohol, a tasteless liquid that is a valued part of many religious and social occasions, is also the cause of much illness and violence.

The other substances of this book—cocaine, nicotine, and opiates—can be smoked, snorted, or swallowed. Alcohol is consumed only as a beverage or as a liquid in cooking. But alcohol makes up for this by having a large range of flavors, preparations, qualities, and prices. Alcohol is unique among the substances discussed in this book in its association with food. The other substances suppress hunger, but alcohol increases the appetite and itself contains calories.

Alcoholic beverages are not difficult to produce and have therefore been consumed in most civilizations. Fermentation of any substance with a high enough sugar content will yield alcohol. The Mayans made balché from fermented honey. The Aztecs fermented agave and made pulque that continues to be drunk in Mexico. Mead was (and still is) made from honey. When infected by a mold, rice can turn into an alcoholic drink, and rice wine is drunk in parts of Asia. The alcoholic beverages of greatest importance to the Western world, and which will be reviewed in this chapter, are those made from grains, grapes, and the sugar cane.

The oldest and best-known alcoholic beverages in Western civilization are beer, produced by the fermentation of germinated barley or other starchy grains, and wine, produced by the fermentation of grapes. Other beverages are more potent because they are distilled. Rum results from the distillation of the liquid that is produced by the fermentation of molasses, which is a by-product of sugar cane cultivation. Whiskey is distilled grain alcohol. Some alcoholic drinks such as gin or absinthe are known less by what is fermented and more by what is added to them as flavorings.

Alcohol has complex effects on the mind and body. Moderate alcohol consumption is pleasurable and enhances creative or social experiences. It is associated with longevity, perhaps because of the beneficial effects of small amounts of alcohol on blood lipids or its ability to lower stress.

Some people drink alcohol in large amounts to become intoxicated. For example, college students drink as much beer as rapidly as possible in drinking contests. Sports fans drink heavily when their team wins; they drink heavily when their team loses. A homeless person drinks mouthwash. This kind of drinking causes havoc. Heavy use of alcohol is an aggravating factor in many illnesses and suicides, and is also harmful to the nondrinker. Drunken drivers injure or kill others, and intoxicated people may be violent. Of the four substances discussed in this book, alcohol is the most dangerous to the unborn.

Beer

Beer is one of the most widely consumed and oldest beverages in the world. It exists in many forms and therefore has many names—beer, ale, lager, stout, and porter. Beer can be made from a number of plants, but since it is most commonly made from barley, that will be the type of beer discussed in this book.

How Beer Is Brewed

"Brewing" refers to steeping a substance in water to infuse the water with the flavors and qualities of that substance. While other popular beverages, such as coffee and tea, are brewed, beer is probably the quintessential example of brewing.

The first step of beer brewing is to convert the barley grain's starch into fermentable sugars. Remarkably, this is done by the grain itself. The barley grains are soaked in water and begin to germinate. Enzymes within the barley soften the outer layer of the seed, and rootlets poke out in preparation for a new plant. At the same time, other barley enzymes break down the starch in the grains to sugars, including maltose. These sugars provide energy for the plant that is about to develop. If the grain does become a young barley plant, the opportunity to make beer has been lost. The brewer must heat the germinating grain at just the right moment to stop the growth of the barley. Once the brewer does that, he has formed malt. The malt, once again, is soaked in water, and "mashing" begins. Although the germination has been halted, enzymes continue the conversion of starch to sugars, and the result is a sweet liquid known as mash or wort.

The wort is boiled with hops. The hops import the characteristic bitterness of beer and also help to preserve it. Yeast is added to the wort, and—finally—fermentation begins. Yeast enzymes change the maltose and other sugars into alcohol and carbon dioxide, and beer is formed. In the twenty-first century, beer is usually filtered to remove yeast and any other solids so that the final product is clear.

Beer in Ancient Civilizations

Beer, a humble drink, has an ancient and distinguished lineage. The domestication and cultivation of barley and other grains occurred in the Fertile Crescent (present-day Iraq, Syria, Lebanon, Israel, Jordan, and parts of Turkey, Iran, and Egypt) (see Figure 1.1). In the many lists of activities that differentiate humans from other animals, agriculture is always included. No other animal species cultivates land. Agriculture began just a few thousand years ago and is one of the most studied and debated activities of early humanity. Beer was present at the beginning of agriculture.

In about 12,000 BCE, populations in the Fertile Crescent stopped their nomadic practices of following after grazing herds. They settled down to cultivate grassy plants and then harvest and cook the grains. This was the beginning of agriculture, a more efficient way of producing food than either nomadic pastoralism or hunting.

The first farming was based on the three "noble grasses," or cereal crops—wheat, rice, and barley. These plants grow, mature, and form seeds each year. The seeds, or grains, are embryos for new plants. Encased in tough husks, they are rich with carbohydrates, proteins, and vitamins—useful for new plants or for hungry animals, including humans. Once the grain is harvested, the tough husk means that the seeds can be stored away for future consumption or for planting. Barley is the most easily grown of these plants (see Figure 1.2).

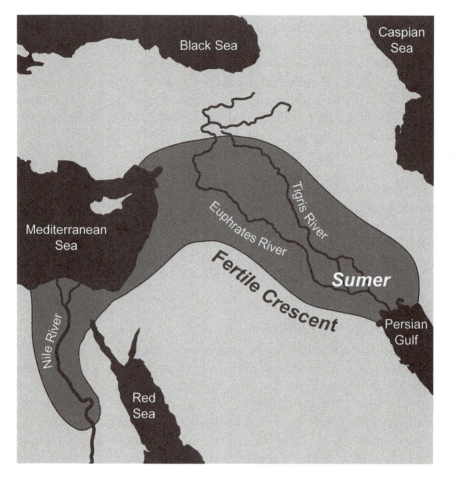

Figure 1.1   Fertile Crescent. (© 2013 Joan M.K. Tycko)

The first creation of a beverage from germinated grains might have happened in Sumer. Sumer was located in Mesopotamia (now known as Iraq), between the Tigris and Euphrates Rivers, and existed for about 3,000 years between about 5000 BCE and 2000 BCE. During this time, the Sumerians developed an efficient agricultural system that freed some Sumerians from the labor of providing food. They had the time and energy to develop other interests, including shipbuilding, sculpting, and carpentry. Cities, such as Sumer and Ur, were born.

The Sumerians, along with the Egyptians, were the first recorded people to develop a written language, using cuneiform script on clay tablets. This script was formed by wedge-shaped reeds that marked wet clay. Perhaps other early cultures had written language, but the Sumerians get

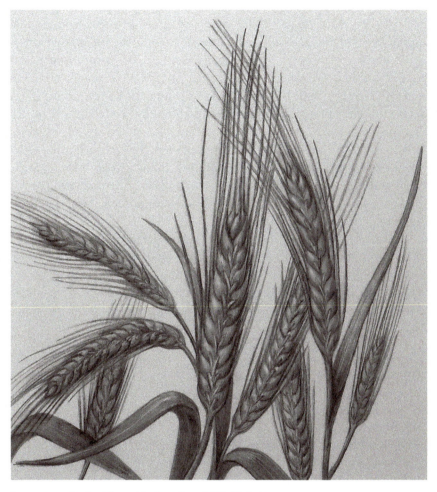

Figure 1.2 **Barley Plant.** (© 2013 Joan M.K. Tycko)

the credit for developing written language because their baked clay tablets have the important attribute of durability.

Much of the Sumerian writing had to do with matters related to agriculture, such as irrigation and land ownership. People counted and measured, and then inscribed their results on tablets. Records on tablets were not subject to the vagaries of human memory, and the tablets could be sent to people far away. Communication no longer depended on physical proximity. Over time, less practical matters such as stories were written down. Cuneiform script was used to record myths and legends, many of which are similar to those described in the Bible. The Sumerians, interested in calculations, also developed a numeric system with 60 as its base.

Barley was the chief grain of Sumer. Dry grains gathered from domesticated barley can be stored for months or years. When harvested barley grains get wet, they begin to germinate. Germinated or sprouting grains are sweeter than the nongerminated grains because the starch turns into sugar. But germinated or sprouted grains cannot be kept for long. They develop mold if they do not grow into plants. The Sumerians discovered that sprouted grains, rather than being thrown away because of incipient moldiness, could be saved by being heated. The Sumerians learned to let barley germinate and then dry the sprouting grains and use them to make bread and beer. Records of Sumerian brewing show that women brewed the beer under the supervision of Ninkasi, a goddess. Almost half of Sumerian grain became ale.[1]

One of the first great literary works was written about the Sumerian king, Gilgamesh, who ruled in about 2700 BCE. A Babylonian version of it, known as the *Epic of Gilgamesh*, was probably written in about 1900 BCE. In this story, Enkidu, a wild jungle boy, becomes civilized when he is introduced to a woman, beer, and bread:

> They placed food in front of him,
> they placed beer in front of him;
> Enkidu knew nothing about eating bread for food,
> and of drinking beer he had not been taught.
> The harlot spoke to Enkidu, saying:
> "Eat the food, Enkidu, it is the way one lives.
> Drink the beer, as is the custom of the land."
> Enkidu ate the food until he was sated,
> he drank the beer—seven jugs!—and became expansive and sang with joy!
> He was elated and his face glowed.
> He splashed his shaggy body with water,
> and rubbed himself with oil, and turned into a human.[2]

Sumer was succeeded by Babylon in about 2000 BCE. The Babylonians integrated the Sumerian numeric system, the cuneiform script, and the habit of brewing beer into their own culture. Beer brewed by the Babylonians was particularly cloudy and thick, and has been described as "edible beer or drinkable bread."[3]

Around the same time, barley was being grown in the rich alluvial lands of the Nile delta. The Egyptians devised efficient irrigation projects that increased agricultural yield. By 3000 BCE, the Egyptian peasants were producing more food than they needed. These surplus calories fueled the development of Ancient Egypt.

The Egyptians developed hieroglyphics at the same time that the Sumerians were developing cuneiform script. The Egyptians also developed an elaborate system of beliefs, many to do with death and the afterworld. They built the great pyramids and tombs of ancient Egypt to safeguard their pharaohs and to provide them with sustenance for their journeys to the next world.

According to legend, Osiris, the god of the underworld and reincarnation, taught the Egyptians how to brew barley into beer. Beer in Egypt was an important drink, although wine was thought to be a more sophisticated beverage. The people who built the pyramids were supplied with generous amounts of beer that provided them with much nutrition.[4]

The Egyptian pharaohs were the first to tax alcohol. They used taxes on beer made from barley to help fund the cost of the construction of pyramids and tombs.[5] Alcohol and taxes have been intertwined ever since.

Beer was highly valued in Mesopotamia and Egypt for its nutritional value and its intoxicating effects. The pyramids are large tributes to the wholesome properties of ancient beer. Beer drunk in those days was not filtered, so it contained the yeast and with the yeast, many vitamins made by the yeast. The cost of a clear beer, as we shall see later, is, for some people, brain damage because vitamins needed by the brain are thrown away. Filtered beer might have led to smaller pyramids.

Beer in Northern Europe in the Middle Ages

Beer became popular throughout northern Europe because of the ease of growing barley in cooler climates. Barley has a short growing season and withstands drought and frost well. Beer is the beverage of Anglo-Saxon and Teutonic peoples.

Beer is also one of the beverages of monasteries. Saint Benedict insisted that monks be able to support themselves and that monasteries be hospitable to travelers. One consequence was that the monks developed the art of beer brewing for themselves and their guests, and then as a source of income. Many monks and nuns became well known for their skill in brewing. Saint Brigid in Ireland was well known for her love of beer. Three men with the name of Arnold have been called saints of beer. Arnold of Metz, Arnold of Soissons, and Arnold of Oudennarde all celebrated beer.

According to one tale, cholera swept through Soissons, a city in northern France, and Arnold (or Arnulf) noticed that those who drank ale were healthier than those who abstained. He brewed his own ale with the help of his crozier and made the sign of the cross over the vat. He convinced the townspeople to drink it and thus saved the community.[6] Arnold of Soissons is also known as the patron saint of hop-pickers.

Hops, the female flowers of the hop plant, were first added to beer in Germany in the eighth century. They balanced the sweetness of the malt and preserved the beer. Beer made from boiled wort and then "hopped" is indeed a safer beverage than water in places with a poorly designed water supply.

The Germans were protective of the quality of their beer. In the 1500s, they passed the Bavarian beer purity law, the *Reinheitsgebot*. This law fixed the price of beer and also regulated the composition of beer—allowing only water, barley, and hops. Other grains were not allowed. Yeast, of course, was also a crucial ingredient, but in those pre-Leeuwenhoek and pre-Pasteur days, the existence of yeast was not known or dreamed of. One reason for this law was to ensure that there would be plentiful supplies of wheat and rye for bakers, and another was to keep the beer free of additives or contaminants. This was one of the first consumer protection laws. Some brewers today claim that their beers are "brewed in accordance with the German Beer Purity Law of 1516."

The belief that beer was a healthy beverage waxed and waned. Christian Heurich, a German American brewer, wrote in his autobiography about a cholera epidemic in 1855 in Vienna:

> A medical congress recommended to the public to stop drinking beer. You can imagine what effect this recommendation had on the breweries. The brewery business was paralyzed, and many employees lost their jobs. As the epidemic grew, many of the former brewery workers became victims of cholera. The remaining brewery workers had very little to do. The cellars were full of beer, and sales were low. As cholera increased in spite of the ban on beer, the remaining brewery workers started to think: "If we have to die, let us die happy." Cholera killed many people outside the breweries who drank water, but those inside the breweries who drank beer were spared. Naturally this did not remain a secret, and the doctors recommended moderate beer drinking.[7]

Beer in England

Beer and its place of drinking—the English pub—has become a well-known part of English culture. Beer was brewed for some centuries in small quantities in the English household. As in Sumer, this was typically done by a woman, known as a brewster or alewife. (A man who brewed ale was a brewer.) The beer was prepared only for the household and typically only lasted for a few days.

This situation slowly changed with the introduction of hops. At first, hops were treated with much suspicion in England, but eventually they were accepted. Hopped beer, which lasted longer than unhopped beer, could now be prepared in larger quantities and for greater numbers of people. Brewing stopped being a household activity. Women were no longer involved, and the brewster was replaced by the brewer.

In seventeenth- and eighteenth-century England, everyone, even children, drank beer throughout the day, beginning with breakfast. This habit changed when tea and coffee, also prepared with boiled water, became available and popular. This may not have been a change for the better, since the nutritional properties of beer were lost. Tea in England was sweetened with sugar, which caused tooth decay.

Taverns became emblematic of England. People would gather to drink beer or other beverages, talk, or play games such as quoits, skittles, and darts. The tavern, or public house, was the heart of the community. Renowned man of letters Samuel Johnson wrote that "there is nothing which has yet been contrived by man, by which so much happiness is produced as by a good tavern or inn."[8]

Beer in the United States

The Pilgrims and Puritans, early European settlers of America, were serious Bible-reading people set on religious freedom for themselves and creating a "city on a hill" to be a beacon for others. Both groups were concerned about the influence of Roman Catholicism on the Church of England and derived many of their beliefs from the Reformation. Their authority was the Bible, and they did not respect the British monarchy or the Pope. The Pilgrims wanted to separate from the Church of England; the Puritans wanted a "purer" form of their religion. The Pilgrims and Puritans fled intolerant England and brought with them their beliefs and many of their habits, including the drinking of cider and beer.

In 1620 the *Mayflower*, containing a crew, settlers, indentured servants, and 40 Pilgrims (or "saints") set forth for Virginia. When they departed from England, they were well supplied with beer.[9] A storm blew them north of their destination. They landed at Provincetown and a few weeks later settled, after a fashion, in Plymouth because they were becoming increasingly desperate about their supplies. Though they were far north of their destination, the journey had been long, and the captain wanted to conserve their supplies for the return journey to England. William Bradford, leader of the expedition, explained that the famous landing at Plymouth Rock was due in part to a fear of running out of beer.

> We had yet some beer, butter, flesh and other victuals left, which would quickly be all gone; and then we should have nothing to comfort us ... so in the morning ... we came to this resolution—to go presently ashore again and to take a better view of two places which we thought most fitting for us; for we could not now take much time for further search or consideration, our victuals being much spent, especially our beer ...[10]

A decade later, the Puritans, known for their gray attire, steepled hats, intolerance, and generally grim attitude toward life, sailed to Massachusetts Bay on the *Arabella*. Perhaps informed by the problems of their predecessors, they were better prepared for the long trip than had been the Pilgrims. They took no chances and carried more alcohol: 10,000 gallons of wine; 14 tuns of fresh water, and 42 tuns of beer (a tun is a large cask that holds about 250 gallons).[11]

Both the Pilgrims and Puritans then took great care to be supplied with alcohol. Their religious seriousness was not the same as opposition to alcohol. Why should they not enjoy their beer? Alcohol (although not beer itself) was mentioned in the Bible repeatedly, and beer drinking was a part of English day-to-day life.

Nor was there opposition to alcohol in yet another American group of religious exiles, the solemn Quakers, who were not well liked by the English Catholics or by the Puritans. William Penn, born into an Anglican family in London, had become a Quaker as a young man and left England to establish a colony friendly to all religious exiles. This colony became Pennsylvania, and one of Penn's first activities was to establish a brewery there. (We shall see later in this chapter that Cotton Mather, as Puritanical a Puritan as ever lived, suggested, when the opportunity arose, that Penn be sold into slavery.)

The objections to alcohol in American life came later and were rooted somewhat in religious beliefs, but not in those of the early settlers. Some Americans may be Puritanical about alcohol, but the Pilgrims, Puritans, and Quakers did not abstain from alcohol.

Early to arrive in North America, beer was quickly exceeded in popularity by other alcoholic drinks, such as hard (alcoholic) cider, rum, and whiskey. During colonial times, hard apple cider was the most popular alcoholic beverage. Apple trees were grown and tended, not for fruit to eat, but fruit to crush, ferment, and transform into hard cider. John Adams, the second president of the United States, drank hard cider every morning when he could.[12]

A later group of immigrants, the Germans, is associated with the resurgence of beer in the United States. The Germans came to the United States in large numbers in the 1800s and brought their taste for beer with them. For example, Heurich, mentioned earlier in the chapter, was born in 1842 in the Duchy of Saxe-Meiningen and emigrated to the United States in 1866. On his journey to America, the ship was quarantined in Liverpool, England, because of a cholera outbreak on board. Remembering the story of the Viennese cholera outbreak, Heurich drank only beer. He did not become ill but was not pleased by the quality of the English beer. He eventually established a successful brewery in Washington, D.C., and brewed beer more acceptable to his palate and, as it turned out, to the palate of the Washingtonians. He became a wealthy and respected municipal citizen.

Many German immigrants settled in the Midwest, where they established large breweries. They brought with them a different method of brewing beer, known as lagering, in which the yeast works at the bottom, rather than top, of the container and at a colder temperature. This method turned out to be better suited for American conditions. In the late 1800s, improved methods of refrigeration and transportation led to an explosion of beer production and consumption. Breweries consolidated and established financial relationships with big-city saloons. By 1915, most of the alcohol consumed in the United States was beer.

Beer drinking then declined in the first part of the twentieth century, for two reasons. It was disapproved of during World Wars I and II because of the strong association with Germany, even though German brewers such as Miller and Anheuser-Busch went to great lengths to emphasize their American patriotism. Also, during the years of Prohibition, many breweries closed.

Beer drinking slowly increased again in popularity in the decades following World War II. Large breweries dominated the American market. The popularity of beer may have also contributed to the end of cider. Cider is rarely drunk now and apples are usually eaten, not fermented. A new development is the popularity of smaller breweries. Microbreweries or craft breweries promise the consumer a local beer with a more interesting flavor than that provided by beer from national corporations.

Conclusion

Beer is part of the beginning of civilization. The development of writing, cities, and theories about life and the afterlife all sprang up with farming and the storing of damp barley. Germinating barley grains did not always have to become new plants or succumb to mold; they could, if treated correctly, and with the help of yeast, lead to bread and beer. Beer helped to build the pyramids of Egypt and to sustain the monasteries in Europe. For Americans, beer drinking is associated with early colonial history and later waves of German immigrants. Beer drinking became less popular during World Wars I and II in the United States, and then once again more popular since the mid-twentieth century.

Wine

Wine is the most aristocratic and complex of all alcoholic drinks—or so say the wine drinkers. Connoisseurs sip wine, appreciate the way it accents and complements food, savor its oakiness and fruit tones, and admire the bouquet. There is a celebratory yet serious aspect to wine; wedding guests toast the bride and groom with champagne.

Wine is important in both Judaism and Christianity. The Bible has many references to wine, beginning with the story of Noah planting a vineyard as soon as dry land appears after the Flood and then becoming drunk. Wine is mentioned often as a subject of praise, but drunkenness is recognized and deplored. The Kiddush is a blessing recited over wine to welcome the Sabbath and Jewish holidays. During Passover, Jewish adults drink four cups of wine. In the New Testament, the story is told of how Jesus turned water into wine at a wedding feast in Cana. Wine is used in the Eucharist, to commemorate Jesus sharing bread and wine with his disciples. During communion, the celebrant consumes a wafer or bread and drinks wine, symbolizing the body and blood of Jesus.

Of all the different kinds of alcohol, wine is most closely connected with the fermented object—the grape (Figure 1.3). There are many varieties of grape vines, but grapes from the grape vine *Vitis vinifera* are best suited for wine making. Grapes from wild grape vines, such as *V. lubrusca*, sometimes have a flat or "foxy" taste. Grape vines grow throughout all temperate climates, but *V. vinifera* grows best in sunny climates with moderate winters and in poor and well-drained soil. They are most commonly associated with Mediterranean and similar climates.

The production of wine depends on people living in a settled place, since vines take at least five years to mature and to produce fruit. Roots

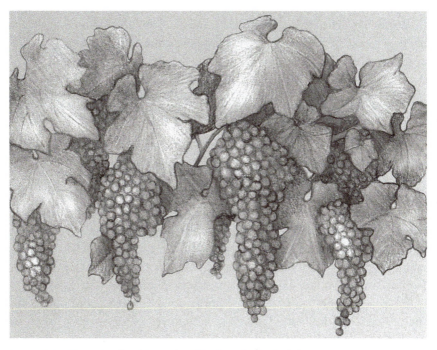

Figure 1.3   **Grape Leaf and Vine.** (© 2013 Joan M.K. Tycko)

deepen, and the grapes develop distinctive flavors over the next couple of decades of growth. Cereals that yield beer, in contrast, are annual crops. Therefore, settlement must be even more stable for wine production than for beer.

How Wine Is Made

The transformation of grapes into wine is simple. Pick grapes off the vine, crush them, and wild yeast (*Saccharomyces cerevisiae*) that live on grape skin will convert the grape's glucose and fructose into alcohol. Yet in this simple process lie a thousand opportunities for disaster.

How can the wine grower ensure that fermentation yields a fine wine and not vinegar? There is much to master. Wine growers make much of the particular piece of land on which the grape vines grow—the terroir. Volumes have been written about which grape vines to grow and how to grow them. The grape grower must learn how to prune the vine, when and how to harvest the grapes, how vigorously to crush the grapes, and which type of yeast to use. The temperature of the process, the decision about what to do with the grape skins, and how to let the wine mature are just a few other topics of concern to all vintners.

Wine today is a clear beverage. It is clarified (or "fined") by agents such as egg white, casein, gelatin, or isinglass—a substance from sturgeon bladder. The sediment is yeasty and rich in B vitamins—but modern wine drinkers do not benefit from this, just as modern beer drinkers get less benefit from their beer than did the Egyptians who built the pyramids.

Wine in Ancient Civilizations

Wine was drunk in Ancient Egypt. Beer drinkers built the pyramids, but the pharaohs and nobility, and those who supervised and directed the workers, drank wine. Even then, drinkers differentiated between different types of alcohol. Egyptians so valued wine that they buried it with the pharaohs so that in the afterlife they would still be able to drink it. The tomb of King Tutankhamen was generously supplied with wine. The wines had different names, depending on the vintners and the terroirs, and were poured into differently shaped bottles. The Egyptians were sophisticated wine drinkers.

Wine was an important part of life in ancient Greece and one of the many ways in which the Greeks saw themselves as superior to those around them. Thucydides, the Greek historian, wrote that "the peoples of the Mediterranean began to emerge from barbarianism when they learnt to cultivate the olive and the vine."[13] Wine was part of the "symposium," during which men gathered in groups to talk and drink. Socrates was the central figure of many symposia and was admired as a man who could drink much wine without becoming obviously drunk. The symposium lives on today in gatherings of scientists or scholars, although wine is no longer an official part of the activity.

In Greek mythology, wine drinking is associated with Dionysus, a son of Zeus. Dionysus taught men how to ferment grape juice into wine and has been depicted as a man with foliage sprouting from his head, as Figure 1.4 shows. Dionysus blurred the boundaries between nature and culture, man and woman, and man and beast. Michael Pollan, in a book about the relationship between plants and humanity, wrote:

> Dionysus brought wild plants into the house of civilization, but by the same token his own untamed presence reminded people of the untamed nature on which that house always rests, somewhat unsteadily ... Wine itself is ... poised on the edge of nature and culture as well as civility and abandon.[14]

Dionysian revels were experiences of ecstasy, intoxication, spontaneity, and loss of control. (In contrast were the calm, rational, and ordered experiences of his brother, Apollo.)

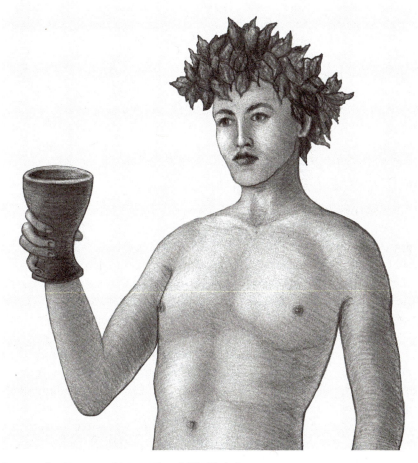

Figure 1.4   **Dionysus.** (© 2013 Joan M.K. Tycko)

The wine drunk by the Greeks would not appeal to the modern oeno-phile. It was pungent, strong, and flavored by pine oils. Greeks always drank their "retsina" diluted with water.

Later, wine became important in the Roman Empire. The Greek Dionysus became the Roman Bacchus. Roman soldiers fighting on the far borders of the empire were abstemious, but back in Rome, the center of the empire, people drank heavily. Pliny the Elder, a Roman author and naturalist, devoted the fourteenth book of his *Historia Naturalis* (ca. 60 AD) to wine and indulged in some editorial comments:

> There is no department of man's life on which more labor is spent—as if nature had not given us the most healthy of beverages to drink, water . . . and so much toil and labor and expense is paid as the price of a

thing that perverts men's minds and produces madness, having caused the commission of thousands of crimes, and being so attractive that a large part of mankind knows of nothing else worth living for.[15]

It was not just the average Roman citizen who drank heavily. Scholars have estimated that about two thirds of the emperors and rulers of Rome between 30 BCE and 220 CE were gluttons and heavy drinkers. Some Roman emperors—such as Nero, Tiberius, and Claudius—were infamous alcoholics.

Wine, Lead, and the End of the Roman Empire

One theory about the end of the Roman Empire is related to wine and lead poisoning. Lead is a soft, heavy metal that, because of its low melting point, resistance to corrosion, and malleability, has been widely used for many years to make objects such as pipes, type for print, and storage vessels. (The Latin word for lead, *plumbum*, is the derivation of our word *plumbing*.) Another property of lead is its sweet taste. Although many peoples in the past used lead, the Romans were the first to use it in large amounts.

The Romans used lead in plumbing and also deliberately in preparation of foods and liquids because of its sweetness. Grape juice or sour wine was boiled down in lead pans to produce a widely used sweetening agent known as *sapa*, which contained some dissolved lead. Sapa was sometimes mixed with wine both to sweeten it and to preserve it. Wine tasted better and lasted longer if it was mixed with sapa. Wine was also contaminated by lead because it was sometimes stored in lead vessels.

This extensive use of lead may have resulted in lead poisoning. Lead poisoning is not a new discovery; it has been recognized for as long as lead has been used. (Currently, it is the most common environmental illness in the United States.) The Greek physician Nikander of the second century BCE knew about it. The Roman architect and writer Vitruvius, who lived in the first century BCE, wrote about the danger of water carried in lead pipes. These warnings were not heeded. The theory to do with the end of the Roman Empire is that because the Roman elite in particular drank a lot of wine with sapa, the ruling classes became lead poisoned and as a result, increasingly ill. Eventually, they were no longer able to rule Rome efficiently. The lead may also have decreased their fertility, so that they had few children on whom to bestow what expertise and authority they possessed. Julius Caesar, for example, had only one child, and his successor, Caesar Augustus, was reported to be sterile.[16,17]

Barbarians from northern climes, perhaps stronger because they were free of lead, destroyed the Roman Empire. The barbarians had no interest in wine; they were well satisfied with their mead and beer. This could have been the end of wine and the triumph of mead and beer were it not for the importance of wine to Christianity. Throughout the Middle Ages, monks continued and developed the art of viticulture, in part because of the importance of wine in communion. (They also continued their interests in brewing beer.) Monasteries were associated with grape vines on the banks of the Rhine and throughout southern France, Austria, Hungary, Switzerland, Italy, and Spain.

Wine and the French: "I am drinking stars."

The French believe that their wine is the beverage par excellence and that its virtues are intimately connected with the essence of being French. Henry Babinski, a French physician, said this about wine and the French (to differentiate them from beer and the beer-drinking "races"):

> L'usage prolongé du vin a certainement contribué à la formation et au développement des qualités fondamentales de la race: cordialité, franchise, gaîté, qui la différencient si profondément des peoples buveurs de bière.
>
> (The long-time use of wine has certainly contributed to the formation and development of fundamental qualities of the race: cordiality, frankness, gaiety, which differentiate them so profoundly from people who drink beer.)[18]

One of the finest wines, associated with French luxury and joie de vivre, is champagne, which was invented by a monk. Dom Pérignon was a blind French Benedictine monk who blended grapes and developed a number of improvements in the wine industry, such as corks and thicker glass. In 1690, he made the first bottle of champagne by having the wine ferment a second time in the bottle. After doing this and sampling the product, he declared, "I am drinking stars." The veracity of this tale is questionable, but such a charming story fits with the effervescent nature of this beverage.

Wine may have its own health benefits, and it is part of the well-known French Paradox, which is the finding of lower rates of heart disease and cancer in wine-drinking nations such as France, Italy, and Spain, despite high fat consumption in those countries. Red wine contains resveratrol, a compound thought to be an antioxidant. However, the validity of the paradox has been questioned, and there is probably not enough resveratrol in red wine to be beneficial.

Even though the French are proud of their wine, French viticulture depends on American grape vines. This is because the roots of French grape vines were irresistible to the sap-sucking root louse *Phylloxera vasta- trix*. This aphid-like insect came from the eastern United States via a ship- ment of grape vine cuttings sent to England or Europe. By the 1860s, this louse had proliferated and sucked the juices out of the roots of the French grape vines and in so doing, ravaged much of the French wine industry. Since many American grape vines were resistant to this louse, the only cure for the French wine industry was to use the resistant American vines. Thus, most French grape vines have been grafted onto American *Phylloxera*-resistant rootstocks. The French were understandably appre- hensive that the foxy taste of American wines would be transmitted from the American roots to the French grapes, but that has not happened. The cause and the cure of the louse disaster were American. The Gallic grape continues to produce fine wine.

Wine in the United States

Wine is not an integral part of American culture or history, but it was savored by many of the Founding Fathers. Benjamin Franklin, John Adams, and Thomas Jefferson—all of them Francophiles—were also oenophiles. They travelled extensively in Europe and appreciated European cuisine. Adams and Jefferson were bitter political enemies, but during their younger years, they shared meals and enjoyed the fine wines of France. Jefferson dreamed of a vineyard at Monticello that could pro- duce wines as fine as those he had drunk with Adams. In Jefferson's post-presidential years, he spent much effort and money on cultivating vines, but he was never able to make wine that could compete with French wine.

Wine is now produced in many American vineyards, particularly in California. Perhaps the Founding Fathers would have thought that these California wines, coming from parts of America unknown to them, are as fine as the prephylloxera wines that they drank in the eighteenth century.

Conclusion

Grape vines are still cultivated primarily in countries with a Mediterranean type of climate, such as Italy, France, California, Chile, and parts of Australia. Those who produce, sell, and drink wine, from the pyramid planners to Dionysus to Thomas Jefferson, have always been convinced of the superiority of this drink to all others.

Rum

Rum is the beverage that results from the distillation of fermented molasses, a by-product of production of sugar from the sugar cane. If beer is everyman's drink and wine is the Frenchman's, then rum is the drink of the English sailor and the swashbuckling pirate of the Caribbean. Rum is also the drink of slavery and mercantilism.

The story of rum is associated with one of the world's cruelest and largest forcible dislocations of people—the Atlantic slave trade. Over nine million people were taken from Africa to work as slaves in the Brazilian or Caribbean sugar plantations, the American cotton or rice fields of the Lower South, and the Chesapeake tobacco fields. This trade transformed the peoples and lands involved and changed the eating, drinking, and smoking habits of much of the world. The indigenous peoples of the West Indies have all but disappeared, as have many of the indigenous peoples of Brazil.

Sugar and Slavery

Saccharum officinarum, sugar cane, is a rapidly growing grass that comes from New Guinea. It can grow as high as 12 feet. Sugar cane needs high heat, abundant rainfall, and a long growing season, so it is found in only a few areas of the world. The thick, solid, and tough stems have a high concentration of sucrose. Sugar cane is a champion at changing sunlight and carbon dioxide into carbohydrates.

Cultivation of sugar spread throughout Southeast Asia and, in about the sixth century CE, Arab traders brought sugar cane to Syria, Cyprus, and Crete. The Portuguese took the cane farther west and introduced it into Madeira, the Canary Islands, the Azores, and West Africa in the fifteenth century. They also brought slaves from East Africa to cultivate sugar in the Canary Islands and the Azores.

Sugar traveled to the Americas because of the marriage of Christopher Columbus to Dona Felipa Perestrello y Moniz, the daughter of a wealthy sugar plantation owner. Columbus learned about sugar and in 1493, he took sugar cane plants to the Caribbean.

The climate of the Caribbean, similar to that of the islands off West Africa, is suitable for growing sugar cane. However, there was little available land, since the Caribbean islands were densely forested. The answer to this problem was obvious—destroy the forests. By the middle of the sixteenth century, sugar cane was grown in large plantations on the tree-stripped islands. Jamaica, Haiti, Cuba, Trinidad, and Barbados became sugar-growing islands. Large forested areas in Brazil also were turned into sugar cane estates.

The cultivation of the plant and extraction of the sugar were difficult. The indigenous Caribbean peoples who might have been conscripted to do the work were few, and fewer still survived the arrival of the Europeans, who were carrying unfamiliar germs and steel weapons. At first, indentured European servants did the work. Later, slaves from the west coast of Africa cultivated and harvested the cane. (This sequence would be repeated on the tobacco plantations.)

Once the sugar cane is harvested, the canes are crushed or mashed into a sweet juice. The juice is boiled, and sugar crystals form. The leftover liquid is molasses. This sweet liquid can be fermented into an alcoholic liquid, and distillation of this liquid leads to rum. Rum quickly became a popular drink associated with the Caribbean and the young sugar cane industry. It was an important part of trade triangles.

Mercantilism and Triangular Trade

An influential European economic theory of the sixteenth and seventeenth centuries was mercantilism. Mercantilists believed that a colonizing power would prosper if she could keep labor costs low, export manufactured goods, and import raw material or cash crops from her colonies. Triangular trade was a form of mercantilism. The idea of a trade triangle is captivating, perhaps because of the pleasing geometric nature of a triangle, but overly simplified. There was always a cat's cradle of trade routes. Nevertheless, we will discuss the "triangles" as they relate to alcohol (and later as they relate to opium).

In the first leg of the triangle, as Figure 1.5 shows, cowry shells, cloth, iron, alcohol, and manufactured goods were sent from England to the west coast of Africa. (Cowry shells are small seashells indigenous to the Indian Ocean near the Maldives and were used as packing material, ballast, and barter.) The alcohol included distilled beverages—first brandy and then rum. Africans had their own grain-based beers and palm wine but grew to prefer brandy and rum.

The cargo was bartered with African slave dealers for slaves. African kings or warlords captured or purchased Africans in the interior and

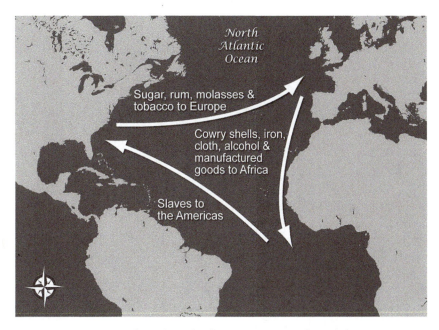

North
Atlantic
Ocean

Sugar, rum, molasses &
tobacco to Europe

Cowry shells, iron,
cloth, alcohol &
manufactured
goods to Africa

Slaves to
the Americas

Figure 1.5   Trade Triangle (with England). (© 2013 Joan M.K. Tycko)

marched them to the west coast, where they were sold to Europeans as slaves. In the second leg of the triangle, slaves were transported across the Atlantic. This sea voyage between the west coast of Africa and either the Caribbean or the east coast of the Americas was the infamous Middle Passage. Slaves were packed tightly in the holds of these ships, shackled, and fed little; they suffered terribly. Inadequate nutrition, filthy drinking water, and poor sanitation led to many diseases, from scurvy to gangrene to dysentery.

The emotions that they went through are difficult to imagine or describe. Some slaves thought that they had been captured by cannibals. Olaudah Equiano in his autobiography wrote:

> When I looked round the ship too, and saw a large furnace of copper boiling, and a multitude of black people of every description chained together, every one of their countenances expressing dejection and sorrow, I no longer doubted of my fate, and, quite overpowered with horror and anguish, I fell motionless on the deck and fainted. . . . I asked if we were not to be eaten by those white men with horrible looks, red faces, and long hair?
>
> . . .
>
> The closeness of the place, and the heat of the climate, added to the number in the ship, which was so crowded that each had scarcely room to

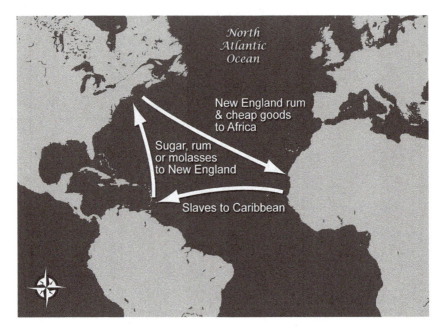

Figure 1.6   **Trade Triangle (with New England). (© 2013 Joan M.K. Tycko)**

turn himself, almost suffocated us. This produced copious perspirations, so that the air soon became unfit for respiration, from a variety of loathsome smells, and brought on a sickness among the slaves, of which many died, thus falling victims to the improvident avarice, as I may call it, of their purchasers. This wretched situation was again aggravated by the galling of the chains, now become insupportable; and the filth of the necessary tubs, into which the children often fell, and were almost suffocated. The shrieks of the women, and the groans of the dying, rendered the whole a scene of horror almost inconceivable.[19]

In the final or third leg, ships carried sugar, rum, or molasses (from the West Indies) or tobacco (from Virginia) back to Europe.

A slightly different form of the triangle formed. In this triangle, shown in Figure 1.6, New England—not England—formed one of the apices. In the first leg, New England sent rum and cheap goods to the west coast of Africa. The second leg was again the Middle Passage. In the third leg, sugar, rum, and molasses were shipped from the Caribbean up to New England. The molasses was fermented and distilled to become New England–made rum. Lumber from New England was used to make casks and provide fuel for her distilleries. (The deforestation of some of the Caribbean islands meant that it was difficult for casks to be made there.)

This second triangle let New England carry on a profitable trade without England taking a cut of any of the profits. In an add-on to this triangle, the French sent molasses from the French West Indies to New England; in return the New Englanders sent their poorest quality cod to the Caribbean.[20]

Merchants made profits at each stage in both trade triangles. Cities such as Bristol and Liverpool in England, and Boston and Newport in America, prospered. The people who worked in the fields growing the sugar and tobacco stayed poor.

Although North American slavery is generally associated with the South, the second triangle illustrates a fact often ignored by New Englanders: the wealth of colonial New England in large part depended on slavery. As well, it was not unusual for slaves to end up in New England, where they became household slaves.

Many of the clergy of New England became comfortable with slavery. Cotton Mather, an influential Puritan minister in New England, wrote to a colleague about some business and included some comments illustrating how acceptable slavery had become, his feelings about non-Puritans, the connection between New England and the Caribbean, and the need for slaves to work in the sugar plantations:

> There is now at sea a ship called the *Welcome* which has on board an hundred or more of the heretics and malignants called Quakers, with W. Penn who is the chief scamp, at the head of them.
>
> The general court has accordingly given secret orders to Master Malachi Huscott, of the Brig *Porpoise*, to waylay the said *Welcome*, slyly as near the Cape of Cod as may be, and make captive the said Penn and his ungodly crew, so that the Lord may be glorified, and not mocked on the soil of this new country with the heathen worship of these people. Much spoil can be made by selling the whole lot to Barbados, where slaves fetch good prices in rum and sugar, and we shall not only do the Lord great service by punishing the wicked, but we shall make great good for his ministers and people.
>
> Master Huscott feels hopeful and I will set down the news when the ship comes back.
>
> Yours in ye Bowels of Christ.
>
> Cotton Mather. [21]

These trade triangles, and many variations of them, continued from the sixteenth century through the eighteenth century, peaking in about 1750. Between nine to 16 million Africans were transported across the Atlantic to Brazil, the Caribbean, and the Eastern Seaboard.

Rum and the Conflict between New England and England

Rum was an important drink in the colonies, but it caused problems with England. New England's ability to make barrels and distill rum was not welcome to the English, since it interfered with the English desire to import raw goods, export manufactured goods, and levy taxes wherever they could.

In 1733, England passed the infamous Molasses Act that taxed rum, molasses, and non-English sugar. Jamaican and Barbadian rum (i.e., rum from British colonies) were exempt from such duties. The goals were clear—to favor English consumption of Jamaican and Barbadian rum, and to discourage purchase of French sugar and New England rum.

The New England colonists were outraged at the interference with their trade. Compliance with the new taxes was unthinkable. Rum and molasses smuggling became widespread throughout the colonies. From the point of view of the New Englander, this was not criminal at all. (Similar opinions would prevail 150 years later during Prohibition.) Visions of freedom from these tax bonds tying the colonies to England began to form.

This was not a small matter for New England. In 1770, rum made up over four-fifths of New England's exports.[22] The rum trade on the coast of West Africa was a New England monopoly. The English taxes were so hated in the American colonies that they helped to cause the American Revolution. John Adams attended a meeting of the Sons of Liberty in 1766 in a distillery where the Sons drank rum, smoked pipes, and plotted rebellion. He later wrote to a friend, "I know not why we should blush to confess that molasses was an essential ingredient in American independence. Many great events have proceeded from much smaller causes."[23]

Rum, among other distilled spirits, played another role in the early history of America. It was an important part of elections. George Washington finished a dismal fourth the first time that he ran for election. In the next election, still trying to become a member of the Virginia Assembly, he ordered 144 gallons of rum, punch, cider, beer, and wine to be delivered to the polling places and to be distributed generously. All of this was for 301 votes. The liquor refreshed, hydrated, encouraged, and rewarded men for voting. Or perhaps it just got them drunk. In any event, the drinkers elected him.[24]

Rum and the Sailor

Rum was an important beverage of the English navy. English sailors had wretched lives, full of danger and deprivation. Pirates and enemy countries often attacked them, and shipwrecks were common. Another problem was that the ships were so small that there was little room to carry much food or water. Diseases were common. The most dreaded was scurvy, which was caused by the lack of fresh fruits and vegetables. Fresh water was difficult to carry because water casks could not be tightly sealed. The water often became contaminated, also causing much illness.

Sailors needed ample fluids for several reasons, one of them being the nature of the food that they did have. Pork, beef, and fish were stored in brine. Biscuits served with salted butter and accompanied by pickled vegetables, oil, vinegar, rice, peas, and oatmeal made up the rest of the diet. Meals were cooked in seawater. The purpose of the salt was preservation of the food, since these were the days before canning or refrigeration.

The salt that preserved the food needed to be excreted. Our kidneys can excrete excess salt, if we have sufficient water. Sailors who already needed large quantities of liquids because of their physical labor and exposure to heat needed more water to excrete the salt that they consumed with their food. Water was safer to drink if it came in the form of alcoholic beverages because the water had been boiled, and alcohol itself had some antiseptic properties.

For a few years, beer was the standard beverage at the start of seagoing voyages. Beer, which was then not filtered, was more nutritious and less alcoholic than it is now. It therefore easily became sour or spoiled and eventually was replaced by wine and rum.

Compared to water, rum was a safe drink. Intoxication may also have made ship life slightly less awful. In some cases, rum was mixed with lemon or lime juice, and this helped to prevent scurvy. This drink was named after Admiral Vernon. In 1740, he introduced a diluted version of rum to the navy. He was known as "old grog" because he wore a grogram cloth coat. The word *grogram* came from "gros grain," meaning a coarse fabric. Various alcohol beverages since then have been known as grog.

The harvesting of sugar cane led to rum, but sugar plays another part in the story of alcohol. Sugar from the Caribbean became an important part of the English diet. It was used in baking and to sweeten tea. Tea (a new drink from China), along with coffee, replaced (to some extent) alcohol in the liquid diet of the English. The English worker stopped drinking beer for breakfast and began to drink sweetened tea at all meals. Some claim that English productivity increased as people switched from alcohol to coffee and tea.

Rum as an Ingredient in Mixed Drinks

Rum has often been used with other alcoholic or nonalcoholic beverages to make mixed drinks, sometimes known as cocktails. In colonial

America, it was common to fashion complicated beverages, often heated, and often with rum as an ingredient. Drink making was inventive in seventeenth- and eighteenth-century New England:

[Flip] was made of home-brewed beer, sweetened with sugar, molasses, or dried pumpkin, and flavored with a liberal dash of rum, then stirred in a great mug or pitcher with a red-hot loggerhead or hottle or flip-dog, which made the liquor foam and gave it a burnt bitter flavor.

Landlord May, of Canton, Mass., made a famous brew thus: he mixed four pounds of sugar, four eggs, and one pint of cream and let it stand for two days. When a mug of flip was called for, he filled a quart mug two-thirds full of beer, placed in it four great spoonfuls of the compound, then thrust in the seething loggerhead, and added a gill of rum to the creamy mixture. If a fresh egg were beaten into the flip the drink was called "bellows-top," and the froth rose over the top of the mug. "Stone-wall" was a most intoxicating mixture of cider and rum. "Callibogus," or "bogus," was cold rum and beer unsweetened. "Black-strap" was a mixture of rum and molasses. Casks of it stood in every country store, a salted and dried codfish slyly hung alongside—a free lunch to be stripped off and eaten, and thus tempt, through thirst, the purchase of another draught of black-strap.[25]

There is a touch of theater here that must have entertained the customers. This was a more rewarding experience than the twenty-first-century habit of flipping open a tab on a beer can taken from a six-pack. The eggs and cream also made a more substantial beverage. The use of a "free lunch" to tempt drinkers would later also be used in saloons.

In the South, Americans drank rum as well as fruit cordials and mint-flavored whiskey. A traveling Englishman described the day of a planter in Virginia just after the American Revolution:

He rises about eight o'clock, drinks what he calls a julep, which is a large glass of rum sweetened with sugar, then walks, or more generally rides, round his plantation, views his stock, inspects his crops, and returns about ten o'clock to breakfast on cold meat or ham, fried hominy, toast and cider ... About twelve or one he drinks a toddy to create him an appetite for dinner, which he sits down to at two o'clock. [He] commonly drinks toddy till bed time; during all this time he is neither drunk nor sober, but in a state of stupefaction ... [When] he attends the Court House or some horse race or cock fight he gets so egregiously drunk ...[26]

During the nineteenth century, the supply of molasses from the Caribbean diminished, due to depletion of the soil and emancipation of the slaves, and whiskey and then beer became more popular in America. A surprising group of people stayed faithful to rum—the temperance workers. More accurately, they stayed faithful to the *word*. The simplicity of the word made it useful for those fond of rhetoric. For example, Carry Nation and others talked about "rummies" whose lives were ruined by "demon rum."

The beverage itself came back into use in the twentieth century as an ingredient of tropical mixed drinks. The daiquiri, for example, is a blend of lime, sugar, rum, and ice. At the Floridita in Havana, made famous by the patronage of Ernest Hemingway, the bartender made drinks, including daiquiris, in this way:

> Constantino's technique involved equal parts precision and flamboyance. He would fill stemmed cocktail glasses with ice to chill them, pour the ingredients (often for several drinks) into a cocktail shaker, and then shake vigorously, reportedly then sending the contents in a great arc from one half of the shaker to the other. He'd empty out the ice from the now-chilled glasses, line these up in a row on the bar, and fill them with a fluid sweep of his arm . . . To watch Constantino was to watch a master craftsman at work.[27]

There is still some mystique to cocktails, but the ready availability of blenders and packaged mixes means that the preparation of a mixed drink no longer has to involve the skill of a Landlord May or a Constantino.

Whiskey

Whiskey is associated with the British Isles, particularly Scotland and Ireland. The word itself comes for the Gaelic word *uisge*, which is a shorter form of the phrase *uisge beatha*, which means "water of life," the term used to describe distilled alcohol.

The spelling of the word and the various names given to this beverage have always been peculiar. The drink is known as *whisky*—no "e"—in Canada, Scotland, and Japan. Because of its connection with Scotland, some kinds of whiskey are known as Scotch. Scotch is now produced in Ireland. Bourbon, a French name, is associated with whiskey produced in Kentucky and Tennessee.

Whiskey is unlike wine, which is associated with one particular fruit (the grape), or beer, which is associated (mostly) with one particular grain (barley). Whiskey, now drunk throughout the world, is associated with many grains. In Scotland and Ireland, whiskey is made from fermented malted barley, but in the United States, it is made from other grains, including that quintessential American grain, corn. In Canada, it is sometimes made, in part, from rye.

Whiskey in the Old World

Monks are thought to have introduced distilling techniques to Ireland and Scotland between 1100 and 1300 CE. The Celts applied the technology of distillation to fermented barley and invented whiskey. Following the sixteenth-century dissolution of the monasteries in England, the monks, who by then had become skilled at the process, had to support themselves and did so by perfecting their art of whiskey making. They often used peat fires to heat and dry the malt. The smoke from the peat fires gave an acrid flavor to the whiskey that is still characteristic of many whiskeys from this area. They learned to age whiskey in wooden barrels or casks. The tannins and other substances in the wood added color and flavors to the whiskey.

Following the Act of Union with England in 1707, new taxes and laws were applied in Scotland. Whiskey began to be taxed. Not surprisingly, and as is a recurrent theme in this book, taxation was hated. The distillers often hid their whiskey, which from their point of view was their own product and had nothing to do with England. The taxmen were known as "excisemen" and were despised. Illicit stills and smuggling became commonplace.

Whiskey in the New World

The story of whiskey in the Americas involves maize and emigration from Ireland and Scotland. Maize, or corn, is a tall grass (*Zea mays*) that grows throughout the Americas and was the basic food plant of the Mayas, Aztecs, and Incans. The high caloric yield of the corn plant meant that not all of the population had to spend their time finding or preparing food, and this allowed people time to develop intricate religions, architecture, roads, and the arts. These civilizations flourished. Maize subsequently became one of the most important grains in the world.[28]

When the English Pilgrims came to North America, they found a land already populated. Corn was a key crop for these communities in the eastern parts of North America. In 1621 Squanto, a Patuxet Native American, may have changed the course of history by an act of generosity. Squanto taught the newcomers how to grow corn. The Native Americans grew their corn along with beans and squash, using the "three sisters method." Corn was a pole for bean vines to climb, the beans fixed nitrogen in the soil, and the sprawling squash vines kept down the weeds while their spines kept away marauding animals.

Squanto's instructions in maize cultivation helped the Pilgrims to survive the harsh winters of New England. Eventually the new Americans taught themselves how to ferment corn, turn it into a mash, and then distill this mash into whiskey. They repaid the generosity of the Native Americans by introducing them to distilled liquors.

The issue of alcohol and Native Americans has always been fraught. When French-Canadian fur traders traveled through what is now Canada and as far south as what is now Missouri searching for beaver pelts, they used beads, guns, ammunition, and whiskey as barter. The results were disastrous for the Native Americans, some of whom drank alcohol for the sole purpose of becoming drunk. Some tribes, alarmed by the violence that resulted, refused to accept alcohol as payment, and various government agencies banned the practice of trading alcohol to the Native Americans, but these efforts were not entirely successful. Although it is difficult to disentangle the effects of whiskey and rum from the other introductions to the New World, such as pigs, cows, dogs, unfamiliar infections, and European understanding of land ownership, many blame liquor, in part, for undermining the cultures of the Native Americans. Similar patterns are found in the interactions between Europeans and other aboriginal peoples.

Although whiskey was known to the first emigrants to New England, another group is usually associated with whiskey in America. Irish and Scottish emigrants brought their knowledge of distilling with them to America. Some of these emigrants had left their homeland once before. England had tried to "settle" Ireland by moving Scottish Protestants to Ireland. During the 1700s, many of these Ulster Scots moved on to America and settled in the Appalachians, as did the Irish.

For most of the 1700s, the Scotch-Irish, as they were sometimes called, planted, cultivated, fermented, and distilled rye and barley to make whiskey, which was their main source of income. Whiskey was bartered for other goods such as sugar, salt, or gunpowder. They must have been delighted to escape from the English and their various laws and taxes. They did, however, still have conflicts with others. They fought Native Americans on the frontier and the English during the Revolution. They were not well regarded by others. They were described as "a set of the most lowest vilest crew breathing—Scotch-Irish Presbyterians from the north of

Ireland." The description is surprising in that these harsh words come from a minister but less surprising when one learns that the minister was from the Church of England.[29]

In 1793, Congress enacted an excise liquor law to raise revenue. This was the first "internal" tax and was proposed by Alexander Hamilton, the first U.S. secretary of the treasury. Hamilton believed in the importance of a vigorous executive branch and the subordination of the states to a strong federal government. He supported the tax as a way of paying down the national debt and of supporting military expeditions against the Native Americans. He established a small "army" of inspectors with enforcement powers.

The Scotch-Irish were fond of their whiskey and distrustful of governments. When it came to their rye whiskey being taxed by the new American federal government, the reaction was predictable. They had fought for the American Revolution but did not sympathize with the new government's need to pay for this revolution. Federal taxes on whiskey were just as odious in western Pennsylvania as they had been in eighteenth-century Scotland.

In 1794, the farmers refused to pay these taxes, and violence raged along the Monongahela River for a couple of years. Tax collectors were assaulted, and farmers who did cooperate with the agents had their barns burned down. Thomas Miflin, then governor of Pennsylvania, refused to call out the state militia. The insurrection was put down by force by President Washington. The Whiskey Rebellion had been brief. The rebellion against taxes continued underground.

Some of the rebels moved farther south and west to Kentucky. In Bourbon County, they began to make whiskey from corn. Some of the whiskey was stored in barrels made from charred oak, and so was born Bourbon whiskey.

The traditions of distilling whiskey and resenting the federal government's taxes and their collectors, known derisively as revenue men, persisted. The whiskey makers continued to ferment corn mash and make moonshine. (The name moonshine comes from the time-honored practice of carrying out illegal activities at night.)

President Washington had fought against the whiskey rebels, but this was a fiscal disagreement only. He was not averse to liquor. Toward the end of his life, he and his Scottish manager built a distillery at Mount Vernon. He grew wheat and rye and then distilled whiskey that he sold. (His 300 slaves did the work.)

Thomas Jefferson, lover of wine and champagne, despised whiskey, or, as it was sometimes called, along with other distilled beverages, ardent spirits. He wrote:

> The habit of using ardent spirits by men in public office has often produced more injury to the public service, and more trouble to me, than any other circumstance that has occurred in the internal concerns of the country during my administration. And were I to commence my administration again, with the knowledge which from experience I have acquired, the first question that I would ask with regard to every candidate for office should be, "Is he addicted to the use of ardent spirits?"[30]

Because it was home-grown, whiskey gradually overtook rum in popularity. Rum depended on the importation of molasses, but whiskey has the advantage that it can be made from locally grown grains. Rum was a drink of the Eastern Seaboard, and whiskey was a drink of the country west of the Appalachian Mountains. By the nineteenth century, whiskey drinking was an important part of American life. It became problematic along the western frontier, where single men in saloons drank heavily and violence often resulted. As noted earlier, beer overtook whiskey in popularity in the late 1800s because of the influx of a new wave of immigrants, the Germans, with different drinking habits.

At the beginning of the twenty-first century, whiskey is becoming a beverage similar to wine in its appeal to connoisseurs. Whiskey sellers promote a concept familiar to wine aficionados—terroir. The terroir for whiskey, however, is not necessarily where the barley (or other grain) is grown. Whiskey terroir can be where the beverage distilled from the fermented barley mash matures or from where the water comes. Distillers boast of the purity of the water from Scotland and Kentucky, for example. Whiskey distillers also complicate matters by maturing their products in different types of casks. The quality of the cask makes the bourbon.

In 2013, a distiller in Islay, an island in the Hebrides between Ireland and Scotland, proud of his Celtic background, described the importance of the locale of whiskey maturation. The distiller used barley that was mashed, fermented, and distilled on the mainland of Scotland but matured in wine casks on Islay. The importance of this is that the casks add subtle flavors from the wine and also allow flavors in from the island air. He described whiskey that matured in Château d-Yquem casks as having a "very distinctive minty note. You're getting the heather fields of Islay—the flavor of wild plants. And there's a lovely oily flavor, from the seas."[31] The distiller is carrying on the tradition started by Celtic monks of a thousand years ago but with more up-to-date methods and language.

Gin—Madame Geneva—The Crack Cocaine of Eighteenth-Century London

Early eighteenth-century England was a country of contradictions and tumult. William III, ruler of the Dutch republic, and his wife Mary, daughter of James II, had seized the British throne from James II in the Glorious Revolution of 1688. (Since then, England has had a constitutional monarchy.) Trade expanded to the West Indies, India, and North America and the arts thrived. Joshua Reynolds and Thomas Gainsborough painted English aristocracy so that these wealthy landowners appear sophisticated, stately, and glamorous. Engravers such as William Hogarth created satiric and less flattering images. Samuel Johnson, James Boswell, Henry Fielding, and Daniel Defoe wrote masterpieces. A liberated and irreverent press documented intense and complicated parliamentary politics. Harvests were good, and wages were high. London was one of the world's liveliest metropolises.

In the midst of this heady time of freedom and wealth occurred the "gin craze." Gin is alcohol distilled from any sort of grain-based fermentation and then flavored with juniper berries. Gin comes from the word *geneva*, a corruption of the French word for juniper—*genévrier*. Dutch gin, known as jenever or genever, became popular. Gin was often drunk by soldiers and gave rise to the phrase *Dutch courage*. Because women so often drank gin it was often referred to, in a sardonic way, as Madame Geneva. Gin was associated with poverty and crime and written about with the same tone that we now use with crack cocaine.

The cause of the gin craze was a confluence of several factors. There was a rural exodus in England in the early 1700s, due in part to the enclosures, in which small farms were joined to form larger and more efficient farms for large landowners. Common grazing areas were lost, and a landless working class emerged. People displaced from rural England poured into London. But the great metropolis was not welcoming. There was no sewage system and no supply of clean water. Jobs were scarce and any actual work often dangerous.

At the same time, several decades of good weather in England had led to excellent grain harvests, so landowners had large quantities of grain to sell. Distillation of fermented grain proved to be a clever way of making money from these too-successful harvests. Good-quality barley was fermented into beer, and poor-quality barley could be turned into gin.

In the 1700s, the English government, wanting to help her landowners and distillers, allowed unlicensed gin production and imposed taxes on imported spirits. Gin became cheap and French brandy expensive. By the middle of the eighteenth century, there were over 15,000 shops or taverns in London where alcohol could be bought, and most of these were gin shops.

Peddlers, often women, bought gin from larger retailers and then resold it in smaller quantities from wagons, carts, or small stalls in the streets. These small business entrepreneurs are analogous to today's street dealers of cocaine or heroin.

Beer drinking, which was associated with centuries of tradition, often took place in groups or among family, in moderation, with meals, and for nourishment. Gin drinking in contrast was often a solitary habit and indulged in with the goal of drunkenness. Gin drinking was blamed for crime, prostitution, and family disintegration.

Gin-drinking women were portrayed as violent, promiscuous, syphilitic, and prone to neglecting, abusing, or killing their babies. A famous case of the day was that of Judith Defour. Defour was a poor single mother living in London whose two-year-old daughter Mary was being raised by the parish. One day, Defour went to visit her daughter and saw that she was wearing new clothes. Defour strangled Mary, stripped her, sold the clothes, and drank the proceeds.

Middle-class Londoners reacted to this and similar stories with panic, despair, and contempt. This was a time of active pamphleteering. Gin and those who drank it were written about with concern by moralists and with glee by wits. The novelist Henry Fielding and the engraver William Hogarth were foremost among those concerned about the effects of gin. In 1751, Henry Fielding, best known for writing the Picaresque novel *Tom Jones*, wrote *Enquiry into the Causes of the Late Increase of Robbers*, in which he described the problems caused by gin drinking and called for sweeping changes in the law:

A new kind of drunkenness, unknown to our ancestors, is lately sprung up among us, and which if not put a stop to, will infallibly destroy a great part of the inferior people. The drunkenness I here intend is . . . by this Poison called Gin . . . the principal sustenance (if it may be so called) of more than a hundred thousand people in this Metropolis.[32]

William Hogarth showed the difference between beer and gin in his companion engravings that illustrated many of Fielding's points. Hogarth's audience was Fielding's "inferior people." The engravings were advertised in this way:

> *On Friday next will be publish'd, Price* 1s *each.* Two large Prints, design'd and etch'd by Mr. *Hogarth*, called BEER-STREET and GIN-LANE. A Number will be printed in a better manner for the Curious, at 1s and 6d each ... As the Subjects of these Prints are calculated to reform some reigning Vices peculiar to the lower Class of People, in hopes to render them of more extensive use, the Author had publish'd them in the cheapest Manner possible.[33]

In *Beer Street*, plump and cheerful people drink tankards of beer, smoke pipes, and paint pictures of happy laborers dancing around a haystack (see Figure 1.7). Two couples flirt. Houses are being built. The only rundown structure is identified by a sign with three balls as a pawnshop. The only thin person is an artist. All in all, a good-humored picture of people relaxing after their work.

In contrast, *Gin Lane* depicts chaos and depravity (see Figure 1.8). The very word *lane* indicates a rundown street. The highest structure is the intact three balls sign of the pawnshop. Falling down buildings form the background. Someone is hanging from the rafters—a suicide? In the center of the picture a drunken woman—perhaps Madame Geneva herself—carelessly drops or throws away her baby into a gin cellar, indicated as such by a flagon inscribed "Gin Royal." Over the cellar is written, "Drunk for a penny, Dead drunk for two pence, Straw for nothing." She is dressed in a careless and provocative way and is picking at a probable snuffbox. Pockmarks on her legs may represent syphilis. Beside her, a dog and a child fight over a bone. On the steps below her, a skeletal man with a dog hungrily eyes a bone. Above her, a woman is being buried; a baby cries beside the coffin. To the viewer's right, another woman forces gin into her baby's reluctant mouth, and a cheerful man skewers a child. (This habit of drugging children would be repeated with opium and "patent medicines" a century later.) To the viewer's left, a workman pawns his tools and a woman her cooking pots, presumably to get money for gin. The general message of this picture is clear. Gin leads to starvation, immorality, and child abuse.

Concern for the children who were treated so badly by their gin-soused mothers was not entirely altruistic. The English middle and upper classes wanted the poor to be fertile and to raise healthy children. They needed a steady supply of cheap, hard-working, and reliable laborers, sailors, and soldiers.[34]

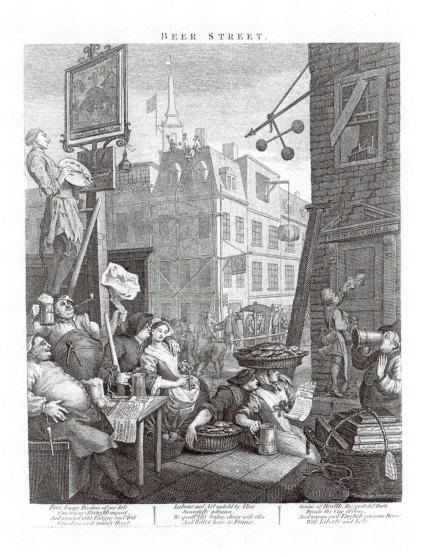

Figure 1.7   **Hogarth's Beer Street. (Wellcome Library, London)**

The government taxed the sellers of gin in an attempt to cut down on gin drinking. The 1736 Gin Act required a £50 license for the sale of gin that most small gin sellers were unable to afford. The result was people selling small quantities of gin and doing so "under the table." The government acted again and passed the Gin Act of 1737, which criminalized gin sellers who did not pay their excise tax and allowed for the payment of informers.

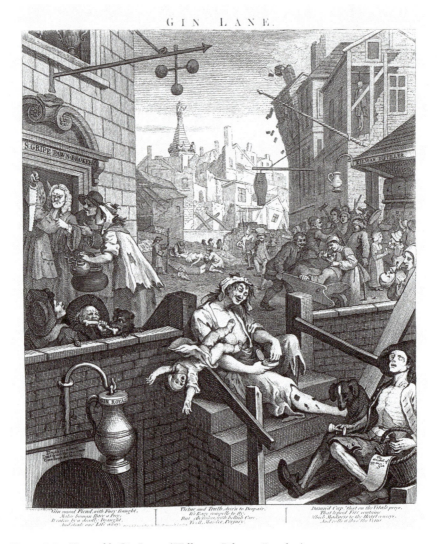

Figure 1.8   Hogarth's Gin Lane. (Wellcome Library, London)

The wealthy London distillers did not go to jail; nor did the middle-class suppliers. But many poor people did. Most of those convicted of selling gin without a license were women. The decision of poor people to sell gin was not necessarily foolish. Women who sold gin did not have to become prostitutes.

Gin sales actually increased. Riots against the government and informers were common. Some informers then devised a new occupation: blackmailing. They visited the gin sellers and took a fee in return for not turning them into the authorities. Informers were then attacked and sometimes killed by mobs.[35] The gin craze, with its widespread defiance of the law, foreshadowed problems in the future with Prohibition in the United States.

The gin craze ended, or people stopped writing about it quite so much, by 1860. Did the work of Fielding and Hogarth have anything to do with it? Perhaps. Another possibility is that when grain harvests failed, distillation of grain alcohol to form gin slowed down.

But gin continued to be associated with the London lower classes and disreputable habits. Although Charles Dickens, in *Sketches by Boz*, took artistic pleasure in describing the miseries of the poor, he explained with compassion why gin continued to be drunk by so many nineteenth-century Londoners:

> Gin-drinking is a great vice in England, but poverty is a greater; and until you can cure it, or persuade a half-famished wretch not to seek relief in the temporary oblivion of his own misery, with the pittance which, divided among his family, would just furnish a morsel of bread for each, gin-shops will increase in number and splendour.[36]

Gin and Tonic

Gin and tonic is the drink of the British colonizers. While gin was associated with the slums of London, the addition of tonic water transformed it into a drink associated with the magnificence of the British Empire. The lower classes drank gin, and the middle and upper classes drank gin and tonic.

The background to the story of gin and tonic is disease. As the British explored, conquered, and moved into tropical areas, tropical diseases, especially malaria, impeded their progress. The only cure for many years was quinine, a substance obtained from the bark of cinchona trees.

The English used quinine to prevent malaria, but quinine by itself is harsh and difficult to consume. As discussed in the opiate chapter, Sir Robert Talbor created a clever medication—quinine, alcohol, and opium—that may have treated the patient's malaria while also encouraging the patient to take the medication repeatedly.

Another way of making quinine easier to consume was to combine it with carbonated water. This formed a bracing drink—tonic water. The addition of gin improved the drink even more. It made for a pleasantly bitter, refreshing, and alcoholic beverage—gin and tonic. Gin and tonic was drunk in tropical countries by the English, who could happily protect themselves against malaria while anesthetizing themselves against the burdens of colonialism.

Tonic water now contains only a trace of quinine, certainly not enough to make it antimalarial. Gin and tonic continues to be a popular beverage, while gin is also part of a sophisticated cocktail, the martini.

Absinthe

Absinthe is a drink of poets, madmen, and murderers. It was medicine for French soldiers and the subject of many paintings. Its essential ingredient is *Artemisia absinthium*, the common wormwood, which grows wild throughout much of the world. Wormwood is toxic to some parasites, hence its name. Absinthe is made by steeping dried wormwood overnight in alcohol along with other herbs such as anise and fennel. Water is then added, and the concoction is distilled. The distillate is a clear green beverage containing about 74 percent alcohol. The biochemical component of absinthe thought to be responsible for its psychotogenic properties is thujone.

A French doctor, Pierre Ordinaire, fled France during the French Revolution and moved to Couvet, a small village in Switzerland. The residents of Couvet drank a local beverage made from wormwood flavored with anise. Ordinaire studied this, modified it, and produced the recipe for modern absinthe in 1792. At his death, he left his secret recipe to two Swiss sisters, who in turn gave it to a Major Dubied, who gave it to his son-in-law Henri-Louis Pernod. Pernod built a small still in Couvet and began to produce absinthe. Absinthe was given to French soldiers during the Algerian war (1844–1847) as a "febrifuge" (a medicine used to lower fevers) and antibacterial agent. The soldiers grew fond of this new substance and brought it home with them.

By 1896, the Pernod factories were producing up to 125,000 liters of absinthe a day. Absinthe was drunk throughout Europe and became a major source of revenue for Switzerland. It eventually crossed the Atlantic, where it took a toehold in New Orleans. (A form of absinthe, Sazerac, is the official beverage of the Crescent City.) However, the center of absinthe drinking was always France. The French market for absinthe was helped by the devastation of the French grape vine rootstocks by the *Phylloxera* louse.

Absinthe is connected with bad behavior and good art, and is discussed later in this respect in the addiction chapter. A complicating factor in trying to ascertain the role of absinthe in causing behavioral problems is the possible presence of other toxins in the beverage. Some absinthe may have contained other substances such as copper salts, methyl alcohol, or antimony. It is also possible that much of the damage attributed to absinthe may have been due to accompanying alcohol abuse. In any event, concern about the ill effects of absinthe grew. In 1890 a British novelist, Marie Corelli, wrote *Wormwood: A Drama of Paris*, in which she wrote:

> The morbidness of the modern French mind is well-known and universally admitted, even by the French themselves: the open atheism, heartlessness, flippancy, and flagrant immorality of the whole modern French school of thought is unquestioned . . . one of those causes is undoubtedly the reckless Absinthemania, which pervades all classes . . .[37]

Absinthe was blamed for a number of murders in Switzerland and France. In 1905, a Swiss man shot and killed his pregnant wife and two children, and then tried to kill himself. Shortly afterward, another man killed his wife with a hatchet and revolver. Both men were heavy absinthe drinkers. These crimes led to much antiabsinthe sentiment. Some thought that much of the antiabsinthe rage in France was fueled by vintners who saw their profits being eroded and by the military who blamed their own failures on absinthe. Absinthe was banned in Belgium in 1906, in Switzerland in 1910, in the United States in 1912, and in France in 1915.

The pendulum has swung, and absinthe is now again available in some countries. The absinthe of the twenty-first century is not, however, the absinthe of Marie Corelli's immoral and flippant fin de siècle Paris, since it contains far less thujone.

Temperance Movements and Prohibition

Alcohol was plentiful in the seventeenth- and eighteenth-century American colonies. Taverns played a prominent role in early American history, and many of the Founding Fathers enjoyed alcohol. There were always people who drank too much, but for the first century of American independence, alcohol was accepted and valued.

Attitudes began to change in the nineteenth century as reform movements spread throughout Europe and North America. Family violence, crime, prostitution, and poverty were blamed on alcohol. Alcoholism was seen as a moral failing. Methodist, Baptist, and Congregationalist clergy were outspoken in decrying the excesses of alcohol drinking.

The importance of wine in Christianity was awkward; they solved this problem by tortuous explanations of the New Testament and declarations that biblical wine was unfermented grape juice.

Organizations to restrict alcohol consumption developed. At first, temperance movements were voluntary and personal. They reflected their name—moderation. Temperance movements promoted personal decisions to stop drinking alcohol. Distilled beverages were more distrusted than beer, cider, and wine. Over time, the movements became more radical. All types of alcoholic beverages were vilified. People were asked to take "the pledge" and renounce alcohol in all forms.

In 1840, six men in Baltimore pledged to stop drinking and formed a group named after the first president. The Washingtonians encouraged each other to stay sober, told tales of their drunkenness, and pledged total abstinence for themselves. They emphasized community, fellowship, and shared storytelling, and soon numbered in the thousands. But within a few years, the Washingtonian movement splintered and then disappeared because of internal arguments.

Meanwhile, others thought that the government should intervene. For almost a century before actual Prohibition, people suggested that the government should ban, or *prohibit*, alcohol. In 1833, the U.S. Supreme Court allowed states to declare themselves "dry" (*dry* in this context means to be alcohol free; *wet* means the opposite). In 1851, Maine was the first state to ban the production and sale of liquor. But this was unsuccessful because there was so much interstate trafficking of liquor.

Many women supported temperance, since they and their children were often injured by alcoholic men. Women lacked financial autonomy, and divorce was rare, so there was little recourse for a woman married to a drunken and abusive husband. In the 1850s, groups of small-town middle-class women protested outside saloons. Sometimes they organized the equivalent of "love-ins," where they prayed.

Susan B. Anthony, the famous suffragette, began her activist career working for temperance but encountered some difficulties. She attended the World's Temperance Society meeting in New York in 1853 and said to a friend, "the brothers will feel very much disturbed at our presence."[38] In fact, the men in the audience hissed and howled to prevent a woman from speaking. Anthony wrote:

> In those early days it was considered gentlemanly to use wine to excess; it was customary and was the law for a husband to take all of his wife's property and use it as he pleased . . . designing men would marry innocent girls

for their money, and almost as soon as the marriage vow was uttered, would waste their wives' dowry in riotous living. . . . I want to ask . . . why when women combine and make a demand they are always laughed at? Women always begin on temperance. Whiskey is the subject thought of by the ladies . . . In New York we got up a petition signed by over 2,800 . . . It was read and laughed at . . .[39]

This illustrated the problems faced by women. Drunken men took their money, sober men did not allow them to talk, and politicians did not listen. Anthony decided that obtaining the vote was the best way to proceed. She turned her formidable energies to the suffrage movement while remaining a supporter of temperance movements.

In 1874, the Woman's Christian Temperance Union (WCTU) was formed and became the largest women' organization of the time. The WCTU took on many other causes such as prison reform, child protection, kindergarten promotion, and elimination of poverty. The WCTU, like the Washingtonians, was weakened by its own good intentions. Members wanted to tackle other causes, and disagreements as to what was the most important issue developed. Many within the movement supported suffrage for women and African Americans as well as abstinence from alcohol—but could not agree on the prioritization of these issues. The WCTU had so many causes that they may have diluted their original message. The WCTU still exists but is no longer as powerful as it once was.

Other forces were at play. Distrust of many of the ethnic minorities flooding into the United States in the late nineteenth century was common. Many of the new Americans—such as the German, Irish, and Italians—were Catholic or Jewish and drank alcohol as part of their day-to-day life or as part of religious ceremonies. Some politicians were apprehensive of declaring themselves wet because they did not want to lose the votes of those with nationalistic and anti-immigrant sentiments. In contrast, Protestant clergy tended to be sympathetic to the drys.

There were other tensions. Southern whites inflamed themselves by creating portraits of whiskey-inflamed blacks assaulting their women. (This is similar to the equally inflated accounts of the powers of cocaine.) The Ku Klux Klan had always hated blacks, immigrants, Catholics, and Jews. They added alcohol drinkers and saloon owners to their list.

The variety of groups supporting the idea of federal prohibition—from Southern Baptists to suffragettes in the Northeast to the Ku Klux Klan was astonishing—and forestalled any cooperation between them. Confessions and appeals to the better nature of humanity had not led to a diminution of alcoholism or helped move the country to prohibition. The Washingtonians and WCTU had raised the issue; another force was to emerge to do the political work.

In 1900, the Anti-Saloon League (ASL) was organized in Ohio and became a powerful political force in the United States. The ASL was a professional lobbying movement. It was based in rural areas, the South, and the Midwest, and was supported by many Protestant clergy.

The ASL cleverly chose the saloon as its object of opprobrium rather than alcohol itself. Saloons—an American semi equivalent of English gin shops—were portrayed as gathering places for drunken, rowdy men that fostered criminality, prostitution, and gambling to the detriment of church and family. The ASL was not actually just against saloons; it was opposed to the consumption of all alcoholic beverages in all places. The name was misleading, clever, and designed to appeal to a wider group of people than might otherwise have been sympathetic to its goals.

Opposition to the ASL was not well organized. The brewers and distillers were unable to form effective opposition without sounding self-serving. They argued amongst themselves. The brewers in particular were hampered by a disinclination for publicity; they were afraid of arousing distrust of German Americans, given the growing unrest in Europe. Many politicians who might otherwise have opposed the ASL were distracted by events in Europe and then by World War I.

Politicians thought that alcohol sales would never be banned because of the federal government's dependence on revenues from alcohol. From 1872 until 1913, there was no income tax, and 90 percent of government revenue came from taxes on alcohol and tobacco.[40] In 1909, Congress passed the Sixteenth Amendment, approving the income tax, and in 1913, this amendment was ratified. With a new source of revenue for the government, a major hurdle to Prohibition had been passed.

Many politicians at the beginning of the twentieth century belonged to the ASL movement, not out of conviction—but out of fear of the ASL. It was not unusual for politicians to be personally wet but to vote dry. The hypocrisy bothered the ASL not at all. They were focused on getting to national Prohibition by whatever means. The ASL movement is credited, or blamed, with developing many political tactics still used today. ASL leaders pressured and blackmailed politicians. They were vindictive to the temperance movement leaders who were not in favor of Prohibition. The ASL, a single-issue movement, supported politicians of any party, as long as they in turn supported the ASL. The dry voting and ASL-fearing or -beholden politicians formed a majority in Congress in 1916.

The entry of the United States into World War I also helped. Anti-German sentiment, and thus antibeer sentiment, increased. Grain was diverted from fermentation to the war effort. Drunken workers seemed unpatriotic. Despite this, politicians in the urban centers of the country and in the Northeast never believed that the ASL would be able to achieve their goal. They had underestimated the strength of the ASL.

In 1917, Congress passed the Eighteenth Amendment to the Constitution, prohibiting "the manufacture, sale, or transportation of intoxicating liquors." This was a surprise to many. In 1919, the National Prohibition Act—known as the Volstead Act after its introducer, Congressman Andrew Volstead of Minnesota—was passed to enforce the new amendment. The amendment went into effect in January 1920. Trafficking and transportation of alcohol became illegal throughout the United States. The Reverend Billy Sunday, a prominent Protestant evangelist, proclaimed:

> The reign of tears is over. The slums will soon be a memory. We will turn our prisons into factories and our jails into storehouses and corncribs. Men will walk upright now, women will smile and the children will laugh. Hell will be forever for rent.[41]

At the beginning of Prohibition, consumption of alcohol, public drunkenness, and alcohol-related crime all decreased. Prohibition was a success. It seemed as though alcohol and all of its attendant problems *could* be legislated away.

Within a few years, though, problems emerged. Americans continued to drink alcohol throughout the 13 years of Prohibition. Instead of drinking beer and wine, they turned to gin and whiskey, in part because stronger beverages were drunk in smaller amounts and so were easier to smuggle and to hide.

A huge market for alcohol still existed, and criminals rushed to supply people with alcohol. The most famous was Al Capone in Chicago. He made millions of dollars and bribed both police and politicians. Police activity used to "catch" bootleggers and their customers was futile, although inventive. Police resorted to wiretapping for the first time. Roy Olmstead, first a policemen and then a successful bootlegger in Seattle who bought liquor from nearby British Columbia, was caught thanks to this new technique.

American crime became better organized and more profitable. Liquor was smuggled into the United States from Canada, Mexico, and the

Caribbean by land, water, and air. The British Redcoats had a difficult time preventing the smuggling of rum into America; so did the American government.

Another problem arising from Prohibition was the poor, and sometimes poisonous, qualities of the illegal alcohol. Moonshine had always been produced in the Appalachians, but now its production increased. Various substances often contaminated it. For example, moonshine was sometimes made in stills devised from radiators. The solder of radiators contained lead, which often leached into the moonshine. Once again, lead, as it had been in Roman times, was a contaminant, and lead-tainted moonshine caused many deaths.

Another poison was methyl alcohol, or methanol. Methanol is also known as wood alcohol because it was often obtained from burning wood. Ethanol (or ethyl alcohol, the subject of this chapter), in contrast, is obtained from the fermentation of grains, so it is sometimes known as grain alcohol. Methyl alcohol has just one carbon atom and two hydrogen atoms fewer than does ethyl alcohol. This small difference has large implications. Formic acid, which comes from methanol, leads to blindness.

Alcohol is used in the manufacture of many substances, such as paint, solvents, and fuels. Industrial alcohol was often stolen by bootleggers during Prohibition and sold as a beverage. To prevent this, industrial alcohol was "denatured," which means that an unpleasant-tasting adulterant or methanol was added. Bootleggers paid chemists to get rid of the methanol, but this job was not always done competently.

People made their own alcoholic beverages. Wine was made at home, ostensibly for religious purposes. Thirsty people or entrepreneurs would fill large containers or bathtubs with cheap alcohol and mix it with flavorings such as juniper berries. The mixture would steep and in a few days, "gin" was ready to drink. Bathtub gin could be produced in a variety of ways but often was quite dangerous. If the alcohol used was denatured, drinkers could become blind or die. Cocktails became more popular, in part to disguise the nasty taste of bathtub gin.

Yet another problem with Prohibition was that of enforcement. ASL members had been brilliant publicists, campaigners, and organizers. They had bullied drinking politicians into supporting Prohibition. Once the Eighteenth Amendment was passed, they must have thought that they had won. But the ASL lobbyists were unable to transfer their vote-getting energy and Machiavellianism to the different art of governing. The implementation of Prohibition needed money. Politicians could be cajoled for votes for Prohibition, but the ASL ran out of steam when it came to convincing them to pay for enforcement. The federal government preferred that the states pay a share, which usually did not happen. As a result of lack of money, federal enforcement was entrusted to agents who were badly paid. The agents were not required to pass civil service exams. They were rapidly hired and poorly trained. They could not have been better chosen from the point of view of the liquor sellers. The agents—along with many office holders—were immediately, frequently, and generously bribed. Enforcement of Prohibition was limited. The ASL, or drys, had won and ended up damaging their cause. Their victory made them look foolish.

Prohibition was not a complete failure. Alcohol consumption did drop during those 13 years. Supporters of Prohibition could point to the weakness of the enforcement rather than the weakness of the idea. Moreover, the ASL actually achieved the goal hinted at by its name. The saloon disappeared (or, at least, became less visible). The ASL had chosen the saloon to attack because it did foster vices, and the loss of the saloon was seen by some as a boon to society.

Overall, however, Prohibition caused many problems, and movements to repeal it sprang up. Henry Ford and John D. Rockefeller Jr. had originally supported Prohibition, hoping that sober workers would have greater productivity, but they turned against it. They were appalled by the lawbreaking. They were also increasingly upset by the income tax and thought that it would be easier to get rid of this tax, or at least lessen it, if the government returned to its earlier source of revenue. As well, many thought that the severity of the Great Depression, which began in 1929, could be lessened by broadening the revenue base and employing the unemployed in the liquor industries. Many hoped for the repeal of both the Sixteenth and Eighteenth Amendments.

One movement to end Prohibition was headed by a woman named Pauline Sabin. A wealthy Republican, she was sophisticated and charming. She was dismayed by the hypocrisy of politicians and the glorification of lawbreakers. She was a foil to the WCTU, which sometimes claimed to speak for all American women.

Franklin Delano Roosevelt was elected president in 1932 and took office in January 1933. On March 23, 1933, he signed an amendment to the Volstead Act that allowed the sale of beer. In December 1933, the Twenty-First Amendment repealed the Eighteenth Amendment. No other amendment has been repealed. The income tax continues.

The lesson of Prohibition can be summed up by the prescient words of Abraham Lincoln. Lincoln himself did not drink alcohol and described liquor as the ". . . angel of death, commissioned to slay if not the first, the fairest born of every family . . ."[42] But Lincoln had a nuanced view of alcohol. As a young man, he sold whiskey. An anecdote from the Civil War is that someone suggested to him that he fire Ulysses Grant because of his heavy drinking. Lincoln replied that the person should find out what Grant was drinking and send a barrel of it to the other Union Army generals. Lincoln's distrust of liquor was surpassed by his distrust of ill-considered legislation. He also said that

> Prohibition will work great injury to the cause of temperance. It is a species of intemperance within itself, for it goes beyond the bounds of reason by legislation and makes a crime out of things that are not crime. A prohibition law strikes at the very principle upon which our Government is founded.[43]

Alcoholics Anonymous

In 1935, two alcoholic men—Bill Wilson, a speculator on Wall Street, and Robert Smith, a physician—formed another temperance movement, Alcoholics Anonymous (AA). They based AA in part on the principles of the Washingtonians and the Oxford Group, a Protestant self-help group popular in the United States at the time.

Wilson and Smith taught that the alcoholic had lost his self-control and that this could be regained by talking to other alcoholics. They developed the well-known principles of the movement: anonymity, fellowship, and reliance on a "higher power." They decided that AA would be decentralized and never depend on the charisma of a central person. AA was not to be a profit-making movement. It would work with "professionals" but not be a "treatment" movement.

AA differs from the earlier prohibitionist movements in that it addresses only the individual alcoholic, not the public. AA does not demand that everyone stop drinking. The principles of AA have been applied to other conditions, and other self-help (or, perhaps more accurately, mutual-aid) groups founded on AA principles have developed. These groups share many features. Members of each group have the same problem, and their goal is to deal with or defeat the problem and combat stigma. Group meetings are free, voluntary, and often involve storytelling. The groups provide support and a sense of belonging and counter the sense of helplessness and hopelessness that accompanies some disorders.

The AA movement is full of paradox. It celebrates both anonymity and fellowship. It is about the shame of alcoholism, and yet the "drunkalog," in which the alcoholic often seems to boast of his or her exploits, is a major part of the meetings. AA encourages the alcoholic to stop drinking yet to focus on his alcoholism. Despite, or because of, the paradoxes, AA is a successful movement. It has lasted while the movements that inspired it, the Washingtonians and Oxford Group, have not, and it has survived the deaths of its two founders.

However, there is no clear evidence of the efficacy of AA. Indeed, some suggest that people who join AA fare worse, in terms of problematic drinking, than those who do not join the organization because AA, by "medicalizing" drinking behavior, gives people an excuse for drinking. The "all-or-none" approach to drinking favored by AA also encourages people not to decrease their drinking but to stop it entirely. This approach is too difficult for some, who might benefit from advice to decrease their drinking. This approach also may lead to people who have a "slip" feeling that they might as well resume binge drinking.[44]

Despite these concerns, most alcoholism experts support AA, and there is much anecdotal evidence of the movement's power. Caroline Knapp, an alcoholic and memoirist, describes in one passage the differences in her life after she started attending AA meetings:

> Abby once asked me to describe a typical evening in my drinking days, and I rolled my eyes and said, "Blah. Exactly the same thing, every night. I'd leave work, get drunk, watch TV, and go to bed."
>
> She asked, "And how about now?"
>
> I thought for a minute, then smiled and said, "Well, now I leave work, go to a meeting, watch TV, and go to bed."
>
> She said, "*Excuse me?*"
>
> But she also understood. The differences are internal, as though a kaleidoscope has shifted, yielding shapes in color instead of black-and-white ... Most nights I end up in a church basement instead of a bar, and even if I don't say a word during a meeting, I have the sense of being in the midst of a human place, where people are actively struggling with their lives, and I almost always leave meetings with a feeling of hope that was foreign in the past.[45]

Once Knapp began to attend AA meetings, she was no longer alone. Rather than spending her evenings drunk, she spent them sober and with a group of people who shared and understood her problem. AA provided Knapp with sobriety, community, and hope.

Effects on the Mind and the Body

How Alcohol Gets into the Body

Alcohol is swallowed and then absorbed from the stomach, small intestine, and colon into the bloodstream. This process is slower if there is food present. Once absorbed, alcohol rapidly spreads to all body fluids and tissues, including the brain, and, in the pregnant woman, the embryo or fetus.

Alcohol is metabolized by the enzyme alcohol dehydrogenase, which is located primarily in the liver. The enzyme removes one hydrogen and thus changes the alcohol into acetaldehyde, a toxic substance. Another enzyme, aldehyde dehydrogenase, changes the acetaldehyde into acetic acid, which in turn is broken down to carbon dioxide and water.

Some people have very little effective aldehyde hydrogenase, so acetaldehyde builds up in large quantities. This is particularly common in people of Asian descent. A person with ineffective aldehyde dehydrogenase may flush, develop a rapid heartbeat, and feel ill if he or she drinks alcohol. This unpleasant reaction may be one of the reasons for low rates of alcoholism in many Asian populations.

Effects on the Mind

Small amounts of alcohol, particularly when consumed with food, decrease anxiety and social shyness. These effects increase pleasure in social interactions and are highly valued. Drinking with meals means that exposure to alcohol is gradual and diluted by other substances. Cocaine increases energy, opiates lessen anxiety, and tobacco calms and distracts, but alcohol, in small amounts, is the most likely, of the four substances, to increase conviviality. Drinking moderate amounts of alcohol with meals with family or friends improves the flavor of the food and the quality of the company. It eases conversation, promotes the flow of ideas, and strengthens the bonds of friendship.

The situation is bleaker for people who drink large amounts of alcohol while also consuming poor diets. The most important nutritional deficiency suffered by alcoholics is lack of vitamin B1, also known as thiamine. The combination of alcohol and a thiamine deficiency is toxic to the brain, and can cause confusion and eventual dementia.

Intoxication

Intoxication is easily recognized and was described by Michael Pollan in this way:

Dionysian revelry, which begins in ecstasy and often ends in blood, embodies this truth: the same wine that loosens the knots of inhibition and reveals nature's most beneficent face can also dissolve the bonds of civilization and unleash ungovernable passions.[46]

The intoxicated person smells of alcohol, speaks in a slurred manner, and is clumsy, irritable, jovial, and confused. The behavior of intoxication is much affected by expectations. In some cultures, intoxication is associated with greater sociability and calm. But in Anglo-American countries, intoxicated people often behave in foolish ways that strike themselves and bystanders as humorous. When associated with bad behavior or "ungovernable passions," the word *drunkenness* is used. Alcohol is more likely than any other substance in this book to lead to a disinhibited state. Some people are prone to boast and laugh about how much they can drink and how drunk they can become.

This kind of childish behavior is due to alcohol's inhibition of the "higher" centers of the mind, particularly those responsible for adult behaviors. The inhibition of inhibition is delightful. The intoxicated person can, temporarily, be free of all of the pernicious and joyless nagging brakes. A psychoanalyst would say that the superego, the part of the mind that always says wait, or no, or think of the consequences, dissolves in alcohol. What a relief to lose that irritating voice!

Another way of describing this is in terms of executive functioning, or thoughtful and deliberate decision making. Executive functioning belongs to the sober.

Intoxication, at least in much of the Western world today, is associated with a tremendous amount of harm. The "irritating voice" that is so pleasant to silence is, of course, useful. Irresponsible people may be happier, but they cause trouble. This is for a number of reasons. Alcohol decreases alertness and reaction time. It is toxic to the cerebellum, a part of the brain that coordinates physical movements. The combination of these deficits leads to the well-known picture of the drunken person lurching about with an unsteady gait and slurred speech. The drunk person at the wheel of a car is more dangerous. The drunk driver does not worry about safe driving and in any event cannot safely maneuver his or her vehicle. Drunk drivers (and pedestrians) are more likely to be involved in accidents than are sober people. At blood levels of above 0.08 milliequivalents per liter, people are considered to be legally intoxicated in the United States and not allowed to drive. (Some countries have decided that any detectable alcohol in the blood leads to inability to drive safely.) The drunk driver often insists that he or she is not impaired. It is not unusual for a person to say, "I'm a better driver when I've had a drink or two; I can handle it." The combination of false confidence, impaired judgment, increased energy, desire to show off, and impaired cerebellum is unique to alcohol.

Violence is also linked to drunkenness. Barroom fights are common. Gin drinking caused so much distress in eighteenth-century London in part because of the violence. The drunken person is easily offended and unlikely to worry about consequences. The intoxicated "super-ego" no longer instructs the person not to hit others. Drunkenness also may be linked to being a victim of violence. The drunk person may be more likely to be provocative or to be an easier target. Violence to oneself, or suicide, is discussed later in this chapter.

Sleep

There is a complex relationship between alcohol and sleep. A "nightcap," or alcoholic drink in the evening, is sedating and decreases the time required to fall asleep. However, there is a dark side to this, in that alcohol disrupts sleep in later parts of the night. Sleep becomes light, fragmented, and no longer refreshing. The disruptive effects may worsen with age. Alcohol withdrawal is associated with particularly severe insomnia. Indeed, sleep may remain disturbed for months to years after withdrawal from alcohol.

Addiction

Addiction to alcohol, or alcoholism, or the decision of people to drink despite the clear harm that it causes, was first seen as an illness by Benjamin Rush, friend of John Adams, signer of the Declaration of Independence, and first surgeon general of the Continental Army. He is sometimes referred to as the father of American psychiatry. His attitudes toward alcohol were complex. He deplored the excessive use of alcohol, particularly distilled liquors. He recommended wine, beer, or opium as alternatives to distilled spirits. As befitting his political activities, he was particularly upset about the effects of alcohol on the new democracy. He hoped to start a temperance movement so that, by the twentieth century, "a drunkard . . . will be as infamous in society as a liar or a thief, and the use of spirits as uncommon in families as a drink made of a solution of arsenic or a decoction of hemlock."[47] He had a personal interest in the subject. His father was an alcoholic, and his parents divorced because of this. His mother's second husband was a distiller.[48]

The theory that alcoholism is a disease was updated in 1960 by E. M. Jellinek, who published a book entitled *The Disease Concept of Alcoholism*. The book was based on responses to a questionnaire filled out by 98 AA members and has been criticized for its small number of subjects.

Alcoholism tends to run in families, even though most children of alcoholics do not themselves become alcoholic. In adoption studies, the most reliable predictor of alcoholism in children is the presence of alcoholism in a biological parent. Children born of nonalcoholic parents who are adopted by alcoholic parents are not at greater risk of developing alcoholism. These observations support the theory that there is a genetic vulnerability to alcoholism.

Cultural factors are important. For example, the habits of drinking with the opposite gender and across generations, drinking with meals, and drinking as part of celebratory or religious rite are all associated with less harm from alcohol. Drinking alcohol with others during meals is common in Mediterranean countries, and this may be why alcohol is less harmful in these countries than it is in countries where it is typically consumed without food. The habit in some communities of men drinking distilled liquors together in bars or pubs is the kind of drinking associated with dangerous alcoholism. Alcohol has been particularly harmful for many indigenous peoples. It is often difficult to tease out biological from sociocultural factors when groups of people have different rates of illness from others, and this is certainly true in this case.

Withdrawal

People with sustained excessive drinking find it extremely difficult to stop drinking, in part because of withdrawal symptoms. Withdrawal is an unpleasant combination of tremulousness, irritability, nausea, vomiting, insomnia, and seizures. The symptoms are usually at their worst two to three days after stopping drinking. At their worst, the symptoms may coalesce into delirium tremens. In this syndrome, the person has a tremor, fever, and rapid heartbeat. Anxiety and visual hallucinations are common. The mortality rate of delirium tremens is high. Withdrawal from alcohol, and not from any of the other substances discussed in this book, can be fatal.

Isolation, Depression, and Suicide

Some alcoholics wear out the patience of their friends, employers, and finally families. Their repeated episodes of intoxication, often accompanied by violent or reckless behavior, fray the fabric of family ties. Their own shame sometimes leads them to desert their families before they are expelled. They become depressed and lose any interest in taking care of themselves. They cannot keep jobs or relationships. They end up living alone or in shelters and become well known to staff in inner-city emergency rooms. If they do not eat well, as often happens with the lonely and poor, they also increase their risk of poor nutrition, which increases their risk of brain damage or dementia.

Alcohol use is associated with suicide because of the links between alcohol and both depression and impulsivity. Mild intoxication is associated with cheerfulness and euphoria, but as a person continues to drink, his or her mood often darkens. If the person becomes addicted to or dependent on alcohol, then more problems set in. Alcohol dependence interferes with relationships and work, which leads to loneliness and poverty, which in turn worsen depression. Depressed people sometimes drink more, and heavy drinking worsens depression. The alcohol intake does not cheer up the person, but it can cause temporary relief from feelings of anxiety and guilt. Depressed people may find it easier to be drunk and numb than to be sober and sad.

While intoxicated, the person can behave impulsively and in ways that are harmful. If the person is not depressed, then the harm may be minor or involved with recklessness that could harm property or others. But a person who is already depressed and drunk loses the inhibitions against self-harm. All of these elements are involved with the high rates of suicide among people with depression who drink too much alcohol.

Effects on the Body

Small amounts of alcohol have long been thought to be healthy. In the past, unfiltered wine and beer contained many nutrients because the vitamin-rich yeast was left in the beverage. Landlord May's flip with its cream and eggs would have slowed the absorption of the alcohol, making drunkenness less likely, and also given the drinker some protein and vitamins. Perhaps this is one of the reasons alcohol drinking was treated with less disapproval in the past. Also, alcoholic beverages were often less likely to be contaminated than other beverages.

Alcohol was often prescribed for its nonspecific effects. Two eminent physicians of the 1800s who were skeptical of most medication, and indeed had little useful medication available to them, did appreciate the good effects of alcohol. Oliver Wendell Holmes Sr. is often quoted as saying, "I firmly believe that if the whole materia medica [medical drugs], as now used, could be sunk to the bottom of the sea, it would be all the better for mankind, and all the worse for the fishes."[49] But he made a few exceptions, including wine. William Osler, another therapeutic nihilist, prescribed gin or whiskey as a stimulant for the aged, including his own mother.[50]

People who have one to two drinks a day do have decreased cardiovascular mortality compared to nondrinkers, possibly due to a change in clotting mechanisms or an increase in high density lipoproteins. (These proteins are thought to remove cholesterol from the blood vessel walls.) But the consumption of three or more drinks a day is associated with high blood pressure, heart damage, and multiple other disorders.

Gut

Alcohol damages many parts of the gut. It irritates the esophagus and stomach, sometimes to the point of bleeding. Alcohol is also associated with acute pancreatitis. Chronic exposure to alcohol is associated with fatty liver and the development of liver failure. Even moderate alcohol intake may increase the risk of liver cirrhosis and liver cancer in those with chronic hepatitis.

Pregnancy

Pregnant women who drink alcohol risk giving birth to babies with Fetal Alcohol Syndrome (FAS) (see Figure 1.9).

A baby with FAS may be smaller at birth than the average baby, and have a small head with small eyes and jaw, flat nose, loss of the usual furrow between the upper lip and nose, and extra skin at the inside edge of the eyes. The baby may also have malformations of organs such as the heart, hands, and feet, and varying degrees of mental retardation. Children with FAS may have learning and attentional difficulties.

The exact causes of FAS are not known. Alcohol and/or acetaldehyde may affect the sperm and egg prior to conception. Many babies born with FAS have been born to women who smoke, use other drugs, and may be poorly nourished. But most of the damage is thought to be due to alcohol or its breakdown product, acetaldehyde, crossing the placental barrier and directly affecting the developing fetus.

FAS has been described in all parts of the world. It is the leading cause of mental retardation in the United States and is preventable. Much of the public's knowledge about FAS has to do with the babies and children with this disorder. As the children grow up, these characteristic features fade somewhat, but their behavioral problems may worsen. Their learning

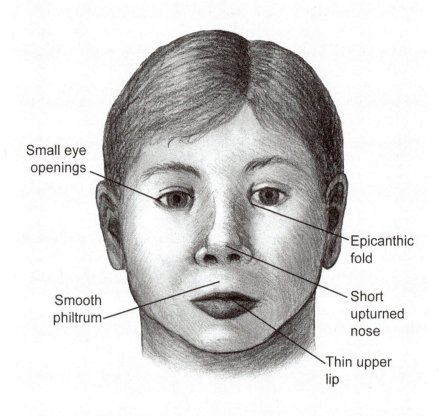

Figure 1.9   **Child with Fetal Alcohol Syndrome. (© 2013 Joan M.K. Tycko)**

disabilities and impulsivity may increase the person's risk for drinking alcohol and having babies themselves in an irresponsible manner.[51]

Malignancy

Alcohol is associated with an increase in the rate of many malignancies, including breast, oral, esophageal, and rectal cancer. Rates of many cancers are increased in people who smoke cigarettes as well as drink alcohol.

Conclusion

Alcoholic beverages have been an important part of most civilizations, and thirst for them and profits obtained by selling them have played a part in much of our history. Used in moderation, alcohol is delightful; used in excess, alcohol is harmful.

Notes

1. Reay Tannahill, *Food in History* (New York: Three Rivers, 1988), 48.

2. *The Epic of Gilgamesh*, trans. Maureen Gallery Kovacs (Stanford: Stanford University Press, 1985), 16.

3. Maguelonne Toussaint-Samat, *A History of Food*, trans. Anthea Bell (Singapore: Wiley-Blackwell, 2009), 163.

4. Tom Standage, *A History of the World in 6 Glasses* (New York: Walker & Company, 2005), 37.

5. Nick Brownlee, *This Is Alcohol* (London: Sanctuary, 2002), 78.

6. Toussaint-Samat, *A History of Food*, 165.

7. Christian Heurich Sr., "My Life, 1842–1934: From Haina in Thuringia to Washington in the United States of America" (English trans., unpublished manuscript, 1985, 6–7), obtained courtesy Bill Lebovich.

8. James Boswell, *Life of Johnson*, ed. R. W. Chapman (Oxford: Oxford University Press, 1998), 697.

9. George F. Willison, *Saints and Strangers* (New York: Reynal and Hitchcock, 1945), 131.

10. Greg Smith, *Beer in America: The Early Years; 1587–1840* (Boulder, CO: Brewers Publications, 1998), 9–10.

11. Willison, *Saints and Strangers*, 131.

12. Alice Morse Earle, *Customs and Fashions in New England* 1893 (repr., Williamstown, MA: Corner House Publishers, 1974), 172.

13. Standage, *Six Glasses*, 52–53.

14. Michael Pollan, *The Botany of Desire: A Plant's-Eye View of the World* (New York: Random House, 2001), 38.

15. Quoted in Harold McGee, *On Food and Cooking: The Science and Lore of the Kitchen* (New York: Scribner, 1984), 428.

16. S. C. Gilfillan, "Lead Poisoning and the Fall of Rome," *Journal of Occupational Medicine* 7, no. 2 (1965): 53–60.

17. Jerome O. Nriagu, "Saturnine Gout among Roman Aristocrats: Did Lead Poisoning Contribute to the Fall of the Empire?" *New England Journal of Medicine* 308, no. 11 (1983): 660–63.

18. Quoted in Griffith Edwards, *Alcohol: The World's Favorite Drug* (New York: Thomas Dunne, 2000), 19.

19. Olaudah Equiano, *The Interesting Narrative and Other Writings*, ed. Vincent Carretta (New York: Penguin, 1995), 55–58.

20. Mark Kurlansky, *Cod* (New York: Penguin, 1997), 80–81.

21. Quoted in Charles William Taussig, *Rum, Romance and Rebellion* (New York: Minton, Balch & Company, 1928), 145–46.

22. Hugh Thomas. *The Slave Trade* (New York: Simon & Schuster, 1997), 328. New England, just like England, liked to export.

23. Taussig, *Rum, Romance and Rebellion*, 68.

24. Ibid., 76–77.

25. Earle, *Customs and Fashions in New England*, 178–79.

26. Quoted in Stephen E. Ambrose, *Undaunted Courage: Meriwether Lewis, Thomas Jefferson, and the Opening of the American West* (New York: Simon & Schuster, 1996), 31–32.

27. Wayne Curtis, *And a Bottle of Rum: A History of the New World in Ten Cocktails* (New York: Three Rivers, 2006), 173.

28. Corn was turned into a drink by many groups in America. The Hopi drank it after it was processed with ash, the Aztecs processed it with lime, and in Peru it was (and still is) fermented and turned into *chicha*. These beverages were mildly alcoholic and not distilled. There is much more about corn in Betty Fussell, *The Story of Corn: The Myths and History, The Culture and Agriculture, The Art and Science of America's Quintessential Crop* (New York: North Point, 1992).

29. Fussell, *The Story of Corn*, 262.

30. Quoted in John Kobler, *Ardent Spirits: The Rise and Fall of Prohibition* (New York: Da Capo, 1993), 33.

31. Kelefa Sanneh, "Letter from Islay: Spirit Guide; Reinventing a Great Distillery," *New Yorker*, February 11 and 18, 2013, 61.

32. Quoted in Jenny Uglow, *Hogarth: A Life and a World* (London: Faber and Faber, 1997), 493.

33. Ibid., 494.

34. Patrick Dillon, *Gin: The Much-Lamented Death of Madam Geneva; The Eighteenth-Century Gin Craze* (Boston: Justin, Charles & Co., 2002), 244.

35. Ibid., 193–200.

36. Charles Dickens, *Sketches by Boz*, 1839. ed. Dennis Walder (London: Penguin Books, 1995), 220.

37. Quoted in Barnaby Conrad III, *Absinthe* (San Francisco: Chronicle Books, 1988), 51. One wonders if the sales of absinthe and tickets to Paris would have increased after the publication of Corelli's novel.

38. Quoted in Lynn Sherr, *Failure Is Impossible: Susan B. Anthony in Her Own Words*, (New York: Times Books, 1995), 46.

39. Ibid., 48–49.

40. http://www.irs.gov/uac/Historical-Highlights-of-the-IRS, accessed July 19, 2013. The income tax has always been unpopular. An income tax was imposed by Abraham Lincoln and his Congress in 1862 to help pay for the Civil War. It was repealed 10 years later. Congress revived the tax in 1894, but the Supreme Court ruled that it was not constitutional.

41. Quoted in Kobler, *Ardent Spirits*, 12.

42. Quoted in Edward Behr, *Prohibition: Thirteen Years That Changed America* (New York: Arcade, 1996), 32.

43. Ibid., 33.

44. Stanton Peele, *Diseasing of America: Addiction Treatment Out of Control* (Lexington, MA: Lexington Books, 1989), 55–83.

45. Caroline Knapp, *Drinking: A Love Story* (New York: Dell, 2006), 271–72.

46. Pollan, *Botany of Desire*, 39.

47. Ian Williams, *Rum: A Social and Sociable History* (New York: Nation Books, 2005), 193.

48. William L. White, *Slaying the Dragon: The History of Addiction Treatment and Recovery in America* (Normal, IL: Chestnut Health Systems/Lighthouse Institute, 1998), 2.

49. Michael Bliss, *William Osler: A Life in Medicine* (New York: Oxford University Press, 1999), 52.

50. Ibid., 108.

51. Michael Dorris, *The Broken Cord* (New York: Harper & Row, 1989), 180.

Additional Sources

Benbow, Mark. "Christian Heurich." In *Immigrant Entrepreneurship: German-American Business Biographies, 1720 to the Present*, vol. 3, Giles R. Hoyt, ed. German Historical Institute. Last modified June 19, 2012, http://immigrant entrepreneurship.org/entry.php?rec=38.

Blocker, Jack S. "Did Prohibition Really Work? Alcohol Prohibition as a Public Health Innovation." *American Journal of Public Health* 96 (2006): 233–43.

Brown, Sally, and David R. Brown. *Mrs. Marty Mann: The First Lady of Alcoholics Anonymous*. Center City, MN: Hazelden, 2001.

Burnham, John C. *Bad Habits: Drinking, Smoking, Taking Drugs, Gambling, Sexual Misbehavior and Swearing in American History*. New York: New York University Press, 1993.

Frankenburg, Frances. *Vitamin Discoveries and Disasters*. Santa Barbara, CA: Praeger, 2009.

Gately, Iain. *Drink: A Cultural History of Alcohol*. New York: Gotham Books, 2008.

Lerner, Michael A. *Dry Manhattan: Prohibition in New York City*. Cambridge, MA: Harvard University Press, 2007.

Mintz, Sidney W. *Sweetness and Power: The Place of Sugar in Modern History*. New York: Viking Penguin, 1985.

Mukamal, Kenneth J. "A 42-Year-Old Man Considering Whether to Drink Alcohol for His Health." *Journal of the American Medical Association* 303, no. 20 (2010): 2065–73.

Okrent, Daniel. *Last Call: The Rise and Fall of Prohibition*. New York: Scribner, 2010.

Rorabaugh, William J. *The Alcoholic Republic: An American Tradition*. New York: Oxford University Press, 1979.

2

Why We Need Water

Alcoholic beverages were often drunk in the past as a safe way of consuming water. Water, so easily taken for granted, is essential for our life. More than half of our body consists of water, and it is crucial for our metabolism. Water seems like a simple substance, but it has unusual properties that can be understood by a brief review of the water molecule.

Properties of the Water Molecule

Each water molecule contains one hydrogen atom and two oxygen atoms. The molecule is V-shaped and polar, meaning that the two hydrogen sides of the molecule are slightly positive and the oxygen side, at the bottom of the V, is slightly negative. Positive and negative electric charges attract one another. This allows the water molecules to form weak hydrogen bonds with each other, as is shown in Figure 2.1. Bonds between molecules in solids, in contrast, are much stronger. The weakness and short life of the hydrogen bonds allow the molecules to change position frequently, letting water flow as a liquid at body temperature.

The polarity of the water molecule also means that it is a good solvent. Indeed, water is known as the universal solvent. The positive or negative parts of compounds, such as salt, or sodium chloride, are attracted to the negative and positive parts of the water molecule. When salt is put into water, the bond between the sodium and the chloride breaks, and the positive sodium ion is surrounded by the negative side of water molecules, while the negative chloride ion is surrounded by the positive side of the water molecules. The salt has been dissolved in the water. The fluidity

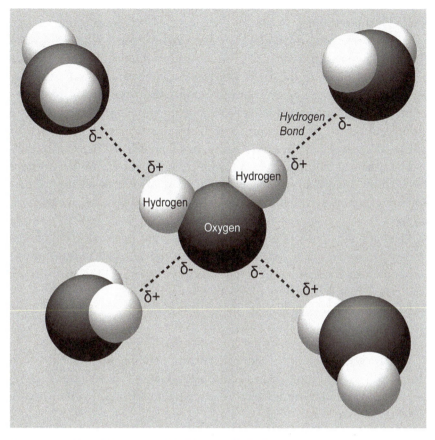

Figure 2.1   **Water Molecule.** (© 2013 Joan M.K. Tycko)

and the dissolving powers of water allow it to carry substances through the body and to facilitate biochemical reactions.

Water Makes Up the Body

Depending on age, gender, and muscle mass, up to two-thirds of our body mass is water. It is obvious that the liquids in our body—such as blood, saliva, and stomach juices—are mostly water. But many of our other "solid" parts are also mostly water. The cells of the body are bathed in watery lymph, and within the cell, organelles are held in the watery cytosol.

Metabolism Depends on Water

The body's metabolism depends on water in many ways. When we eat food, saliva and juices in the stomach and small bowel break down the food. The blood supply to the gut picks up the breakdown products such as carbohydrates and distributes them to the cells, where they are "burned" along with oxygen to produce energy. The oxygen comes from air that is inhaled into the lungs. Oxygen does not dissolve well in blood, so it is carried by hemoglobin in red blood cells to the rest of the body's cells. Carbon dioxide, a waste product of the burning, does dissolve in blood and is transported from the cells by the capillaries and then the veins, to the alveoli of the lungs, where it is then exhaled out of the body.

The situation is different when the body burns proteins. When proteins are used for energy, ammonia compounds are formed as waste products and are excreted by the kidneys as urea that dissolves in water to form urine.

The body uses water in other ways. When water evaporates, or changes from a liquid to a gas, it absorbs heat. Therefore, when we sweat, some of our body heat changes liquid water into water vapor, and in this way we cool down, that is, we lower our body temperature.

Water and Diarrhea

We also use water to excrete other waste products. Food that is not absorbed into the bloodstream, other breakdown products, and bacteria are excreted through our bowels. Feces contain water, especially when in the form of diarrhea.

Here are two of the terrible ironies of life. One of the causes of diarrhea is pollution of drinking water by feces. People ill with cholera, for example, can excrete up to 20 liters of fluid a day. It is not difficult to imagine the results of an outbreak of cholera in a community without adequate sewage treatment. Diarrhea increases the need for water, which increases the amount of diarrhea, which increases the contamination of water, which leads to more diarrheal illnesses in more people. This is a vicious fecal cycle. If a person is sweating because of a high fever, the problem becomes worse. The other irony is that water is generally helpful for life, but this extends to the life of an unwanted microorganism. Water can be easily contaminated by microorganisms.

Contaminated water became a particular problem with the development of agriculture a few thousand years ago. The human population increased, and people and their domesticated farm animals began to live together in settled areas. This meant that disposal of human and animal waste and acquisition of clean water became more difficult; the transmission of infectious diseases became easier.

Where Do We Get Our Water?

We get the water we need from a variety of sources, such as fruit and vegetables. But this is not enough, and we usually have to drink additional quantities of fluids. The amount of water we need varies according to the water and salt content of food, the temperature of our body and surroundings, the functioning of our kidneys, the water content of our feces, and our activity level. Most of us need about two to three liters a day. We can survive without food for a few weeks but not without water for more than a day or so.

Dehydration

Without enough water, a person becomes dehydrated. The dehydrated person is tired and thirsty. As the dehydration continues, the person stops making urine and becomes poisoned by his own waste products. Sweating stops and blood pressure drops. In severe cases, the person can become confused and then comatose. Severe dehydration can be fatal.

Safety of Alcohol

The need for water explains some of the popularity of alcohol in the past, since drinking alcoholic beverages is a way of consuming water. The chemical formula for alcohol (or, more specifically, ethanol) is CH_3CH_2OH. The –OH, or hydroxyl, group is polar. This means that alcohol itself is a solvent. For example, as is reviewed in the opium chapter, it dissolves opium to form laudanum. Alcohol and water, two polar substances, mix well.

There are advantages to drinking water with dissolved alcohol. It is better to drink an alcoholic beverage than contaminated water because the preparation of many alcoholic beverages, particularly beer or distilled beverages, involves boiling that kills bacteria. Alcohol itself is a mild antiseptic.

The safety of alcoholic beverages was described in the chapter about alcohol. In eleventh-century France, the Bishop of Soissons noted that people who drank ale did not become ill with cholera. Eight centuries later, John Snow, the anesthetist discussed in the chapter about pain, investigated an outbreak of cholera in London. He tracked the outbreak down to a well supplied by the Broad Street pump. Workers in a brewery close to the pump did not develop cholera because they got their water from a separate well and because of the safety of the beer that they drank. Snow himself did not drink alcohol, but he did always boil his drinking water. Beer-drinkers stayed cholera-free during an epidemic of cholera in mid-nineteenth-century Vienna. These examples attest to the superiority of beer over water during a cholera outbreak.

The popularity of laudanum described in the opium chapter was also due in part to the problems of infectious diarrhea. During an epidemic of dysentery, drinking laudanum was a way of drinking clean water, decreasing diarrhea, and lessening misery.

Other fluids, such as milk, are even more easily contaminated than water because the rich supply of nutrients in milk encourages the proliferation of microorganisms. Pasteurization of milk prevents the spread of tuberculosis and other diseases, but before this invention, milk was often a dangerous beverage.

Another reason to drink alcohol was to avoid drinking water with too much salt in it. Our kidneys can excrete salt, but they do this by excreting water along with the salt. If we drink water that is very salty, we excrete more water than we ingested along with the salt. People who drink ocean water become dehydrated. Sailors drank rum because there was no salt (or bacteria) in rum.

For many centuries, drinking alcoholic beverages was a safe way of consuming an adequate amount of water. Alcoholic beverages were safer than contaminated or salty milk or water. In the developed world, we now have the luxury of clean water, either from the faucet or from plastic bottles. This privilege was not always available in the past, and in much of the underdeveloped world today, people continue to have limited access to clean water.

3

Fermentation

Sweet but cloying grape juice changes to a complex and subtle wine. Heavy lumps of dough become a frothy batter. Bubbles rise to the surface of liquids and burst open, releasing tantalizing aromas. This transformation of fruits and grains to alcohol and carbon dioxide is fermentation. It is the work of yeast, a one-celled fungus.

Yeast was discovered not in a scientist's laboratory, but in a draper's shop. In seventeenth-century Holland, the Dutch cloth merchant Anton van Leeuwenhoek used magnifying glasses to count the threads in cloth. He was among the first to realize that there was more to be seen than what was visible to the naked eye. Driven by curiosity to look into everything in and around him, he devised new methods for grinding and polishing tiny spherical or curved lenses. He perfected the simple microscope. Others were using a compound microscope (a microscope with two lenses), but Leeuwenhoek's skill at grinding single lenses let him see with greater precision. He also took great care with lighting. He achieved magnification of several hundred times and began to examine everything around him.

With wonder and excitement, he described what he had found in some lake water:

> I now saw very plainly that these were little eels, or worms, lying all huddled up together and wriggling; just as if you saw, with the naked eye, a whole tubful of very little eels and water, with the eels a-squirming among one another: and the whole water seemed to be alive with these multifarious animalcules. This was for me, among all the marvels that I have discovered in nature, the most marvelous of all; and I must say, for my part, that

no more pleasant sight has ever yet come before my eye than these many
thousands of living creatures, seen all alive in a little drop of water, moving
among one another, each several creature having its own proper
motion . . .[1]

He described bacteria in scrapings from his teeth and teeming animal
life in pond water. He used dyes such as saffron. (The use of dyes must
have come naturally to a draper.) We will discuss dyes again when we
review the work of an Italian physician, Camille Golgi. In 1680,
Leeuwenhoek was the first person to see and to describe yeast, the one-
celled factories. But the time was not yet right to make a connection
between yeast and alcohol.

In the eighteenth century, Antoine Lavoisier, the great French chemist,
deduced that fermentation produced alcohol and carbon dioxide. He
thought that alcoholic fermentation was a chemical reaction that did not
involve living organisms. Later scientists worked out the chemical formula:

glucose ($C_6H_{12}O_6$) $\rightarrow$ ethanol ($2C_2H_5OH$) + carbon dioxide ($2CO_2$) +
energy

In 1835, Charles Cagniard de la Tour in France and Theodor Schwann
in Germany examined deposits in beer vats and saw yeast cells multiply-
ing. The connection between yeast and fermentation had tentatively been
made.

Disputes over fermentation became part of a long-running debate
about vitalism, the theory that there is something specific to living things
not found in the inanimate world. Vitalism could seem mystical or religious, and inimical to laboratory research. Vitalism received a blow in
1828 when Friedrich Wöhler synthesized urea from inorganic compounds. Urea is a molecule formed from proteins and is found in urine.
Urea was thought of as a compound formed only in the body, but
Wöhler's work changed that concept.

Wöhler worked with Justus von Liebig, an eminent German chemist
who studied metabolism, the process by which organisms live and grow
by consuming other materials.[2] Liebig and Wöhler agreed with de la
Tour and Schwann in thinking that yeast was involved in fermentation.
However, they did not think that the yeast had to be *alive* to carry out
the fermentation.

Meanwhile, Louis Pasteur, the distinguished French scientist, was also
developing an interest in fermentation. Pasteur began his life as a chemist

but, like Leeuwenhoek, became enchanted by the world of microorganisms. While working at Lille University in northern France, he was approached by the local beet sugar industry that also made beer. The industry had lost control of beet sugar fermentation and was producing undrinkable, sour beer. Pasteur investigated the Lille beet sugar fermentation problem thoroughly and, while so doing, made one of the discoveries for which he is famous.

In 1860, he demonstrated that live yeast ferments sugar to produce alcohol, carbon dioxide, and energy. Alcohol is the by-product valued by drinkers, and carbon dioxide is important for bakers because it leavens the bread. Energy is the product of interest to the yeast. Pasteur had discovered that the activities of the tiny organisms first described by Anton van Leeuwenhoek in 1680 were responsible for fermentation.

Pasteur also realized that the fermentation process could be contaminated by unwanted yeast varieties or other microorganisms such as bacteria. Bacteria had infected the beet juice at Lille and ruined the fermentation. Pasteur learned that the activity of yeast and other organisms could be stopped by heating so that the product is not ruined by unwanted fermentation or other microbial activity. This solved the problem at Lille. Heating wine, beer, or milk to a temperature that is high enough for a long enough time to kill unwanted microorganisms is now known as pasteurization.[3]

Pasteur's theories of fermentation were not accepted by his German colleague Liebig. Pasteur and Liebig shared an expertise in chemistry and an interest in the borders between life and nonlife. But they fought intensely about the nature of fermentation. Professional competitiveness and national pride were involved.

Pasteur, a deeply conservative Catholic Frenchman, was a vitalist. In opposition to him were many scientists, including Liebig, who saw themselves as more scientific and rational. They believed that fermentation was a chemical process, while Pasteur believed that it depended on the ineffable qualities of life. In some ways, Pasteur might be said to have had an old-fashioned approach.

Liebig and Wöhler, fortified by Wöhler's ability to synthesize organic molecules in the laboratory, believed that biochemical reactions did not require life. They argued that fermentation, for example, did not have to rely on living organisms. Liebig thought that decomposing organic material transmitted its "vibrations" to the fermentable sugar, changing the sugar into carbon dioxide and ethanol.

After the deaths of the antagonists, Eduard Buchner made an observation in 1897 that settled this dispute. This was a by-product of work he was doing to help his older brother, Hans.

Hans Buchner was an investigator in the new science of immunology. Eduard helped his older brother develop techniques to break down the membranes of microorganisms and then to preserve the inner material of the cells. Since the two were working in Munich, a brewing town, yeast was a readily available microorganism on which to experiment. Eduard first froze and then thawed the yeast, but the cell membranes survived this brutal treatment. He tried direct grinding in a mortar with equally poor results. Then he ground yeast down with sand and was finally able to rupture the cell membranes. He pressed out a cell-free extract and then used sugar as a preservative. To his surprise, he saw fizziness. Without having planned to, the younger Buchner had shown that sugar could be changed into alcohol and carbon dioxide by something in the cells, even though the cells had been killed. The telltale bubbles proved that a cell-free extract could indeed ferment. This has been called the experiment that initiated biochemistry. Liebig and Wöhler had been correct. Living cells were not required. Eduard Buchner received the Nobel Prize in Chemistry for this discovery in 1907.

But Pasteur was also correct. Fermentation is a miraculous event, both chemical *and* vital. There is no contradiction. Enzymes within the yeast facilitate chemical reactions that change sugar and water to carbon dioxide and alcohol. The fact that the enzyme can be taken out of the cell and remain active is remarkable. But the cell produces the enzyme.[4]

The driving curiosity of Leeuwenhoek (an untutored draper), the genius of Pasteur, and the willingness of Eduard Buchner to help his older brother all led to answers to the question that must have occurred to many since the Mayans enjoyed balché and Aztecs pulque. These men, with the help of others, showed that honey, fruit, and grains change into alcohol through the machinations of live yeast.

Notes

1. Daniel J. Boorstin, *The Discoverers* (New York: Vintage, 1983), 330-31.
2. Liebig described many chemical reactions in plants and animals. He pioneered artificial fertilizers and devised a distillation apparatus, the Liebig condenser. He may have been the first chemist to make—or to use a more scientific word, synthesize—chloroform. He realized that a by-product of the brewing process, spent yeast, had nutritional value. He thus is responsible for marmite, a

pungent but nutritious spread made up of concentrated brewer's yeast. He also invented the bouillon cube.

3. Pasteur's brilliance was not limited to this. He discovered that crystals in nature could be right handed or left handed, disproved the idea of spontaneous generation, and discovered vaccines for anthrax and rabies.

4. Yeast cells, despite their seeming simplicity, have a rich array of enzymes and are also able to synthesize other substances, including some B vitamins essential for our health. Yeast synthesizes B1 (thiamine), B2 (riboflavin), B3 (niacin), B5 (pantothenic acid), B6 (pyridoxine), B7 (biotin), and B9 (folic acid). In the past, yeast and its many B vitamins were not removed from alcoholic beverages, so these beverages were more nutritious than they currently are. In the twenty-first century, wine and beer are filtered, or "fined," to clarify the beverage. The clear drink, although perhaps more esthetically pleasing and more stable, is less nutritious.

4

Distillation

Alcoholic drinks are made by yeast fermentation of a sugar. This miraculous process is not strong enough for the thirst of many, since fermentation is a self-limiting process that stops when the alcohol content of the beverage reaches 14 or 15 percent. Distillation is a way of "improving" on the work of the yeast and increasing the alcohol content of the beverage. In this chapter, we will explain how distillation works. Curiously, several common words in the English language come from this process, and the derivation of those words will also be explained.

The secret of distillation lies in the different boiling points of alcohol and water. Alcohol has a lower boiling point (78 degrees Celsius) than water (100 degrees Celsius). Heating a liquid that contains both alcohol and water to a temperature between these values allows alcohol, but not water, to evaporate. The heating must take place in a closed vessel to avoid loss of the alcohol vapor. A "still" is a piece of machinery that heats the liquid and then captures and condenses the alcohol vapor.

(The differentiation between the freezing points of alcohol and water also allows for the production of stronger alcoholic beverages. If apple cider is placed in freezing temperatures, the water freezes and the alcohol remains as a liquid. This highly alcoholic beverage is known as applejack.)

Distillation in one form or another has been practiced since the time of the Babylonians. Arabic and Persian chemists mastered the art in the eighth and ninth centuries CE. In the twelfth century CE, alchemists developed the science further and were able to separate one liquid from another.

One story about the derivation of the word *alcohol* is that it is related to distillation and the manufacture of cosmetics. Men and women have often used pigments or colors to make themselves more attractive or more frightening. The use of color to accentuate the eyes has been particularly important. One of the most widely used pigments in the past was the rare metal antimony. The Arabic word *al Kohl* referred initially to a fine black powder, antimony, which was used to color eyelids.

The word *al Kohl* gradually came to refer to something very fine, the refined products of distillation, or the essence of any material. Paracelsus used the word to refer to the essence of wine in the sixteenth century and eventually, according to some etymologists, the word became *alcohol*.

Remnants of this idea can be found in words we use today. The use of the word *spirits* to refer to distilled beverages is a reminder of the belief that distillation separated the dross from the otherworldly. The alcohol first produced was sometimes known as *aqua vitae*—the water of life. Distilled drinks were sometimes referred to as *ardent spirits* as a way of emphasizing their strength and burning quality.

Distillation cannot yield pure alcohol, since some water and other substances inevitably evaporate along with the alcohol. What is condensed with the ethanol depends on the source of the alcohol and the nature of the distilling process, and it will lead to a distinctive beverage.

The alcohol content in distilled beverages is sometimes described as "proof." This comes from the practice in the eighteenth century of ensuring the strength of the rum given to British sailors. It was "proved" by pouring it on gunpowder. If the liquor was not watered down, the gunpowder could ignite if exposed to a spark. Proof now refers to the alcoholic strength of a liquor, which is twice the percentage by volume of alcohol present. (The word *proof* is also used to describe the viability of yeast in baking.)

Distillation is a way of overcoming the "natural" inability of yeast to produce highly alcoholic beverages. As discoveries go, an argument can be made for this one ranking with the invention of gunpowder, the cigarette, or crack cocaine in terms of its harmfulness. Drunkenness is more easily achieved with distilled beverages. The distiller, from the point of view of the temperance movement, is more clever than spiritual.

5

Alcohol and the Adams Family: The Scourge of Intemperance

Alcohol played an important role in the Adams family, an eminent family of the American Revolution. Some in this family were maltsters and others were brewers, and many enjoyed cider and ale. But some Adams family members were destroyed by alcohol.

Samuel Adams was born in Boston in 1722. He was from a Puritan family; his father was a successful and wealthy brewer. Adams ran his father's brewery but lacked his father's skills in this area. He was an equally unsuccessful tax collector. He found his métier in politics and became one of the most vocal of the colonists who argued against taxation without representation. He was a founding member of the Boston Sons of Liberty, a group of American patriots who met in taverns. Sam Adams, who had a genius for publicity, developed the symbol of the liberty tree and orchestrated much of the public enthusiasm for the American Revolution.

In 1770 during a confrontation between the British military and Bostonians, five colonial citizens were killed. Sam Adams quickly named this incident the Boston Massacre and used it to stir up public feeling against the British soldiers. In a demonstration of commitment to law and order, his second cousin John Adams (who supported Sam Adams) successfully defended the British troops in the subsequent trial.

Sam Adams and others became increasingly outraged at the English taxes and then the monopoly of the East India Company. On December 16,

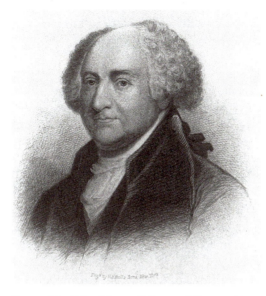

Figure 5.1   **John Adams. (Library of Congress)**

1773, about 100 Bostonians dressed as Mohawk Native Americans boarded three ships, the *Dartmouth*, the *Eleanor*, and the *Beaver*, and threw 342 chests of tea into Boston Harbour.

This act was not per se against taxes, since the tea at that time was not taxed. But the tea was cheap and interfered with the business of American tea smugglers. The tea also represented the power and monopoly of the East India Company and the English Crown. Adams turned this event into an iconic symbol of colonial independence and tax protests—the Boston Tea Party.

Although John Adams had argued in defense of the British soldiers during the Boston Massacre in an admirable display of impartiality, he was, of course, committed to American independence and became second president of the United States (see Figure 5.1). As far as we know, he had no particular problems with alcohol. During his years in Europe as a diplomat, he and his political rival, Thomas Jefferson, savored fine wine. He was fond of hard cider, at that time the most popular alcoholic beverage in the colonies. He was proud of his apple orchards on his farm in Quincy, Massachusetts. Whenever he could, he drank a tankard of hard cider before breakfast.[1]

He married Abigail Smith, daughter of a clergyman. Her brother, William, was an alcoholic. Abigail's younger sister Elizabeth had a son,

William, who also became an alcoholic. Charles Francis Adams, John and Abigail's grandson, later noted:

> The Smith blood seems to have had the scourge of intemperance dreadfully applied to it. Yet the first example of the race whom I know of, was an exemplary clergyman. A son, grandchildren in two branches and great grandchildren have defied all the efforts of the most careful education. Here have been the causes of the bitterest sorrows of our family.[2]

John Adams is known as a crusty and bad-tempered man—especially when compared to the smooth and charming Jefferson. But Adams was an exemplar of kindness and consideration when it came to his marriage to Abigail. Their letters to each other are candid and tender. He addressed her as "my dear Partner." Anxious concerns for their children permeate their correspondence.

They had five children, two of whom became alcoholics. John and Abigail's son Charles began life as a charming, amicable boy who was loved by all. When he went to Harvard as a student, he began to drink heavily. He was plagued by alcoholism and debt. John Adams "renounced" him and described him as "a mere rake, buck, blood, and beast."[3] He destroyed all of his son's letters and papers. His rage and disgust reflect the turmoil, misery, expense, and embarrassment that heavy drinking can cause to family members. Charles died in 1800 at the age of 30.

Charles's younger brother, Thomas, also began his life well. But a few years later when he went to Harvard, he became a lazy, rowdy young man who gambled and drank heavily. He married and had seven children but was unable to provide for them. He and his family were an ongoing burden to his parents.

John and Abigail's first son, John Quincy, had a different career. A sober man in every sense of the word, he was a diplomat, the sixth president of the United States, and a Massachusetts congressman who was an outspoken antislavery advocate. Yet he did not escape from the problems of alcoholism. He had to care for Thomas's family, and two of his own three sons also became alcoholics.

The differences between John, John Quincy, and some of their sons are striking. Being sons of the president of the United States conferred no protection. Perhaps the expectations placed on the sons who could not manage to become successful themselves were intolerable.

In the spirit of Abigail Adams, who famously reminded her husband to "remember the ladies," the question of alcoholism among the female

Adams family members should be considered. Some of the Adams women were rebellious and openly unhappy about their lives, but we know nothing about any episodes of alcohol abuse. Perhaps they had less access to liquor. Perhaps some women did succumb to alcohol, and this was just too awful to document.

Brewing provided Sam Adams's family with a respectable income, and Sam used taverns as a meeting place to hatch various plots against the British. Modern-day commerce has honored this by naming a Boston beer after him. His second cousin John, the second president, enjoyed wine and hard cider, which seems to have been nothing but good for him. In contrast, several in the Adams and Smith families had their lives ruined by alcoholism. Alcohol was both a blessing and a curse to this family.

Notes

1. Alice Morse Earle, *Customs and Fashions in New England*, 1893 (repr., Williamstown, MA: Corner House Publishers, 1974), 172.

2. Paul C. Nagel, *The Adams Women: Abigail and Louisa Adams, Their Sisters and Daughters* (Cambridge, MA: Harvard University Press, 1987), 10.

3. Paul C. Nagel, *Descent from Glory: Four Generations of the John Adams Family* (Cambridge, MA: Harvard University Press, 1983), 79.

6

Patent Medicines, Lydia Pinkham, and the Great American Fraud

Patent Medicines

Patent medicines occupy a colorful and contentious place in the history of medicine and substance use in nineteenth-century England and the United States. The word *patent* applies to the shape of the bottle, the "brand" of the medicine, or promotional materials, and rarely to the actual formula of the "medicine." Patent medicine was not medicine as we understand it today. It was often a mixture of alcohol, cocaine, and opiates with some herbs. One of the most profitable and well known of these mixtures was made by a Quaker schoolteacher, Lydia Estes Pinkham.

Pinkham and other people marketing patent medicines contrasted themselves frequently and favorably to the medical profession. This was not difficult to do in the 1800s, since the doctors of that time had no antibiotics or other effective medication. If a person went to a doctor, he or she ran the risk of the doctor prescribing a treatment that usually was not helpful. Physicians were likely to prescribe calomel (mercury), bleed the person, or perform a risky surgical procedure. Physician fees were high. Buying patent medicines was cheaper and sometimes safer than seeing a doctor.

Patent medicines were sometimes made and sold by alternative practitioners who had expertise in herbal medicines. Some alternative practitioners were homeopaths who used very small amounts of drugs, and others were naturopaths who used a variety of natural remedies such as sunlight or massage.

Three of the best-known alternative practitioners were Samuel Thomson, Sylvester Graham, and Lydia Estes Pinkham. Samuel Thomson was a New Hampshire farmer who believed that medical treatments could be found in plants. He promoted herbs as being "natural" and aligned with the body's own tendencies toward health. "Thomsonians" also believed in a Jacksonian or democratic style of practice in which people did not have to turn to experts to treat themselves. Thomson used 60 to 65 different herbs and drugs, and wrote self-help books. He had a great effect on many practitioners, particularly in the South. John Pemberton, the inventor of Coca-Cola, was briefly a Thomsonian. Another was the unfortunately named Albert Isaiah Coffin, who took Thomsonian teachings to England. In his lectures, he mocked the pretensions of physicians and attributed more powers to them than perhaps they had:

> ... the licensed to kill enters the house of sickness, and, at the bedside, takes in charge, with the authority of law, his exclusive right over the prostrate victim, whose blood he draws, whose frame he tortures, whose bowels he secretly poisons, and whose disease he cures, or at his will, prolongs: but kill or cure, his charge is made, in amount wholly at his discretion ... thousands perish under their hands who otherwise would have survived ... mercury, opium, alcohol, and the use of the lancet are of themselves sufficient to account for the speedy depopulation of a world ...[1]

Sylvester Graham, a Presbyterian minister from Connecticut, began his career as a temperance worker but then branched out to advocate for greater health, not just sobriety, for Americans. He urged his followers to avoid doctors, medicine, meat, and white bread. His name lives on in Graham crackers.

Lydia Estes Pinkham, a teacher from Massachusetts, was similar to Thomson and Graham in her belief in "natural" cures. She invented, advertised, and sold a "Vegetable Compound," that became one of the best-known and most successful patent medicines. She was an innovative and successful marketer of patent medicines and an early American woman entrepreneur. Her life and career illustrate many themes common to patent medicine and shed some light on the temperance movement.

Lydia Estes Pinkham and Her Family

Lydia Estes, born in 1819, was raised in a Quaker family in Lynn, Massachusetts. Quakers, known for their abstemiousness and sense of

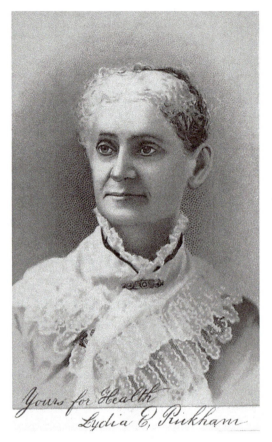

Figure 6.1   Lydia Pinkham. (Hagley Museum and Library)

egalitarianism, were among the earliest abolitionists. They were also entrepreneurial. At the age of 16, Estes was a member of the Lynn Womens Anti-Slavery Movement. She became a schoolteacher and was active in the free-thinking and independently minded community of Quakers in Lynn. She befriended Frederick Douglass, the former slave who became a leader of the abolitionist movement, and taught his wife to read. Lydia Estes married Isaac Pinkham in 1843, and together they had four children.

In the frenzied years of the early 1870s, Isaac Pinkham speculated in real estate. He bought land and several properties and became wealthy, although he was heavily mortgaged. In 1873, Jay Cooke's banking house in New York failed, and the Panic of 1873 ensued. Banks, the stock market, and house prices crashed. Credit froze. Isaac Pinkham had bankrupted his family. He collapsed, and the welfare of his family was left to his wife.

Lydia Estes Pinkham had always made home remedies, based on Thomsonian herbal theories, and had distributed them to friends and family. Her famous Vegetable Compound consisted of a number of herbs such as black cohosh, false and true unicorn root, and chamomile, all dissolved in alcohol. The compound contained 15 to 18 percent alcohol, making it a potent alcoholic beverage. She claimed that the alcohol was used "solely as a solvent and preservative." She was following in the footsteps of Thomas Sydenham and Robert Talbor of seventeenth-century England, whose somewhat similar compounds are described in the opiates chapter. The compound was also sold as alcohol-free tablets, but this was not the big seller that the liquid came to be.

Her sons encouraged her to sell her remedies rather than just giving them away to friends and neighbors. After some resistance, she began to do so in early 1875. All four children and their spouses eventually became involved in the business. Her sons originated many of the advertising ideas, which is where the genius of the Pinkham family lay. Whether the compound was effective is not clear; the advertising certainly was.

The Pinkham family distributed thousands of leaflets and cards. The cards sometimes had inspirational messages or showed beautiful landscapes. One of the Pinkham sons, Will, had a different idea, and spent $60 of the $84 that he had received from a wholesaler on a single day's advertising in the *Boston Herald*. His family cried when he told them this.[2] But Will Pinkham had spent the family's money wisely. In the late 1800s, much newspaper advertising had to do with products supposed to promote health or treat illness. Newspapers were in an alliance with patent medication manufacturers, and all profited handsomely. Newspaper advertisements were effective.

Pinkham retained her early interest in teaching and improving the lot of others. She wrote a brief folder, *Guide for Women*, which described female physiology in simple terms. Her sons distributed this and other educational material with the Vegetable Compound.

In 1879, Dan Pinkham realized that his mother's countenance was the best possible advertisement. The Pinkhams did not patent her formula or her process, but they did patent her trademark—her portrait (see Figure 6.1). Her compound was promoted with slogans such as "Only a woman can understand a woman's ills." Her wise, kind, reassuring, and maternal picture accompanied many products.

The advertisements were a constantly changing series of promises. They promised cures for all female complaints, including prolapsed uteri, menstrual cramps, weakness, nerves, tumors, and kidney problems. Some women may have used the tonic to treat "menstrual irregularities," possibly a euphemism for unwanted pregnancies. Women were assured that the Vegetable Compound was safer, more private, and more natural than seeing a (male) doctor.

The Pinkham Company promoted the idea of free and nonmedical advice to its customers. The company encouraged women to write in with their problems and promised, "Men NEVER see your letters." Pinkham contrasted her free advice to the expensive services offered by physicians. She asked, "Do you want a strange man to hear all about your particular diseases?"[3] Since so many women's complaints were gynecological and since all gynecologists then were male, these arguments had great appeal.

But Pinkham and her company were not entirely high-minded, and they did not refrain from using other approaches to make sales. In her book about Pinkham, Sarah Stage gives examples of three inspired advertisements:

> A FEARFUL TRAGEDY, a Clergyman of Stratford, Conn, Killed by His Own Wife, Insanity Brought on by 16 Years of Suffering with Female Complaints the Cause. Lydia E. Pinkham's Vegetable Compound, The Sure Cure for These Complaints, Would Have Prevented the Direful Deed.

Another advertisement stated:

> "I am not Well enough to Work." How often these significant words are spoken in our great mills, shops, and factories by the poor girl . . . Standing all day, week in and out . . . the poor girl has slowly contracted some deranged condition of her organic system . . .

Pinkham did not neglect more economically fortunate women:

> Women Who Brave Death for Social Honors. In the midst of one of the most brilliant social functions of the season, a noted society woman started suddenly from her chair with a scream of agony . . . the distinguished Physician told her anxious husband that she was suffering from an acute case of nervous prostration brought on by female trouble, and hinted at an operation. Fortunately, a friend advised her to try Lydia E. Pinkhams

Vegetable Compound. The result was that she escaped the surgeon's knife and today is a well woman . . .[4]

This combination of high-mindedness and the willingness to terrify poor and wealthy women (and their husbands) while castigating male physicians was successful. The Lydia E. Pinkham Medicine Company became a multi-million-dollar business. Pinkham died at the age of 64 in 1883. Her company lived on.

Pinkham's Company after Her Death and the Great American Fraud

Many patent medicine companies were fraudulent. Companies sold alcohol-containing compounds as cures for alcoholism. Opiate-containing preparations were promoted as cures for opiate addiction. Perhaps most infamously, patent medicines were associated with the desire to keep the baby quiet. A woman gave her baby a remedy that contained alcohol or opium, and the family slept better.

The patent medicine makers were protected by the newspapers, since the newspapers profited from their advertisements. Much of the newspaper advertising then had to do with products claiming to promote health or treat illness. Just as there was little regulation of the production of products, there was little regulation of what companies could say in their advertisements. Patent medicine companies sought national markets, and their advertising helped support the growing number of newspapers. The interests of these companies were well publicized and supported.

(Several decades later, advertisements for cigarettes would fill the newspapers and also perhaps affect what newspapers would publish about cigarette smoking.)

There was a famous "red clause"—so called because it was prepared in red ink—in which the newspapers agreed to cancel their contracts if patent medicines were infringed upon by state or federal laws. This clever move further encouraged newspapers to lobby on behalf of keeping patent medicine companies free from regulation.

Nevertheless, some journalists began to investigate these companies and their advertisements. Because of its success, Lydia E. Pinkham's company got much attention from these journalists. Between 1904 and 1907, in a series of articles in the *Ladies Home Journal*, lawyer and writer Mark Sullivan wrote about patent medicines. He noted the death of Lydia Pinkham, which was not acknowledged by the company. Even though she had died in 1883, the company continued to advertise that Mrs. Pinkham read and answered all questions sent to her. The title of one of his articles was "How the Private Confidences of Women Are Laughed At."[5] Sullivan also wrote about the cozy arrangement between patent medicine companies and the newspapers.

Edward Bok, editor of the *Ladies Home Journal*, also enjoyed mocking the close connection between the Woman's Christian Temperance Union (WCTU) and Lydia E. Pinkham's company. Bok polled a sample of the WCTU and reported that 37 of 50 members regularly took patent medicines that were highly alcoholic.[6]

The most famous of the muckrakers was Samuel Hopkins Adams, who in 1905 published a 10-part series called "The Great American Fraud" in *Collier's Weekly*, describing the worthless and often addictive substances in patent medicines. Adams, who had a hyperbolic pen to match that of Coffin, wrote that the practice of selling cough syrups containing opium and cocaine "stupefies helpless babies, and makes criminals of our young men and harlots of our young women."[7] The American Medical Association—doubtless happy to have an ally in its competition with the patent medicine makers—distributed over 150,000 copies of these articles.[8]

The muckraking journalists had little influence on sales, but they did affect legislation. Pushed on by these reformers and by Upton Sinclair's novel *The Jungle*, which describes the filth of the Chicago meatpacking industry, legislators passed the federal Meat Inspection and Pure Food and Drug Act of 1906. Interstate commerce in mislabeled and adulterated drugs was prohibited. Truthful labels on patent medicines were mandated. If the patent medicines contained alcohol, cocaine, or opiates, they had to say so. If the labels were truthful, they obtained a "number" from the federal government that served as a guarantee of the medicine meeting some production standards but not of being effective or safe. This act was the beginning of federal involvement in food and medication.

The hope was that this precursor to the more modern concern with transparency would help the informed consumer turn away from patent medicines. Yet this act turned out to be a gift to patent medicine makers. The Pinkham and other companies boasted that their products, because the labels were truthful, were "guaranteed" by the Food and Drug Act. The company, for the first time, noted the inclusion of alcohol but continued to advertise that the Vegetable Compound cured all medical problems. Sales soared.[9]

There was a temporary hitch when the government noted that the Vegetable Compound was really nothing but flavored alcohol. It did not have enough of the vaunted herbs to be considered anything other than an alcoholic beverage and therefore should have been taxed as such. The Pinkham Company responded by increasing the amount of herbs in its compound, but this overstretched the dissolving properties of alcohol. In some cases bottles exploded, and in many cases customers complained of sludge at the bottom of bottles. Eventually, these problems were fixed.

The government finally cracked down on misleading advertising. The company again rose to the challenge by increasing their use of testimonials. The testimonials substituted for the advertisements and documented the miseries to which female flesh is susceptible. This is a typical letter:

> June 26, 1901.
> I will write and let you know how much good Lydia E. Pinkham's Vegetable Compound has done me.
> I cannot express the terrible suffering I have had to endure. I was taken last May with nervous prostration; also had female trouble, liver, stomach, *kidney* and *bladder* trouble. I was in a terrible condition. The doctor attended me for a year, but I kept getting worse. I got so I was not able to do any work. Was confined to my bed most of the time, and thought I would never be able to do anything. People thought I would not live.
> I decided to try your medicine. I have taken twelve bottles Vegetable Compound and cannot praise it too highly, for I know it will do all and even more than it is recommended to do. I tell every suffering woman about your medicine and urge them to try it ...[10]

During Prohibition, sales of patent medicines continued. Some people turned to these medicines as a way of legally buying alcohol. The Pinkham Company was at its most successful during these years.

Slimy Serpents

When Franklin Delano Roosevelt was elected president in 1932, he ended Prohibition. Another reform advocated by the New Dealers was a tightening of the 1906 Pure Food and Drug Act. The patent medicine companies reacted predictably. They claimed that drugstores would be "sovietized" by the federal government, which was a "powerful sinister machine." The politicians responded in kind, claiming that "every slimy serpent of a vile manufacturer of patent medicine is right now working his wriggling way round the Capitol" and that "the consumers of this country are being raped."[11]

In 1938, after a heated five-year battle, Congress passed a new Food, Drug, and Cosmetic Act. This act stated that labels on the medicine had to identify the drug, indicate how it should be administered, and list possible adverse effects. Companies were required to submit evidence of the safety of their products.

Eventually, the Pinkham Company failed. Legislation such as the 1938 act may have interfered somewhat with the product, but other factors were also at play. The prestige and credibility of the medical profession increased with the advent of antibiotics. Another reason for the failure was a common problem in family companies: succession. There were disputes between family members that lasted for decades and that were highly profitable for lawyers. The business was sold to a pharmaceutical company in the 1960s, and the manufacturing plant was moved from Massachusetts to Puerto Rico.

Conclusion

Was the Pinkham family consciously fraudulent? Lydia Pinkham was a teacher and fervent supporter of free speech and abolition. She was a hard worker who supported her husband and children. It is difficult to believe that this good Quaker woman would consciously manipulate people. Did she and her children know that many people bought her Vegetable Compound because of the alcohol? Did they themselves drink it for the alcohol? Pinkham and her family believed in her remedies. She was a temperance worker from her early days, as was Graham. She did not think that drinking her alcoholic compound was the same as drinking liquor. When her sons became ill, she advised liberal use of her remedies, so she cannot be accused of hypocrisy. The company did deceive the public in not announcing her death, but they probably believed that they were doing the correct thing. Perhaps her family had become intoxicated by the fame and success of their Vegetable Compound. We can search the trademark picture of Lydia Pinkham for the answers but are only rewarded by her Mona Lisa smile.

Notes

1. S. W. F. Holloway, "The Regulation of the Supply of Drugs in Britain before 1868," in *Drugs and Narcotics in History*, ed. Roy Porter and Mikuláš Teich (Cambridge: Cambridge University Press, 1995), 83-4.

2. Sarah Stage, *Female Complaints: Lydia Pinkham and the Business of Women's Medicine* (New York: W. W. Norton & Company, 1979), 37.

3. Paul Starr, *The Social Transformation of American Medicine* (New York: Basic Books, 1982), 128.

4. Stage, *Female Complaints*, 146–49.

5. Starr, *Social Transformation*, 130.

6. Stage, *Female Complaints*, 167.

7. Samuel Hopkins Adams, "The Subtle Poisons," *Collier's Weekly*, December 2, 1905, 16.

8. Starr, *Social Transformation*, 131.

9. Stage, *Female Complaints*, 178.

10. Project Gutenberg's Treatise on the Diseases of Women, by Lydia E Pinkham, 1901. Available at www.gutenberg.org/files/29612/29612-h/29612-h.htm (accessed July 20, 2013), 53.

11. Thomas Hager, *The Demon under the Microscope* (New York: Harmony, 2006), 229–32.

7

Carry Nation: Hatchetation against Saloonacy

Carry Nation was the most famous person in the battle against alcohol in pre-Prohibition America because of her vandalism. Ridiculed throughout her life and afterward, she was innovative and determined in her efforts to abolish the drinking of alcohol in the United States.

She was born Carrie Amelia Moore in Garrard County, Kentucky, in 1846. She changed her name several times throughout her life and eventually chose to be known as Carry A. Nation.[1] (Her second husband's name was David Nation.) She grew up in the Midwest, which was then plagued by bloodshed—interracial violence, the Civil War, and later the Jaybird-Woodpecker war. Her father, George Moore, had been a well-to-do Kentucky gentleman who owned slaves and who lost much of his fortune in the various conflicts of the time. Her mother was an odd woman, possibly ill with bipolar disorder, who spent her final years in an insane asylum. Her mother treated Carry badly, often neglecting her. The family, and later Carry herself, led a peripatetic existence, never quite settling down.

In 1853, Carry's family moved to Danville and the next year to Woodford County, both in Kentucky. In 1856, the family moved again, this time to Belton, Missouri. Three years later, Carry was sent to boarding school in Independence, Missouri. In 1861, she and her family moved to Texas, and one year later they were back in Missouri.

Charles Gloyd, a physician, moved into the family's house as a boarder in 1865, and two years later, at the age of 20, Carry married him. He was

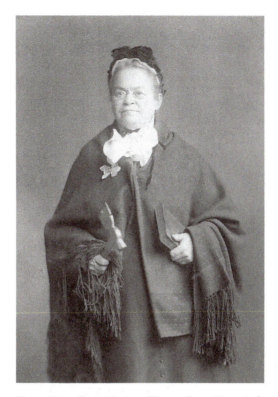

Figure 7.1 **Carry Nation. (Kansas State Historical Society, Kansas)**

drunk at their wedding. She left him several months later because of his alcoholism. Their daughter Charlien was born in 1868. Gloyd died shortly afterward.

To support herself and her daughter, Carry became a teacher. In 1874, she met David Nation, a widower with children of his own. He was a lawyer, Civil War veteran, minister, and newspaper editor. The two married and in 1877, the blended family moved to Brazoria County, Texas, to grow cotton. They were unsuccessful and moved to Richmond, Texas, where Carry Nation ran a hotel. In the summer of 1884, she attended a Methodist revival meeting and began to experience visions. Five years later, the family moved to Medicine Lodge in Kansas, where David accepted a position as a minister.

Carry joined the Woman's Christian Temperance Union in the mid-1890s and became president of the Medicine Lodge chapter. She became a jail visitor and saw that while many men were imprisoned because of alcohol-caused problems, they could still get alcohol while in jail. This seemed wrong and, upset by the easy availability of liquor, she organized a march on the biggest saloons in Medicine Lodge in 1894.

The family moved again in 1896 and homesteaded in the Cherokee Strip in Oklahoma Territory. In this wild part of the country, where there were clashes between Native Americans and whites, outlaws and vigilantes, Carry Nation began an active preaching and philanthropic career. In 1899, the family returned to Kansas, and she continued her reforming efforts by helping the town's poor people. She interfered with her husband's job by sometimes interrupting his preaching. She became increasingly angry about saloons, of which Kansas had many.

The temperance movement was gaining strength at the time, yet so was opposition and "work-arounds." Kansas had been legally "dry" since 1880, but Kansan authorities tolerated saloons that were well supplied with liquor from surrounding "wet" states. There was little will to control saloons in Kansas, since the owners were often politicians or closely connected with them. Some saloon owners paid regular fines that were a revenue source for the local government. The saloons were bastions of male leisure, privileges, alcohol consumption, and sometimes prostitution and gambling.

Men enjoyed the easygoing atmosphere of saloons. Saloons offered companionship, free food (salty to encourage beverage consumption), and sometimes a place to cash checks or pick up mail. Women saw saloons as places where men caroused and drank away their money. But the opinions of women mattered not at all. Married women could not own property themselves, so women had little economic clout. Women could not vote, so politicians ignored them.

Carry Nation continued to be infuriated by the mockery and disrespect of the law. She opposed the consumption of any and all amounts of alcohol but focused her efforts (as did the successful Anti-Saloon League) on the saloons. In early 1900, she marched on saloons in Medicine Lodge and in Kiowa. She compared herself to those biblical figures who fought against wrongdoers—Deborah who urged Barak to attack Sisera, David who brawled with Goliath, Esther who struggled against Haman, and even Jesus who expelled the money changers from Herod's Temple. She also compared herself to the abolitionist John Brown, in that she was setting free those enslaved by alcohol. She "smashed" saloons, meaning that she vandalized them. She flung bricks at mirrors and windows, and damaged casks of alcohol.

She made one of her most renowned forays in the winter of 1900, when she traveled to Wichita, where there were many saloons. The most elegant was the Carey Hotel Bar, which had a 50-foot cherry wood bar, brass rail, and cut-glass decanters. A huge Venetian glass mirror hung over the bar. With an iron rod, she smashed all of it. She threw rocks at an oil painting called *Cleopatra at her Bath* and altogether caused almost $3,000 dollars of damage. She was sent to jail and calmly noted that the bar owners who were lawbreakers should be the ones put in jail.

The next year, she returned to Wichita and with other women singing hymns such as *Onwards Christian Soldiers*, she attacked a saloon with a hatchet. Once again, she was jailed and then released on bail. A few weeks later, she traveled to Enterprise, Kansas, where she smashed up more saloons. Between 1900 and 1905, she was arrested some 30 times. David divorced her.

Nation was a whirlwind of destruction, but she was also involved in more peaceful activities. She edited and wrote most of a newsletter, *The Smasher's Mail*. She also wrote an autobiography, *The Use and Need of the Life of Carry A. Nation*, which went through several editions, as well as a temperance play, *The War on Drink*. She began another paper, *The Hatchet*. She printed her own publications. She helped those hurt by the violence and neglect of heavy drinkers by establishing the Home for Drunkards' Wives and Children.

She became widely known for her activities and writings, and toured the Chautauqua circuit in northeastern United States. She used her lecture-tour fees, along with sales of water bottles and souvenir hatchets, to pay her jail fines. She visited Canada twice in 1904, spoke at the provincial parliament in New Brunswick, and was arrested. In 1908, she attended the National Prohibition Party convention as a delegate. Later that year, she traveled to Scotland, took the opportunity to smash a mirror in the ship bar, and traveled and spoke throughout the United Kingdom. In 1909, she smashed up whiskey barrels in Topeka and again was taken to jail.

She was verbally adroit and took some pleasure in manipulating her own name. In 1903, she legally changed her name from Carrie Amelia Moore Gloyd Nation to Carry A. Nation. She wrote:

> ... There are just two crowds, God's crowd and the Devil's crowd. One gains the battle by "can" and the other loses by "can't" ... I do not belong to the "can't" family. When I was born my father wrote my name Carry A. Moore, then later it was Nation, which is more still. C.A.N. are the initials of my name, then C.(see) A. Nation! And altogether Carry A. Nation! This is no accident, but Providence.[2]

She used her sharp tongue against her enemies. She described drinking men in clubs as "well dressed, gold fobbed, diamond studded rummies that are more hateful than those behind the prison bars, their bodies a reeking mass of corruption."[3] Facing charges of malicious destruction of property, she asked the judge to amend the charges to read "destruction of malicious property."[4] She named three trusty hatchets Faith, Hope, and Charity. She coined the punning term "hatchetation" to describe her activities in saloons.

Although Nation is known today for her opposition to alcohol, in her mind tobacco was an equal offender. As well as railing against smoking, she would sometimes jerk cigars and cigarettes out of men's mouths. She was horrified by the smells and appearance of tobacco. A devout Christian, she did not hesitate to reprimand priests and ministers who smelt of tobacco. She described the odors of tobacco in her usual colorful language:

> I can prevent a man from spitting in my mouth, but I cannot avoid his smoke. A man seems to think that he is free to project his stinking breath in my face on the street, in hotels, in sleeping cars, coaches—indeed, in every public place. Now I would as soon smell a skunk. There is some excuse for the skunk; he can't help being one. But men have become so rank in their persons from this poisonous odor that they almost knock me down as they pass me. And when I say, "Man, don't throw that awful stench in my face," he answers, "You get away." I reply, "If I smelled as badly as you do, I would be the one to get away."
>
> Oh, the vile cigarette! What smell can be worse and more poisonous? I feel outraged at being compelled to smell this poison on the street. I have the right to take cigars and cigarettes from men's mouths in self-defense, and they ought not to be allowed to injure themselves. . . . I believe it ought to be a crime to manufacture, barter, sell or give away cigars, cigarettes and tobacco in any form.[5]

Carry Nation was not celebrated by all women. On one occasion, a group of women physically attacked her. Some temperance women viewed her with unease and were embarrassed by her. In turn, she disapproved of the costly clothes of many women and rebuked them for wearing "dead corpses" of birds in their hats and whale-boned corsets.[6]

When she likened herself to great figures of the past, perhaps she was not so hyperbolic. Her smashing of whiskey barrels is similar to the smashing of tea barrels by the American patriots in Boston in 1773. There are similarities between her pouring whiskey into the street and the dumping of opium into streams organized by Lin Ze-Xu in China 1839 (described in the opium smoking chapter). Her saloon smashing was actually braver than the activities of the former groups of men. She did not disguise her identity by dressing up as a Mohawk Native American, she did not have the support of authorities, and she often acted by herself and risked and sustained physical assaults.

The comparison to the activities of the American patriots may strike some as farfetched. Yet the similarity between saloon-smashing women and the Boston Tea Party patriots was first made by Abraham Lincoln.[7] Her references to women of the Bible, easily mocked, are similar to claims made on behalf of other women. In the midst of his battle against slavery, the sober John Quincy Adams supported the ability of the Grimké sisters to submit a petition to Congress. Their petition was sneered at, but Adams reminded Congress of the biblical examples of Miriam (prophetess and sister of Aaron and Moses), Deborah, and Jael who killed Sisera.[8]

Nation understood how to manipulate the press, make money, and get attention for her cause. She was fearless in her attempts to help women and children who she saw as being hurt by drunken husbands and fathers. She was clever, brave, and humorous. Many contemporaries found her inspirational and described her as kind and charismatic.

Others see a crazed and moralistic harridan who made her cause look foolish. The censorious pen of history has not treated her kindly. Her extravagant comparisons of herself to biblical figures seemed immodest, and she was easily parodied. In his history of the temperance movement, Pegram wrote that her "violent actions and bizarre personal behavior lent an unwelcome air of fanaticism and even burlesque to the determined moral activism of American women."[9] In a book about Prohibition, Behr describes her as the "wildest, maddest, most frenzied crusader . . . unbalanced and out of control . . ."[10]

Carry Nation had a life of contradictions. She began her life in a wealthy family that became impoverished and nomadic. Her mother was, at the least, difficult, and her own daughter had a variety of poorly defined disorders. Her first marriage ended in the death of her alcoholic husband, and her second marriage ended in divorce. She emerged from these blows to become a champion of sobriety. An advocate of temperance, she was not temperate in her activities or language. A deeply religious and conservative person, she reveled in her jail stays and gloried in her property damage.

Carry Nation died in 1911. Had she lived just another eight years, she would have seen her cause win with the beginning of Prohibition. But this was a Pyrrhic victory. Outlawing of alcohol throughout the United States made it clear that sobriety cannot be legislated. Prohibition was repealed in 1933. Perhaps it is just as well that Nation never lived through the debacle of Prohibition. On the other hand, drinking habits in the United States *did* change, and saloons, the main object of her opprobrium, did indeed disappear. Many share her disgust at secondhand smoke. Perhaps this would have pleased her.

Notes

1. Carry Nation changed her name often. I have followed one of her biographers, Fran Grace, and used "Carry Nation, Nation, or Carry" throughout.

2. Mary Ann Blochowiak, " 'Woman with a Hatchet': Carry Nation Comes to Oklahoma Territory," *Chronicles of Oklahoma* 59, no. 2 (1981): 137.

3. Carry A. Nation, *The Use and Need of the Life of Carry A. Nation* (n.p.: Hard Press, ca. 1906), 158.

4. Fran Grace, *Carry A. Nation: Retelling the Life* (Bloomington: Indiana University Press, 2001), 152.

5. Nation, *Use and Need*, 153.

6. Grace, *Cary A. Nation*, 150.

7. Thomas R. Pegram, *Battling Demon Rum: The Struggle for a Dry America, 1800–1933* (Chicago: Ivan R. Dee, 1998), 58.

8. William Lee Miller, *Arguing about Slavery: John Quincy Adams and the Great Battle in the United States Congress* (New York: Random House, 1998), 318–22.

9. Pegram, *Battling Demon Rum*, 111.

10. Edward Behr, *Prohibition: Thirteen Years That Changed America* (New York: Arcade, 1996), 40.

8

Cocaine

The leaf of the coca bush that grows in the valleys of the Andean Mountains is an important part of life in these areas. The introduction of this honored leaf to Western society was followed by chemical advances that resulted in the isolation of cocaine, an alkaloid molecule, which is the active ingredient of the coca leaf. (An alkaloid is a bitter-tasting chemical found in plants and other organisms.) This story involves the Spanish discovery and then destruction of the Incan Empire, explorers, the need for local anesthesia, and the young, ambitious Viennese doctor Sigmund Freud. While cocaine is one of the most feared substances of abuse today, the coca leaf continues to be revered in the Andes.

The Coca Plant

Erythroxylon coca (sometimes spelled *Erythroxylum coca*) is an evergreen plant that grows to about two or three meters in height (see Figure 8.1). The plant, referred to as a small tree, or a tall bush or shrub, lives from 50 to 100 years. This is different from many of the other plants discussed in this book, such as the cereals, tobacco, and poppies, which are annuals. The coca plant is similar to the grape vine in its longevity and to tobacco in that the leaf is the important part of the plant. About 1 percent or less of the coca leaf is cocaine. Coca grows in valleys within the tropical mountainous regions of South America in Peru, Bolivia, Ecuador, and Colombia.

The leaves of the coca plant can be harvested several times a year. At times, herbicides are used to destroy coca plants in attempts to encourage coca farmers to grow other crops. But the farmers have difficulty growing

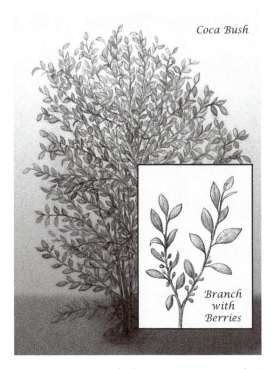

Figure 8.1   **Coca Bush.** (© 2013 Joan M.K. Tycko)

other crops as profitably, so the plant continues to be grown throughout large areas of South America.

History

The Use of Coca in the Andes

Coca leaves have probably been chewed for at least 8,000 years in South America.[1] We know little about the pre-Incan Native American Andeans, except that they were masterful stone carvers. Numerous artifacts have been found in which figures have cheeks bulging with what is thought to be coca leaf.

Coca has been particularly associated with the Incas. The Incas began as a tribe in the Cusco area (now in Peru) in the twelfth century. Under the leadership of Manco Capac, they formed a small city-state and over the next several hundred years began to assimilate many other tribes. The Incan Empire lasted from about 1200 to 1600 CE. At its height, it comprised 12 million people and stretched out over 2,500 miles along the

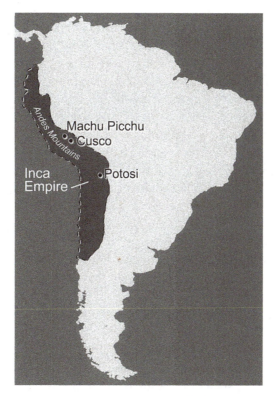

Figure 8.2   **The Incan Empire.** (© 2013 Joan
M.K. Tycko)

Pacific coast of South America from present-day Ecuador to Chile (see
Figure 8.2). The emperor was sometimes known simply as the Inca.

Messages between all parts of this large empire were carried by men running on a 3,250-mile network of well-maintained roads carved into the
Andes. Some of the paths were cobbled. Causeways, bridges suspended by
ropes, stairways, and switchbacks allowed the runners to cross marshlands,
rivers, and mountain peaks. Culverts drained the roads, and retaining walls
maintained their integrity. Along the roads were villages and relay posts.

The messages themselves were recorded by knotted-string devices
known as *quipu*. This form of communication was used throughout the
Andes but most notably by the Incas. Only a few quipu still exist, and,
unlike Sumerian cuneiform tablets, they have never been deciphered.

The runners traveled long distances, often on sharp inclines, in severe
cold and searing heat, and in the relative hypoxia of high altitudes. The
messengers chewed coca leaf to give them more energy and endurance,
to cope with the weather and the altitude, and to control their hunger.

The Incan Empire accomplished many other engineering feats, and all without the wheel or domesticated animals that could carry people or heavy burdens. (The Andean llama and alpaca were domesticated but could carry little weight.) Their main achievement was Machu Picchu, built in the fifteenth century at an altitude of 8,000 feet. It is set in a remote mountainous area and consists of about 200 buildings, many perched on precipices. Granite blocks cut with bronze and stone tools form the buildings. No mortar was used. Terracing and irrigation reduced erosion and increased the area available for cultivation of potatoes and maize (or corn). It is usually assumed that coca leaves were used by the laborers to allow them to work in the harsh climate and high altitude of Machu Picchu. In a somewhat similar way, beer was used by the people who built the pyramids in Egypt.

Coca was also a part of religious rituals and celebrations of the Incan culture. For example, priests and supplicants were allowed to approach the Altar of the Inca only if they had coca leaf in their mouths. In the pre-Incan and Incan eras, only men chewed coca leaf.

Coca leaf in the pre-Incan and Incan eras, and in much of Andean South America today, is chewed in a particular way. Coca leaves are formed into a "wad" of coca leaf placed between the gum and cheek. Lime-rich materials such as seashells are mixed in with the coca leaf to free the cocaine alkaloid from the rest of the leaf. The cocaine in the coca leaf is diluted by many other substances in the leaf, some which may be nutritious. Coca leaf is sometimes steeped in hot water to form coca tea, a beverage that may help to overcome altitude sickness.

The Conquest of the Incas and the Spanish Greed for Silver

In the fifteenth century, Spanish explorers and soldiers crossed the Atlantic searching for gold, spices, and trade opportunities. They also coveted silver, which was often used as currency because of its durability and portability. The Spanish mined silver in their own country for about 1,000 years; used it for trade with other countries; and wanted more. They were also intent on the conversion of the "heathens" and were often accompanied by priests and friars. They explored, conquered, and exploited much of what is now Mexico, Central and South America, and the Caribbean.

One of the most famous Spanish explorers was Francisco Pizarro, who led a small number of Spanish conquistadors to the Andes. They arrived in 1532 and by the next year, this group of less than 200 men was fighting the far more numerous Incas. The Spanish had horses, steel, and guns, all unknown to the Incas. The horses, larger than the llamas and alpacas, carried Spanish cavalry, armed with lances or swords and protected by armor and helmets. Some soldiers used a harquebus, a primitive kind of rifle, which created thunderous noises. The Spanish carried with them other deadly weapons that were terrifying because they were invisible and inaudible—germs. Illnesses such as smallpox and measles swept through the Andean population like a scythe. The Incas were further hobbled by the depredations of their own civil war and attacks from their own Andean enemies. The Spanish triumphed.

Following their victory, the Spanish pursued their primary aim of getting gold and silver from this newly discovered land. This mystified the Andeans, who valued these soft, malleable, and lustrous metals for their beauty, and crafted ceremonial items and jewelry from them. The Spanish began by holding the Incan emperor, Atahualpa, hostage and demanded that his subjects fill rooms with all of their gold and silver objects. Then the Spanish melted down all of the gold and silver objects and killed Atahualpa.

To us, this seems like deceit and looting, but Pizarro would not have seen it this way because he would have known about the Treaty of Tordesillas of 1494. In this agreement, the Spanish and Portuguese divided the world along a line running longitudinally just west of Cape Verde. Brazil, Africa, and Asia went to the Portuguese; the rest of the Americas to the Spanish. Therefore, Pizarro was only taking what he believed belonged to his country.

Coca and Silver Mining at Potosí

After this looting—it is impossible for a twenty-first-century author to use another word—had finished, the Spanish looked for more silver. They found large quantities in mines throughout Mexico and even more in the Incan Empire. Thick veins of silver ran through a 300-foot outcropping, Cerro Rico (rich hill), rising from a flat plain in what was then Peru but is now Bolivia. The plain is located at an altitude of 13,400 feet—much higher than Macchu Picchu at 8,000 feet, and roughly the same height as Chamonix in the French Alps. (Denver, in comparison, is located 5,280 feet over sea level.)

Cerro Rico and the plain on which it sits are unfriendly places. The thin air makes work difficult. Crops grow badly because of the poor soil, marked temperature swings, intense sunlight, and short growing season. Despite these brutal conditions, the Spanish organized a huge effort to extract silver, and in 1545 founded the mining city of Potosí on this forbidding plain. They conscripted the Native Americans to do the work.

Native American Andeans dug out the silver-containing ores by hammer or pick axe, and then crushed them to a powder. They mixed the powder with a variety of materials, including mercury, much of it mined in Huancavelica in Peru. The resulting slime was spread in a one- or two-foot-thick layer on a patio, a shallow enclosure. The Andeans mixed the slime with their feet so that the mercury and silver formed an amalgam. The mixture was then washed of all impurities. The mercury-silver amalgam was heated, the mercury was driven off, and pure silver was left behind. Many of the workers must have been poisoned by their exposure to mercury, one of the most toxic metals.

At first, the widespread use of the coca leaf among the Andean people shocked the Spanish. The Bishop of Cusco outlawed coca, declaring that it was an agent of the devil. (Nicotine, too, had been deemed to belong to the devil.) But the Spanish realized that they could get more work and silver from the Andeans and supply them with less food if they gave them coca leaf to chew. The Spanish also realized that the coca leaf could be taxed. After further consideration, the bishop reversed his understanding of the ownership of the coca leaf and declared it to be divine.

Coca leaf, while helpful in controlling workers' fatigue and hunger, was of no use against the other problems that afflicted the Andeans, such as malnutrition, silicosis, tuberculosis, and pneumonia. As the veins close to the surface became exhausted, the mining shafts became deeper, longer, and more perilous. Sometimes the shafts collapsed or were flooded. Coca leaf did not protect miners against either accidents or mercury poisoning. Miners died at early ages. Perhaps as many as 600,000 miners died at Potosí mining silver for the Spanish.[2] Because of the high mortality rate, it became increasingly difficult to find workers. Just as happened on sugar and tobacco plantations, slaves were brought over from Africa to do the work.

In the sixteenth century, the Native Americans and African slaves in the New World were producing three quarters of the world's silver,[3] much of it from the Cerro Rico. Beginning in 1574, a mint at Potosí converted the rich deposits of silver into great quantities of coins. A Spanish dollar, or peso, was worth eight reales. (A reale was a unit of currency in Spain.) Many of the famous "pieces of eight" were Potosí coins.

Immigrants came to Potosí from all parts of Europe to make their fortunes. At its peak, in the early to mid-seventeenth century, the city of Potosí was the most populous in the Western Hemisphere, consisting of about 160,000 inhabitants. In comparison, London had a population of 130,000; Amsterdam 80,000; and Seville and Venice 150,000 each.[4]

The city had churches, monasteries, and convents. Like other frontier towns, it also was home to dance halls, brothels, and gambling dens. There was friction between different ethnic groups. For example, violence between Basque and Castilian immigrants continued from across the Atlantic. Within the short period of a century or so, there were repeated cycles of inflation, deflation, and market crashes.[5]

Once the silver had been mined and minted, llamas and mules carried the silver coins across the mountains on a several-week trek to the Pacific coast. Ships took the silver up to the western coast of Panama, from where it was transported over the isthmus to the Caribbean coast.

The path across the isthmus and through the jungle was narrow and muddy. The jungle was full of rock-throwing monkeys, snakes, bats, and hostile Native Americans. The mule trains were often attacked by escaped Native American and African slaves. Mosquitoes transmitted malaria and yellow fever. The silver that reached the east coast of the isthmus was loaded onto galleons in the port city of Cartagena in what is now Colombia. These galleons joined other treasure-carrying ships at Havana to travel in convoys across the Atlantic.

The silver attracted the attention of the English adventurer Francis Drake, who began his nautical career by sailing with his relative John Hawkins, collecting slaves in Africa and selling them to Spanish colonists in return for Caribbean produce. Drake attacked a mule train carrying the silver from the mines in Peru, and he also attacked Cartagena. Drake was a hero to the English and was knighted by Queen Elizabeth I in 1581. He was a pirate to the Spanish. Galleons loaded down with Potosí silver were often plundered by Spain's other European rivals, the Dutch and French.

Much silver was lost to shipwrecks and piracy, but even so, by the 1590s, nearly 3 million kilos of silver traveled across the Atlantic each year. Silver also traveled across the Pacific to Manila in the Philippines, where it was traded for Chinese products, such as porcelain. Some silver traveled south along the Rio de la Plata (river of silver) into Argentina. Portuguese sailors took it to Lisbon, where they traded it for what was needed in Peru, including slaves from Africa.

Potosí silver and cheap labor funded the Spanish monarchy in its wars against the French, Dutch, English, and Turks. But the influx of precious metal had no intrinsic value. In fact, the silver may have triggered inflation and the eventual collapse of the Spanish Empire. Some historians argue that Spain eventually foundered because it depended on gold and silver, rather than agriculture or industry.[6]

Other consequences of the silver mining were environmental. Some of the mercury used in the mining process was recovered, but much was lost via spills and evaporation, and by being washed away. Experts have estimated that much of the mercury—previously sequestered within the earth—is now in the air, rivers, and oceans, where it can poison more people.[7]

Another environmental problem was the loss of trees. The areas around Huancavelica were deforested because charcoal was needed in the mercury mining process. Potosí itself was above the tree line, but trees from the surrounding lower areas were cut down to produce timber to support mine shafts and to make wooden axles for grinding mills. Wood was also used as fuel to roast the ore, heat the amalgam, and then reheat and fashion the silver into ingots or coins.[8]

Coca and European Explorers, Mountain Climbers, and Runners

South America appealed to Europeans interested in more than just gold and silver. Adventurers of all sorts journeyed to this new continent and often came across coca leaf in their explorations. The German geographer and naturalist Alexander von Humboldt traveled in South America from 1799 to 1804; described the geography, flora, and fauna, including the coca leaf; and noted the leaf's energizing effects. William H. Prescott, an historian, never traveled to South America but did review the notes and books of others. In his best-selling accounts of the Spanish conquests, he described the wondrous effects of the coca leaf.

Exploration of South America was also fueled by the European interest in colonizing Africa and Asia. Malaria was prevalent in these areas, so the Europeans were eager to find a cure for this debilitating illness. Cinchona grows in roughly the same areas of South America as does coca and its bark is the only natural source of quinine, a safe and effective treatment for malaria. Europeans hunting in the mountains of South America for cinchona used coca leaves to boost their energy. One of these explorers was Sir Clements Markham, the patron of Robert Scott's two expeditions to the Antarctic, president of the Royal Geographical Society, and Incan historian and linguist. In 1860, he was searching for the healthiest cinchona plants:

> To keep up with his Indian porters, Markham had adopted the native habit of chewing coca. Like many an explorer since, he found it produced an

"agreeable soothing feeling" and meant he could abstain from eating food for long periods. More important, it enabled him to climb steep mountain-sides "with a feeling of lightness and elasticity."[9]

A few years later, it was being used in Europe for similar reasons. Another vigorous and adventurous British enthusiast was Sir Robert Christison, the president of the British Medical Association and personal physician to Queen Victoria. In 1875, at the age of 78, he climbed Ben Vorlich, a small Scottish mountain, and gave the credit to coca leaf.

In the late 1800s, some race walkers chewed coca leaf to improve their performance.[10] This was one of the earliest examples of "doping" athletes and is a reminder of how Incan messengers used coca leaf. The ability of coca to help people walk long distances is also reflected in one of the current slang names for cocaine—Bolivian marching powder. By the mid- to late 1800s, coca leaf was known throughout Europe as a useful way to increase energy and endurance.

Vin Mariani and a Statue of Liberty That Could Have Been Taller

In the late 1860s, a Corsican pharmacist, Angelo Mariani, created a drink composed of coca leaves marinated in Bordeaux wine and named it Vin Mariani. The combination of alcohol, coca leaf, and the advertising skills of Mariani was successful (see Figure 8.3). Mariani was a brilliant publicist and one of the first salesmen to use celebrities to help him sell his product. Celebrities of the day such as Jules Verne, H. G. Wells, and Thomas Edison endorsed the wonders of this drink. Vin Mariani was associated with great productivity, or at least a sense of productivity. The only way that Ulysses Grant was able to finish his memoirs may have been his use of Vin Mariani. Frederic-Auguste Bartholdi, the architect who designed the Statue of Liberty, said that if he had used Vin Mariani at the time, the statue would have been several hundred meters in height. Most surprising was the endorsement of Pope Leo XIII.[11]

Drinkers of Vin Mariani described it as soothing and energizing.[12] It was considered a healthy beverage. The combination of alcohol and cocaine, however, leads to the formation of cocaethylene, which is more toxic to the heart than cocaine or alcohol alone. Was Vin Mariani harming those who drank it? Probably not, since there was almost certainly not enough cocaine in the Vin Mariani to lead to enough cocaethylene to cause heart damage. Those who drank the wine after the coca leaf had been steeped in it consumed only a small amount of cocaine diluted by

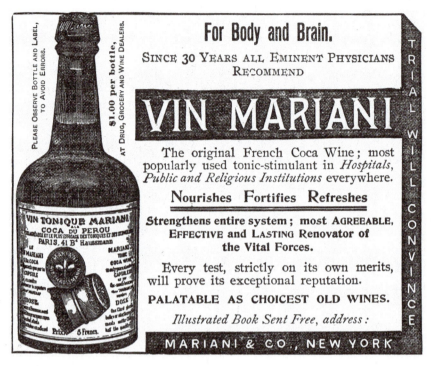

Figure 8.3 **Advertisement for French Coca Wine.** (© Corbis)

many other substances. Were the Vin Mariani drinkers becoming cocaine addicts? Again, probably not, since coca leaf consumed by mouth is less addictive than cocaine that is injected, smoked, or snorted. Vin Mariani was not a particularly powerful or addicting beverage.[13] Mariani was a stronger publicist than drink maker.

Coca-Cola, the American Drink

Many entrepreneurs tried to create their own forms of Vin Mariani, the most successful of which was developed in the United States. John Stith Pemberton was a pharmacist who obtained a medical degree from the Southern Botanico Medical College in Forsyth, Georgia. This was a medical school that followed the teachings of the herbalist Samuel Thomson. Pemberton fought in the Civil War as a Confederate soldier, was wounded, and then possibly became a morphine addict. Once the war was over, Pemberton used his training in botanical medicine to create and sell many herbal medicines. Pemberton read about the European and British enthusiasm for coca leaf and was impressed by the mountain climbing of the 78-year-old Christison. In 1881, he concocted a beverage using wine, coca leaf, and kola nut extracts containing caffeine, and named it French Wine Coca. He marketed it as a patent medicine and claimed many properties for it, including the ability to treat morphine addiction, or morphinism. He may have treated his own morphine addiction with his French Wine Coca.[14]

In 1886, alcoholic drinks were briefly banned in Atlanta. Pemberton removed the alcohol from French Wine Coca and then added sugar and more caffeine. He announced his creation of a "valuable Brain Tonic and a cure for all nervous affections."[15] The exact recipe was a secret and continues to be so, but he did boast about the coca leaf. He also made it carbonated. This became Coca-Cola, the archetypal American temperance drink. Pemberton hinted at its special powers and advertised it as a panacea for all illnesses. His bookkeeper, Frank Robinson, came up with both the name and the Spencerian script. The beverage became popular.

In 1887, Pemberton became ill and decided to sell the rights to his invention. He sold his secret formula to several people, thus leading to much confusion. But eventually Asa G. Candler took over the product. Candler gave away coupons for free drinks and gave storeowners who sold it gifts bearing the Coca-Cola brand. He began to sell it in bottles. Eventually, Coca-Cola became the world's dominant soft drink.

Around the turn of the century, people became aware of the harm that could be caused by cocaine. In the South, some landowners gave black sharecroppers cocaine in an attempt to decrease the food the workers consumed.[16] This is reminiscent of the Spanish using coca leaf to extract more work from the Peruvian silver mine workers.

An unpleasant myth emerged. Newspapers were fond of stories of black men, crazed on cocaine, attacking white women and filling mental asylums.[17] The stories were sensational and false. Nonetheless, the presence of coca leaf in Coca-Cola became an embarrassment.

In 1903, the Coca-Cola Company began to use decocainized coca leaf and added more sugar. Coca-Cola ran into surprising trouble with the U.S Bureau of Chemistry (later to be known as the Food and Drug Administration) because of this decision. In a confusing court case, head of the U.S. Bureau of Chemistry Harvey Wiley, using the 1906 Pure Food and Drugs Act, prosecuted Coca-Cola for false advertising. He charged that Coca-Cola did not contain coca leaf and kola nut when the name implied both. He also charged the company with adulteration of the drink by adding caffeine.

In other words, Coca-Cola was in trouble, not because they used coca leaf, but because Wiley thought that they did not. In his zeal to protect the American public, Wiley sometimes went off the rails of common sense. This strange case with the odd name, *The United States vs. 40 Barrels and 20 Kegs of Coca-Cola Syrup*, continued from 1909 to 1914. Eventually the company decreased the amount of caffeine while doubling the amount of decocainized cola leaf and kola nut. The bureau had succeeded in increasing the contribution of the coca shrub to Coca-Cola.

For several decades, Maywood Chemical Works in New Jersey removed the cocaine from coca leaf imported from Peru and sold it to pharmaceutical companies. At times, Coca-Cola needed more coca leaf than was needed to provide cocaine for legitimate medical reasons, and at those times, processing of coca leaves was done under the supervision of federal agents who destroyed the cocaine.

Coca-Cola has been the most successful version of Vin Mariani. Other patent medications fashioned at about the same time are quaint relics, while Coca-Cola is a worldwide symbol of American enterprise. Coca-Cola has benefited from the secret combination of ingredients, aggressive marketing, and its alliterative name. It has come far from the days when a Civil War veteran stirred up a potion in a kettle at home that he could sell as a tonic and cure for morphine addiction.

Isolation of Cocaine

In 1855, German chemist Friedrich Gaedcke extracted the active ingredient of the leaf, and named it *erythroxyline*. Albert Niemann also extracted this substance in 1859 as part of his Ph.D. thesis work and named it *cocaine*. Niemann was a student of Wöhler, who also had a role to play in the working out of fermentation. Niemann's work and his choice of name for the coca leaf alkaloid have been better known than Gaedcke's work.

Coca leaf had never been a good traveler because it easily became moldy. In contrast, cocaine traveled easily and had the advantage of being a uniform product. Pharmaceutical companies used the work of Niemann and Gaedcke to turn cocaine isolation into a commercial enterprise. One such company was Parke-Davis, an American herbalist company. In the early 1880s, it began to market products made from coca leaf extracts. In Germany, Merck was pursuing much the same course.

Until 1884, coca leaf and cocaine had small markets as stimulants and as an ingredient in Vin Mariani. Because of the discoveries of three Austro-German physicians, other markets for cocaine developed.

Cocaine Is Marketed as a Treatment for Addiction, Asthma, Fatigue, and Pain

A German army physician, Dr. Theodor Aschenbrandt, was looking for ways to boost the performance of German soldiers and obtained pure cocaine from Merck. In 1883, he reported that cocaine increased the physical endurance of the soldier subjects. This report attracted the attention of a young Viennese physician, Sigmund Freud, who suggested that cocaine was a safe way to increase energy and to treat addiction to opiates. (This is described in greater detail in the chapter about Freud and cocaine.) Freud talked about cocaine with one of his colleagues, Carl Koller, a young Viennese doctor studying ophthalmology. The ability of cocaine to produce local anesthesia fascinated Koller.

At that time, cataracts were removed without any anesthesia. Patients suffered terribly. All surgery is unpleasant, but surgery on the eyes is terrifying. Ophthalmologists needed a numbing drug that acted quickly but briefly and did not injure the delicate tissues of the eye. Koller tried many different drugs in the laboratory with no success.

He then decided to try the new drug mentioned to him by Freud. He experimented on the eyes of frogs. Cleverly, Koller "cocainized" one eye of a frog but not the other and determined that the cocainized eye was indeed numb. In 1884, Koller cocainized his and a colleague's eyes and found that they could press on their corneas and push pinheads into them painlessly.[18]

A Heidelberg ophthalmologic congress was about to take place. The 27-year-old Koller had not even finished his ophthalmology training. He was too poor to travel from Vienna to Heidelberg. A colleague, Josef Brettauer, attended the congress and on September 15, 1884, described and demonstrated to the world how Koller numbed the cornea.

Koller had not been the only physician to think that cocaine could be useful for eye surgery. Physicians in Peru and Russia had also suggested this use for cocaine but today get no credit for their work. This is because they lived far from medical centers, did not pursue their ideas, or published their findings in obscure journals. Koller was young and poor but lived in the hub of medical discoveries—middle Europe—and he published his findings in a prestigious German-language ophthalmology journal. His discovery spread throughout the Western world rapidly.

Many individuals and companies used his findings. William Halsted, a surgeon in New York and then Baltimore, developed the usefulness of cocaine further by administering it as regional anesthesia. (His subsequent

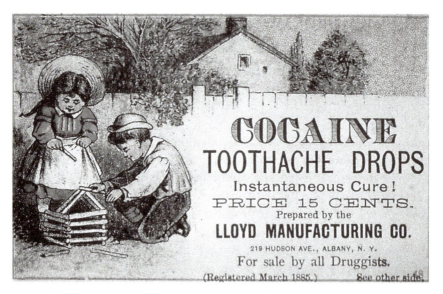

Figure 8.4   Cocaine Toothache Drops. (National Library of Medicine)

addiction is described in a separate chapter.) Pharmaceutical companies saw the opportunities in cocaine. It was marketed, for example, as a safe treatment for toothaches (see Figure 8.4).

The advertisement for "cocaine toothache drops" in Figure 8.4 shows two well-dressed children in pleasant surroundings concentrating intensely on building a log house. They seem to be well behaved and not to be displaying any signs of toothache or of being "high" on cocaine. The advertisement would convince anyone that cocaine tooth drops were effective and safe for everyone, including angelic children.

In the late 1800s and early 1900s, coca leaf and then cocaine were also used in Europe and North America as tonics or cures for addictions, colds or fevers. In 1885, Parke-Davis marketed cocaine in a tonic that, in their words, would be able to "supply the place of food, to make the coward brave, the silent eloquent and to free the victim of alcohol and opium habit from their bondage."[19] In 1887, the official remedy of the United States Hay Fever Association was declared to be cocaine.[20] Parke-Davis sold coca cheroots and coca cigarettes in which cocaine was smoked. The company also sold small kits containing syringes and powdered cocaine so that customers could inject the substance.[21] Cocaine was a legal and socially acceptable way of lessening pain from some surgical procedures and toothache, and also dealing with fatigue, asthma, or addictions.

Cocaine in the Twentieth Century

Popular newspapers and "muckrakers" in the United States became increasingly concerned about a connection between cocaine use and criminal behavior. Cocaine was injected and snorted in the underworld. As noted earlier in this chapter, much of the concern was blatantly racist. In 1914, President Taft named it "Public Enemy Number One." Sheriffs in the South asked for higher-caliber guns because they claimed that black men under the influence of cocaine were immune to normal bullets.[22]

Cocaine traveled from the underworld to more well-to-do urban communities. In the early twentieth century, snorting cocaine powder became popular among the wealthy and the Bohemians in Europe and the United States.

For unclear reasons, the use of cocaine in the United States and in Britain then decreased. A possible reason is the emergence of the new synthetic drugs, the amphetamines, which might have replaced cocaine because they were cheaper. Cocaine itself was no longer needed as a local anesthetic because of the introduction of synthetic drugs such as novocaine.

Beginning in the 1960s, drug abuse authorities began to pay more attention to the amphetamine black market, and—perhaps as a result—cocaine reappeared. The reappearance has also been linked to the increasing use of marijuana and hallucinogens in the 1960s, and the belief of many young Americans that it was safe to use illegal drugs.

Cocaine powder was snorted once again, as it had been in the 1920s, this time by Wall Street financiers in Manhattan and Hollywood stars in Beverly Hills. Its high cost elicited comparisons to fine champagne. People wore silver or gold cocaine spoons around their necks as a way of boasting about their use. For a few years, it was seen as relatively safe, and even some drug experts were unalarmed.

The Development of Free Base and Crack Cocaine

The coca cheroots and coca cigarettes sold by Parke-Davis were never very popular because cocaine powder, or the salt known as cocaine hydrochloride, melts at about 197 degrees Celsius. Above this temperature, the molecule degrades. Therefore, heating cocaine powder actually destroys it.

However, cocaine in the form of *free base* melts at about 89 degrees Celsius and then boils, leading to an inhalable aerosol. The structure of the cocaine molecule does not change. When smoked, free base cocaine vaporizes, and cocaine reaches the brain in a few seconds.

Cocaine hydrochloride is changed from a salt into a base by removing the hydrochloride molecule.[23] This is done by using any number of products, such as ammonia. Cocaine and ammonia seem like an unlikely combination, but it was widely used in Hollywood. Julia Phillips, the Academy Award–winning producer of the *Sting*, wrote about her experiences with cocaine hydrochloride and then free base. As befits a movie producer, in some striking vignettes she describes making free base. At first, she prepared free base by

> ... dissolving the raw product in water, mixing it with a small amount of any household cleaner that has ammonia in it, then drying and rolling around in a Melita coffee filter. It makes hard little rocks ...[24]

A friend of hers tells her not to do this because of the toxicity of ammonia. He shows her how to use ether, and she is fascinated:

> Walter takes me through the steps for his method. First dilute the coke in water ... Then add an equal amount of anhydrous ether ... Then the tiniest bit of ammonium hydroxide, to precipitate a reaction ... Now screw on the cap, and shake it up ... Luminescent crystals start to grow. When everything turns white on the plate, and Walter pronounces it dry, he scrapes it with an industrial razor and produces a pipe. This pipe has nine thousand screens in it, to keep the base from melting down the stem when lit ...[25]

This was a dangerous technique because ether is flammable. In the early 1970s, baking soda (or sodium bicarbonate) was discovered as a safer way of preparing free base cocaine. The mixture of cocaine powder and baking soda is heated until small chunks of free base cocaine form. This way of changing the salt into a base was safer than using ammonia or ether.

Free base cocaine made with baking soda was first known as rock cocaine. It became better known in the 1980s in New York as crack cocaine. The name crack comes from the crackling sound that the heated substance makes. The first medical reports of what would be a major social, health, and crime epidemic came from the Bahamas. The Bahamas was a convenient stopping point for cocaine being sent from Colombia to the eastern United States. Free base cocaine was associated with violence and psychiatric problems.[26]

Free base made with ammonia or ether was eclipsed by crack cocaine. Crack cocaine required no chemistry or cooking skills. It was cheap, easy to prepare and smoke, and addictive. It rapidly infiltrated America's poor urban communities while cocaine powder remained a drug of the wealthy.

Crack cocaine was associated with inner cities, minorities, and violence. Newspapers reported that women on crack cocaine no longer cared for their children. The depiction of the crack-crazed woman using drugs during her pregnancy and then neglecting her addicted baby once born was similar to the portrait of gin-drinking women by Hogarth or the story of the baby killer Judith Defour.

Snorting the powder was associated with wealth and irresponsibility; smoking crack cocaine was associated with violent crime. This differentiation was crude and inaccurate, but powerful.

In 1986, the 22-year-old basketball star Len Bias died after using cocaine. Bias may have died from an overdose of cocaine powder and alcohol, not crack cocaine, but at the time, the public perception was that yet another young person had died because of crack cocaine. This may have stimulated passage of the American Anti-Drug Abuse Act of 1986. Possession of five hundred grams of cocaine or five grams of crack triggered a five-year mandatory minimum sentence. Possession of five thousand grams of cocaine or 50 grams of crack automatically meant a 10-year mandatory minimum sentence. Sentences were doubled if the offender had a prior felony conviction. Parole was not an option. The hope was that tough laws and mandatory minimum sentencing would stop the epidemic of crack cocaine use. Conservative and liberal politicians alike believed that this approach would save the inner cities from the menace of crack cocaine.

The 100-to-1 disparity between powder cocaine and crack cocaine meant, since crack cocaine was so available and cheap, that poor people with small amounts of crack made up a disproportionate share of the people jailed for drug offenses. Another way of looking at this was that the wealthy snorted cocaine with impunity, while the poor—often African Americans—were jailed for smoking crack cocaine.

Two years later, the American Anti-Drug Abuse Act of 1988 made all those even indirectly involved in crack cocaine sales subject to these sentences. So people who were "lookouts" (typically youngsters) could also be considered co-conspirators and sentenced harshly.

Whether these mandated sentences affected crack cocaine use is not clear. Most authorities in the twenty-first century think that they did have a terrible effect on inner cities by putting so many young men in jail. The combination of easy money associated with crack cocaine along with high rates of incarceration was associated with decreased investment in education and legal employment in some minority communities.[27]

Eventually, in 2010, Congress somewhat reduced the powder cocaine–crack disparity in sentencing from 100-to-one to 18-to-one. Crack cocaine is still thought to be more dangerous and addictive than powder cocaine, although the evidence for this is not conclusive.

Cocaine is often used with other substances. Cocaine and opiates form a "speedball" that can be sniffed or injected. Cocaine speeds the person up, and the opiate calms the person down. The combination of cocaine and alcohol appeals to many. Vin Mariani contained coca leaf dissolved in wine. Coca-Cola mixed coca leaf with, at different times, alcohol, sugar, or caffeine. Patent medicines often contained combinations of drugs. Some of these combinations, such as high doses of cocaine and alcohol, or the injected speedball, are reported to be particularly harmful.

Cocaine and International Crime

After World War II, cocaine began to be smuggled out of South America by gangsters and politicians. Manuel Noriega, for example, was a politician involved in smuggling cocaine. Noriega was born in Panama and enlisted in the Panamanian army. He received more military training in the United States and worked closely with the Central Intelligence Agency (CIA). He was military dictator of Panama from 1983 to 1989. His relationship with the United States deteriorated amidst charges of drug laundering and abuse of human rights. In 1989, the United States invaded Panama and captured Noriega. He was convicted in Miami in 1992 on counts of drug trafficking, racketeering, and money laundering. France extradited him in 2010 and convicted him of murder and money laundering.

Noriega had been a close colleague of Pablo Escobar, the creator of the Medellín drug cartel. Escobar bought cocaine paste in Bolivia and Peru, refined it, and then smuggled the cocaine through Panama into the United States with the help of Noriega.[28] Escobar has been accused of arranging the murder of several Colombian supreme court justices. There was brutal competition between him and his competitors, the Cali cartel, which led in the early 1990s to the deaths of over 50,000 people in Colombia.

Cocaine also influenced politics in Nicaragua. During the struggle of the Sandinistas, a socialist political party, against the Nicaraguan government, the CIA formed alliances with "contras," anti-Communists, who were also cocaine smugglers. An American government investigation, headed by then senator John Kerry, reported that Oliver North, then a member of the National Security Council staff at the White House, and other senior officials worked with contras and others, such as Manuel Noriega, who welcomed a cover for their smuggling work. The CIA investigated itself and reported that it had indeed worked with known drug traffickers during the years of the war in Nicaragua.

Some journalists have accused the CIA of knowing that Nicaraguan-based contras were smuggling cocaine into Los Angeles as crack cocaine and using the profits from this enterprise to support their struggle.[29]

The destruction of coca plants and cocaine processing labs in Colombia and elsewhere as well as the interdiction of cocaine shipments led to the product becoming more expensive. This makes smuggling cocaine more profitable and stimulates trade.[30]

Drug cartels are efficient and profitable businesses. They do not have to worry about accountability to stockholders, lobbyists, or voters. Because they often operate as dictatorships or autocracies, they can be nimble; they do not have to be slowed down by regulations or have their directives lost in bureaucratic swamps. Profits are immense. Cocaine (and heroin) drug lords do not have expenses such as taxes or advertising although they do have to spend money on bribery and elimination of the competition.

The peasants or farmers who grow coca stay poor. The couriers of drugs, known as mules, and street vendors risk jail or death. The large-volume traffickers become wealthy. They may give money to the poor and sometimes are celebrated as "Robin Hood" philanthropists. Escobar, for example, remains a hero to the poor people of Medellín, where he built churches and sports facilities. However, the wealth and viciousness of these smugglers does not guarantee them immunity or long lives. Noriega is, as of 2013, in prison, and Escobar was killed in a shootout in Medellín in 1993. The drug lords live in opulence but only for as long as they can avoid their competitors or the government.

Effects on the Mind and Body

How Cocaine Gets into the Body

There are a few ways cocaine can get into the body and then the brain, and the effects differ according to the preparation and route. Chewing coca leaves or drinking coca tea gets cocaine to the brain rather slowly, and the results are mild and prolonged. Snorting cocaine powder gets it into the brain faster. It gets into the brain fastest and causes the most intense rush by using it intravenously or by smoking crack cocaine. The rush is short lived.

Effects on the Mind

Intoxication

Cocaine does not reduce anxiety in the way that the other three substances discussed in this book do, but it does lead to a sense of intense pleasure. Cocaine increases arousal, sexuality, energy, and attentiveness. Fatigue disappears, and the person feels euphoric. These effects are far more pronounced with cocaine than with coca leaf. Messengers in the Andes chewed coca leaf and ran along knife-edge high mountain ridges with confidence and alertness, but they were probably not intoxicated.

Snorting, injecting, or smoking cocaine leads at first to euphoria. But this can quickly change to irritability, suspiciousness, and rage. Cocaine can also be associated with hallucinations—hearing, seeing, or feeling things that are not really there. Injecting or smoking crack cocaine is the route most commonly associated with the development of paranoia and hallucinations. The person may feel that bugs or parasites are crawling under his or her skin. Users sometimes pick at their skin, trying to get rid of the hallucinated "cocaine bugs." Some users also develop repetitive and compulsive behaviors or extreme anxiety.

Addiction

The perception of cocaine as an addictive drug is recent, since there are none of the physical withdrawal signs that are so clear in withdrawal from alcohol and opiates. Not everyone who uses cocaine becomes dependent on it, but many of those who use high doses by snorting, injecting, or smoking it do indeed become addicted. Cocaine addicts experience intense misery, somnolence, and craving for cocaine when not using it. As described elsewhere, this is thought to be related to changes in dopaminergic pathways that may take months to readjust. During this time, the person will experience prolonged anhedonia—the inability to experience pleasure.

Effects on the Body

Nose

Using the nose to snort cocaine powder can damage the nasal tissues. This is partly due to blood vessel constriction, which is directly due to the cocaine, and partly due to chemical irritation from adulterants. The cocaine may also impair the movement of the cilia, which move the mucus blanket along the interior of the nose. Cocaine can destroy the turbinates or palate and lead to perforations of the nasal septum. The anesthetic effects of the cocaine mean that much damage can be done without the person noticing.

Heart and Blood Vessels

Cocaine constricts, or narrows, the blood vessels, causing high blood pressure and decreased blood supply to the heart. The heart beats faster. Cocaine has been associated with heart attacks and disturbances in the rhythm of the heart rate, known as cardiac arrhythmias. Len Bias probably died from a cardiac arrhythmia. If used for a long time, cocaine damages the muscles of the heart. Using cocaine while drinking alcohol may increase the risk of damage to the heart.

Pregnancy

Cocaine use during pregnancy may increase the risk of miscarriage, preterm birth, birth defects, and perhaps growth delay. Some babies may be born dependent on cocaine and be "jittery." Experts suspect that these babies may develop learning difficulties as they grow older. Fears that there would be a generation of desperately ill "crack babies" may have been unfounded or exaggerated.

Conclusion

In the twenty-first century, Potosí is now part of Bolivia. Young Bolivian men continue to work in the mines in Potosí. The silver veins are mostly exhausted, but there are other metals, such as tin, to extract. The miners still chew coca leaf to help them withstand the atrocious conditions, and they still die too early. Dynamite is used now, which makes the work easier but more dangerous. Cerro Rico is riddled with mining shafts, and the top has collapsed. Tourists can visit the mines and buy the miners gifts such as alcohol, coca leaves, and small sticks of dynamite.

Coca leaf itself continues to be honored in the Andes. Many Andeans continue to chew coca leaf as a mild stimulant, and the coca plant itself is an integral part of Andean culture. However, coca leaf, in the more dangerous form of cocaine, is still exported from the Andes and neighbouring regions to far-away countries to lead to wealth, misery, and crime, similar in some ways to Potosí silver. A boomtown mentality persists with regard to cocaine, as it did with silver, with criminality, fortunes made and broken, and wide swings in price. The coca leaf seems fragile in compari-son to silver, but it has outlasted this element as an important part of the region's economy.

The presence of Coca-Cola throughout the world is an evocative reminder of the days when coca leaf was thought to bring youthfulness, vigor, and freedom from pains, aches, and morphinism to its users. For many, coca leaf, when refined to yield cocaine, is now associated with medical problems and addiction.

Notes

1. Tom D. Dillehay et al., "Early Holocene Coca Chewing in Northern Peru," *Antiquity* 84, no. 326 (2010): 939–53.

2. Henry Hobhouse, *Seeds of Change: Six Plants That Transformed Mankind*, rev. ed. (New York: Shoemaker & Hoard, 2005), 337.

3. Jason W. Moore, " 'This Lofty Mountain of Silver Could Conquer the Whole World': Potosí and the Political Ecology of Underdevelopment, 1545–1800," *Journal of Philosophical Economics* 4, no. 1 (2010): 59.

4. Ibid., 60.

5. John Demos, "The High Place: Potosí," *Common-Place* 3, no. 4 (2003): 1–6.

6. David Landes, *The Wealth and Poverty of Nations* (New York: Norton, 1999), 171–73.

7. Jerome O. Nriagu, "Mercury Pollution from the Past Mining of Gold and Silver in the Americas," *Science of the Total Environment* 149 (1994): 167–81.

8. Moore, "Lofty Mountain," 63.

9. Mark Honigsbaum, *The Fever Trail: In Search of the Cure for Malaria*. (New York: Farrar, Straus and Giroux, 2001), 118.

10. Steven B. Karch, *A Brief History of Cocaine* (Boca Raton, FL: CRC Press, 1998), 19.

11. Dominic Streatfield, *Cocaine: An Unauthorized Biography* (New York: Picador, 2001), 60–61.

12. In a similar way, laudanum, the combination of alcohol and opium, a different combination of drugs, was extremely popular for many years as an uplifting and soothing beverage.

13. Karch, *Brief History*, 28–29.

14. Mark Pendergrast, *For God, Country, and Coca-Cola: The Definitive History of the Great American Soft Drink and the Company That Makes It*, rev. ed. (New York: Basic Books, 2000), 25.

15. Ibid., 31.

16. Ibid., 87.

17. Streatfield, *Cocaine*, 141.

18. Koller was not alone in his use of frog eyes. George Wald, the Nobel Prize–winning scientist who discovered much about the retina, experimented on the eyes of 300 frogs to discover vitamin A (retinol). The large bulging eyes of frogs are irresistible to experimenters.

19. Hobhouse, *Seeds of Change*, 308.

20. David F. Musto, *The American Disease: Origins of Narcotic Control*. expanded ed. (New York: Oxford University Press, 1987), 7.

21. Karch, *Brief History*, 89.

22. Streatfield, *Cocaine*, 142–43.

23. The cocaine hydrochloride is "reverse-engineered" back to a chemical base. Cocaine exists as a base in one of the earlier steps in the production of cocaine from the coca leaf. See footnote 28.

24. Julia Phillips, *You'll Never Eat Lunch in This Town Again* (New York: Random House, 1991), 358.

25. Ibid., 359–60.

26. James F. Jekel, et al., "Epidemic Free-Base Cocaine Abuse. Case Study from the Bahamas," *Lancet* 327, no. 8479 (1986): 459–62.

27. Philippe Bourgois, *In Search of Respect: Selling Crack in El Barrio* (New York: Cambridge University Press, 1996), 318–27.

28. To isolate cocaine from the coca leaf, the leaf is pulverized and mixed with solvents, such as kerosene, and then bases and acids so that cocaine can be precipitated out. The result is a putty-like substance known as paste. It can be smoked and in that way is similar to free base cocaine, but it is not yet fully refined.

29. Alexander Cockburn and Jeffrey St. Clair, *Whiteout: The CIA, Drugs and the Press* (New York: Verso, 1998), 277–315.

30. Alfred W. McCoy, *The Politics of Heroin: CIA Complicity in the Global Drug Trade*, 2nd rev. ed. (Chicago: Lawrence Hill, 2003), 446–60.

9

Sniffing Cocaine, Heroin, and Tobacco

People who sniff or snort drugs use the nose as a gateway to the body. The nose is a deceptively designed entrance. The external nose is a small and unimportant part of the organ. The real work of the nose takes place behind what we can see and feel. The nose is a symmetrical structure that is divided by the septum, a layer of cartilage and thin bone, into two nasal cavities. From the wall of each cavity protrude three strange and largely unknown bones, the turbinates. They are horizontal bones, stacked above each other, that look like three chubby fingers. These odd bones, shown in Figure 9.1, are crucial to breathing comfort and efficiency.

The turbinates are lined with a membrane that is covered with a blanket of damp mucus that warms and humidifies the incoming air. The air is thus "conditioned" before it travels to the alveoli of the lungs, where the important oxygen and carbon dioxide exchange takes place. Some inhaled molecules go directly to the olfactory organ in the brain to be "smelled." The mucus on the turbinates also filters the air and traps small particles. Cilia, which are thin whip-like projections of the cell wall, move the mucus with the particles to the back of the nose, where there is an opening to the esophagus, so some sniffed or snorted substances are swallowed and go to the stomach.

Because of the scrolled or whorled construction of the turbinates and their ample blood supply, much blood flows through the nose. This arrangement can be subverted for the purpose of drug administration.

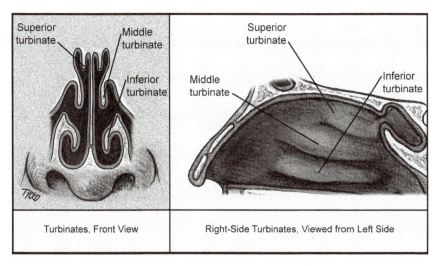

Figure 9.1   **Turbinates.** (© 2013 Joan M.K. Tycko)

Sniffed or snorted drugs do not go to the lungs or, for the most part, to the gut, but are absorbed through the thin turbinate membranes directly into the bloodstream. They thus bypass the usual route, which is through the stomach, intestines, and liver. This standard route is slow because it involves the body's safety checks. Swallowed drugs are processed, or metabolized, by cells in the liver and intestine. Most of the sniffed or snorted drugs avoid what is known as first pass—or hepatic (liver)—metabolism and hence reach the brain more rapidly and unchanged than if they were swallowed.

Cocaine

Cocaine is probably the drug most frequently thought of with respect to the nose. The user puts the cocaine on a mirror or other flat surface, chops it into a fine powder, makes "lines" of the powder, and then uses a rolled-up piece of paper to snort the powder into one nostril while holding the other nostril closed. The powder is absorbed through the turbinates into the blood stream. The turbinates are, however, designed to condition inhaled air and not to absorb this drug. They can be hijacked for this purpose, but at a cost. Cocaine constricts the blood vessels, which leads, over time, to a decreased blood supply and damage to the nose.

Additionally, adulterants in the cocaine can irritate the mucous membranes. The cocaine may also impair the activity of the cilia. Because cocaine is an anesthetic, severe damage can take place before the person is aware of it. Some people who snort cocaine can develop a hole in the septum, known as a septal perforation.

Heroin

Heroin, when available as a pure powder, can also be sniffed or snorted. This way of using heroin has the advantage of not involving needles or injections. Sniffed heroin does not reach the brain for 10 or 15 minutes and because of this, sniffing heroin is not as addictive as other ways of using the drug.

Tobacco

Christopher Columbus was astonished when he saw Native Americans smoking and sniffing tobacco. He had seen neither activity before his journeys to the New World. We are more familiar now with *smoking* tobacco, but *sniffing* tobacco was popular in the eighteenth century in Europe. The person would pick some tobacco powder, known as snuff, between his or her fingers, put it in his or her nose, and then sneeze it out. This odd habit became fashionable, and for some years, it was a particularly aristocratic habit. In England, Queen Anne and Queen Charlotte used snuff. Artisans, including jewelers, enamellers, silversmiths, and goldsmiths, created ornamented snuffboxes that were symbols of wealth and good taste.

Snuff is well known to anatomists and medical students because of a curious indentation in the wrist. When the thumb is extended outward, a small hollow between tendons can be seen. Some people put snuff in this hollow; hence it is known as the "snuffbox."

Sniffing tobacco has now been eclipsed by the habit of burning tobacco and inhaling it. We are used to people doing this by smoking cigars, pipes, or cigarettes. Why do people smoke through their mouths and not through their nostrils? We inhale air through our nostrils to humidify and warm it, which might make smoking through our nostrils rather than our mouth more comfortable. We do not smoke through our nostrils because although the nostrils can *flare* they cannot *pucker* as the mouth can. The *orbicularis oris* mucles in the lips act as a sort of sphincter that allows the lips to form a tight seal on the cigarette, allowing great suction power on the cigarette—the nostrils are not so agile. Hence, there is not as much power in the nostrils as there is in the mouth to draw on the cigarette or to hold onto a cigar or pipe.

A related difference between sniffing powders through the nose and smoking through the lips is aesthetic. As Humphry Bogart and Bette Davis demonstrated, smoking cigarettes can seem elegant and sexy. Sneezing after sniffing snuff or holding a rolled up piece of paper to one's nostril to snort cocaine seems undignified rather than sophisticated.

10

William Stewart Halsted

William Stewart Halsted is one of the most important figures in the history of American surgery. He devised regional anesthesia, a way of numbing a body part without interfering with consciousness. He invented new surgical procedures and techniques, and he improved surgical education. Yet he was addicted to morphine and possibly cocaine throughout his career.

Halsted was born in 1852 in New York City to a wealthy family, the oldest of four children. Halsted had a privileged education, attending Phillips Academy in Andover, Massachusetts, and then Yale College. He obtained his medical degree from Columbia University in New York in 1877. This was not as good a medical education as it sounds today because in the late 1800s, medical education and practice were quite backward throughout the United States, particularly when compared to that in Europe. In many American medical schools, students did not even have to be high school graduates. They were not expected to attend lectures, dissect cadavers, or examine patients. Aware of the inadequacies of his medical education, Halsted traveled to Austria and Germany to continue his education. He remained impressed with German medicine for the rest of his life. He returned to New York to become a successful physician. He was hard working and ambitious, and became adept at dissections and a master of anatomy. He also formed an important friendship with William Welch, a pathologist who would later help to create the Johns Hopkins School of Medicine.

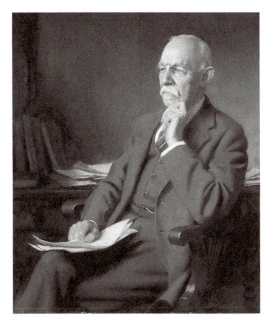

Figure 10.1 **William Stewart Halsted. (Alan Mason Chesney Medical Archives of the Johns Hopkins Medical Institutions)**

Halsted was an adventurous and fearless surgeon with such self-confidence that he was willing to treat the illnesses of family members. While he was working in New York, his younger sister bled heavily after delivering a baby, and he transfused his own blood into her. This was one of the first blood transfusions. Almost unbelievably, he operated again on another family member. In 1882, his mother became ill and on her kitchen table in the middle of the night, he removed her gallbladder. This was one of the first gallbladder surgeries in the United States. Halsted's operations on his sister and mother were hazardous. Most physicians do not operate on their own family members, let alone with unproven techniques. Yet Halsted saved the lives of both women and advanced the art of surgery.

Halsted's career course changed trajectory after Koller's 1884 work in Vienna with cocaine. Dentists and eye surgeons—those men who inflicted great pain on their patients and who often could not bear it—began to apply cocaine directly to teeth and eyes to numb them. Halsted took the next step and injected cocaine into the *nerves* that carried sensations from the area about to be operated on. This was the beginning of regional anesthesia. For example, he injected cocaine into an area in the face just under the eye. Cocaine applied here numbs the nerves carrying sensation from the upper jaw and made dental extractions less painful.

Halsted then used cocaine deftly and successfully in multiple other procedures. Together with his New York medical students, he expanded the uses of the drug. Halsted's work increased the number of operations, both dental and otherwise, that could be performed with local anesthesia. Halsted showed that cocaine interfered with the transmission of sensation but not with the control of muscles. It did not interfere with consciousness. The patient who received an injection of cocaine was conscious, followed any instructions of the surgical team, and felt no pain.

Halsted could not have known it at the time, but injected or snorted cocaine is different from cocaine consumed by mouth because of its quick onset of action. Halsted, with some of his colleagues and students, began to sniff cocaine powder. Many of these young doctors, including Halsted, became addicted to cocaine. Crippled by his addiction, Halsted was unable to work, and it seemed that his medical career was about to end.

Halsted's friend Welch became aware of Halsted's problems and came up with a clever solution. In the spring of 1886, Welch and some other friends chartered a schooner. Welch went with Halsted to the Caribbean and back to try to keep him away from cocaine. This two-month trip might have been pleasant, but it was not therapeutic. Since Halsted took a generous supply of cocaine with him and stole drugs from the ships doctors' cabin, this expensive maritime cure did not work.

Halsted was subsequently hospitalized twice at the Butler Hospital, a psychiatric hospital in Providence, Rhode Island, and was possibly the hospital's first cocaine addict. His first hospital stay lasted from May to November 1886, and the second one lasted from April to December 1887. During these lengthy hospitalizations, he received much of what we would call occupational therapy: gardening, music, and walks around the beautiful grounds. His medical colleagues gave him respectful and kind advice.

There were no medicines then to treat addiction. But physicians always like to do *something*. At some point, Halsted's biographers think that an adventurous physician may have used morphine to treat Halsted's cocaine addiction. This would not have been that unusual, since many patent medicines then sold as cures for addiction contained morphine. Freud and others thought that cocaine could treat morphine addiction so it is not surprising that a Butler physician would have tried the reverse. Perhaps this idea came from Halsted himself.[1, 2]

The hospitalizations were as pleasant and as unhelpful as the Caribbean cruise. Welch was not aware of the therapeutic failure and thought that Halsted was discharged from his second Butler stay cured. Not so. Halsted continued to use cocaine and now morphine as well.

Meanwhile, Welch was becoming more involved with a new institution in Baltimore. Johns Hopkins, a Baltimore Quaker merchant, was an entrepreneur who had invested in railroads and banks. Some of his business involved alcohol. For example, he traded some of his goods for moonshine, rebottled it, and sold it as Hopkins' Best.[3] Through his railroad and financial investments, as well as his alcohol sales, he became wealthy. At his death, Hopkins left his fortune to be used to establish a university and medical school in Baltimore.

The task was taken up by John Shaw Billings, a surgeon who designed the entire Hopkins Hospital and its medical school. The medical school was to be different from other American medical institutions of the time. Johns Hopkins would be a not-for-profit school that admitted only qualified students. Laboratory work and bedside teaching, rather than just lectures, would be emphasized. The Johns Hopkins Hospital opened in 1889 and was followed four years later by the Johns Hopkins University School of Medicine.

Billings hired William Welch to be one of the founding physicians. Welch, too, had studied in Germany and was determined to create a medical school and hospital to rival German institutions. Welch recruited his old friend Halsted in 1886 to join him in the newly formed pathology laboratory. The other two physicians, making up the "Big Four" of Johns Hopkins, were William Osler and Howard Kelly. Within a few years, most of the medical advances in American medicine came from Baltimore.

In 1889, Halsted became temporary chief of the department of surgery, a year later surgeon-in-chief, and then two years later professor of surgery. Halsted developed the (now outmoded) technique of radical mastectomy—in which the entire breast and surrounding tissue including part of the armpit—were removed to treat breast cancer. Until Halsted, there was no treatment for breast cancer. Women often did not come to medical attention until the cancer involved the whole breast, at which point the physician felt helpless. Halsted, using his formidable knowledge of anatomy and attention to detail, was able to remove the entire breast and associated tissue safely and at least make the woman more comfortable for some time.

He introduced the use of rubber gloves into surgery to help an operating room nurse who had developed dermatitis, probably due to her exposure to mercuric chloride, then used as an antiseptic agent. (He later married the nurse with the sensitive skin.) He improved hernia and thyroid surgeries. He propagated the art and science of safe surgery by scrupulous aseptic technique, gentle handling of the tissues, and attention to stopping blood loss. A pioneer in medical education, he started the first formal surgical residency training program in the United States and developed the idea of surgical residencies in which residents took on more responsibility as they matured. He established experimental laboratories.

Welch had gathered about him a group of brilliant men. They demonstrated what has been called the "contagious companionship of excellence."[4] But Welch had gambled when he asked his friend to come to Baltimore.

During his long tenure at Johns Hopkins, Halsted remained a mysterious figure. He was moody, irritable, and shaky in the afternoons, and then mysteriously revived in the evenings. He was sarcastic and a loner. He was often unpredictably absent. He was predictably absent from Hopkins every year from May to October. For two of these months, he stayed at his wife's family home in the mountains of North Carolina. For the rest of the time, he traveled throughout Europe. These European jaunts were usually solitary.

Historians now think that some of his peculiarities were due to his drug addiction. We know that his addiction to morphine never remitted because of the revelations of his colleague, William Osler. Osler had written an account of the "inner history of the Johns Hopkins Hospital" in a small black book that he then sealed. He intended it to be read at the 100th anniversary of the Johns Hopkins hospital in 1989. However, it was opened and published in 1969, on the eightieth anniversary. Osler wrote that Halsted had continued to use large amounts of morphine while at Johns Hopkins.[5]

There is no corresponding "proof" that he continued to use cocaine, although this seemed possible to some of his colleagues. William Welch thought so, as did Harvey Cushing, the great neurosurgeon and perhaps the most outstanding of Halsted's students.[6, 7] But we know tantalizingly little about the details of his drug abuse. Did he ever use cocaine and morphine together? (This would have been similar to the risky speedball.) Where did he buy the drugs? Halsted was using these drugs well before the Harrison Act, and there was less opprobrium attached to them. Did he buy them "on the street"? Did a physician prescribe them for him? Did he buy them from pharmaceutical companies? Perhaps he bought supplies on his summer trips to Europe. Was his use of either cocaine or morphine, or both, responsible for his afternoon dips in mood? Was he searching for a cure or was he indulging in drugs in the summers?

Cushing and others have suggested that Halsted's struggles with his addictions were responsible for his strength of character and his creativity in establishing the first American school of surgery.[8, 9] Others have wondered how much more he could have achieved if he had been drug free.[10]

Halsted never talked or wrote about himself or his addictions. Other physicians were enthusiastic about cocaine anesthesia, but Halsted never boasted of his discovery and seemed to avoid the topic as much as possible.

Halsted had immense self-confidence, which allowed him to experiment with new treatments and to operate on his sister and mother. He was not interested in self-disclosure. He revealed much about anatomy; he explored the secrets of the body; he journeyed through the sensory nerves, the muscles, and blood supplies—but he did not explore his own psyche. Or perhaps he did but chose not to lay it open on the operating table of history.

Notes

1. Gerald Imber, *Genius on the Edge: The Bizarre Double Life of Dr. William Stewart Halsted* (New York: Kaplan, 2000), 80.

2. Howard Markel, *An Anatomy of Addiction: Sigmund Freud, William Halsted, and the Miracle Drug Cocaine* (New York: Pantheon, 2011), 142.

3. Kathryn A. Jacob, "Mr. Johns Hopkins," *Johns Hopkins Magazine* 25, no. 1 (1974): 13–17.

4. Wilder Penfield, "Halsted of Johns Hopkins: The Man and His Problem as Described in the Secret Records of William Osler," *Journal of the American Medical Association* 210, no. 12 (1969): 2215.

5. Ibid., 2214–18.

6. Imber, *Genius on the Edge*, 346.

7. Markel, *Anatomy of Addiction*, 238–9.

8. Penfield, *Halsted of Johns Hopkins*, 2215.

9. Markel, *Anatomy of Addiction*, 239.

10. A. Mark Clarfield, "Book Review: Genius on the Edge; The Bizarre Double Life of Dr. William Stewart Halsted," *Journal of the American Medical Association* 303, no. 17 (2010): 1756.

11

Sigmund Freud and Cocaine

Sigmund Freud was born in Moravia in 1856 to a Jewish middle-class family. At the age of 17, he began to study medicine at the University of Vienna and by the age of 26, he was a physician. Although this sober intellectual is better known now for his theories of the unconscious and the development of psychoanalysis, for a short time he promoted cocaine to his friends, family, and other physicians. His enthusiasm for cocaine played an important part in an opthalmologist's discovery of cocaine as an anesthetic and in his own perception of the importance of dreams.

In the spring of 1884, the 28-year-old Dr. Freud was concerned about the health of his friend, Ernst von Fleischl-Marxow, another physician. While performing an autopsy, Fleischl-Marxow had infected his right thumb, which subsequently had to be amputated. Following the surgery, he developed painful nerve growths, known as traumatic neuromas, at the site of the amputation. He began to use morphine to control the pain and became addicted to this drug.

At the same time, Freud was reading about the work of a German army physician, Dr. Theodor Aschenbrandt. Aschenbrandt gave pure cocaine provided by the German pharmaceutical company Merck to soldiers, and their endurance improved. Freud also read reports from other physicians suggesting that cocaine cured morphine addiction. In April 1884, Freud encouraged Fleischl-Marxow to try cocaine, the substance that had helped the soldiers and addicts, to build up his strength and to fight the morphine addiction.

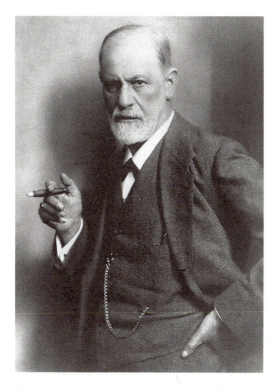

Figure 11.1 **Sigmund Freud with a Cigar. (© Corbis. By permission of The Marsh Agency Ltd on behalf of Sigmund Freud Copyrights)**

Freud also bought some cocaine from Merck and began to use it himself; he took it by mouth. It energized him and lifted his spirits. He performed laboratory experiments to try to determine whether cocaine increased muscular strength or reaction time. He mailed some to his fiancée for her use. He read as much as he could about the drug, including reports from Parke-Davis (an American pharmaceutical company). He wrote "Über Coca" (On Coca) and in July 1884, it was published in a Viennese medical journal, *Centralblatt für die gesammte Therapie*. In this rapidly written article, he described the plant and the Incan myth of how Manco Capac, the son of the Sun-God, had brought coca to mankind as a gift from the gods. He reviewed the work of many scientists, most now unknown, who had experimented with cocaine. He described its effects on many systems of the body. He was most impressed by its mild stimulant and antidepressant effects. In this enthusiastic paper, he wrote:

> The psychic effect of [cocaine] consists of exhilaration and lasting euphoria, which does not differ in any way from the normal euphoria of a healthy person ... Long lasting intensive mental or physical work can be performed without fatigue ...[1]

He recommended cocaine as a treatment for morphine or alcohol addiction. In the final paragraph of the paper, he noted its possible use as a local anesthetic, but this seemed to be almost an afterthought, as he did not emphasize this or develop the idea.

Freud also recognized the hypersexuality that cocaine can cause. In June 1884, he wrote a suggestive letter to his fiancée in which he stated that under the influence of cocaine, he would be "a big wild man with cocaine in his body."[2]

While Freud was taking a vacation with his fiancée in September 1884, one of his colleagues, Carl Koller, with whom Freud had talked about cocaine, used the drug to anesthetize first the eyes of animals and then his own and colleagues' eyes. Koller developed painless cocaine-assisted cataract surgery and was celebrated internationally for this. Freud felt that he had been cheated out of this discovery but clarified who was really to blame: "I may here recount, looking back, that it was my fiancée's fault if I did not become famous in those early years."[3]

In 1885, Freud, now understanding the analgesic properties of cocaine, tried to treat trigeminal neuralgia, a painful condition affecting a facial nerve, with injected cocaine but was unsuccessful, perhaps because of his lack of surgical expertise and skill.[4] He continued to take cocaine by mouth, mainly as a stimulant when depressed or anxious, for the next few years. For example, he casually described how he took some cocaine when anxious about a meeting with the great French neurologist Charcot.[5]

Meanwhile, Fleischl-Marxow had begun to inject cocaine.[6] He was perhaps the first person to describe cocaine-associated tactile hallucinations; he felt snakes creeping over his skin. Fleischl-Marxow lived for the next six years, still suffering terrible pain from his neuromas. Freud had hoped that the cocaine would help his friend stop using morphine, but this did not happen, and Fleischl-Marxow continued to use morphine with cocaine. He died in 1891, addicted to both drugs.

Freud had witnessed his friend's addiction to cocaine but seems not to have worried that this could happen to others. Other physicians, however, were alarmed by increasing numbers of people who *did* become addicted to cocaine. Eventually, in 1887, Freud warned against the use of cocaine by morphine addicts and against the injection of cocaine. He implied that in the absence of these two conditions, cocaine was safe.

The story becomes more complicated with the involvement of another medical acquaintance, Wilhelm Fliess, an ear-nose-and-throat doctor. Fliess believed in "vital periodicity" and that the nose was not only the center of the face, but also the center of human physiology and that there was an important "reflex nasal neurosis." He and Freud became intimate friends and wrote lengthy and confessional letters to each other. There is much in this correspondence about "biocycles" and the nose.

Freud no longer used cocaine by mouth, but he and Fliess frequently used "cocaine paint" as a paste in their own noses. They sometimes cut out small growths from each other's noses. In January 1895, eight years after he had warned against its use with morphine and four years after the death of Fleischl-Marxow, Freud wrote to Fliess describing his use of cocaine:

> I must hurriedly write to you about something that greatly astonishes me; otherwise I would be truly ungrateful. In the last few days I have felt quite unbelievably well, as though everything had been erased—a feeling which in spite of better times I have not known for ten months. Last time I wrote you, after a good period, which immediately succeeded the reaction, that a few viciously bad days had followed during which a cocainization of the left nostril had helped me to an amazing extent. I now continue my report. The next day, I kept the nose under cocaine, which one should not really do; that is, I repeatedly painted it to prevent the renewed occurrence of swelling; during this time I discharged what in my experience is a copious amount of thick pus; and since then I have felt wonderful; as if there had never been anything wrong at all . . .[7]

Six months later he wrote to Fliess that "I need a lot of cocaine."[8]

He and Fliess collaborated in the care of one of Freud's own patients. Emma Eckstein was a young woman with a number of problems, including menstrual discomfort and frequent nosebleeds. Some historians have thought that Freud encouraged her to use cocaine to treat her nasal problems.[9] She made little progress, and Freud consulted with Fliess, who decided that Eckstein needed surgery on the turbinates of the nose to treat her "nasal neurosis." Fliess traveled from Berlin to Vienna in early 1895 to operate and then returned to Berlin. The results are described by Freud in a vivid and revealing letter in March 1895.

Dearest Wilhelm,

Just received your letter and am able to answer it immediately. Fortunately I am finally seeing my way clear and am reassured about Miss Eckstein and can give you a report which will probably upset you as much as it did me, but I hope you will get over it as quickly as I did.

I wrote you that the swelling and the hemorrhages would not stop, and that suddenly a fetid odor set in, and that there was an obstacle upon irrigation. (Or is the latter new [to you]?) I arranged for Gersuny to be called in; he inserted a drainage tube, hoping that things would work out once discharge was reestablished; but otherwise he was rather reserved. Two days later I was awakened in the morning—profuse bleeding had started again, pain, and so on. Gersuny replied on the phone that he was unavailable till evening; so I asked Rosanes to meet me. He did so at noon. There still was moderate bleeding from the nose and mouth; the fetid odor was very bad. Rosanes cleaned the area surrounding the opening, removed some sticky blood clots, and suddenly pulled at something like a thread, kept on pulling. Before either of us had time to think, at least half a meter of gauze had been removed from the cavity. The next moment came a flood of blood. The patient turned white, her eyes bulged, and she had no pulse. Immediately thereafter, however, he again packed the cavity with fresh iodoform gauze and the hemorrhage stopped. It lasted about half a minute, but this was enough to make the poor creature, whom by then we had lying flat, unrecognizable. In the meantime—that is, afterward—something else happened. At the moment the foreign body came out and everything became clear to me—and I immediately afterward was confronted by the sight of the patient—I felt sick. After she had been packed, I fled to the next room, drank a bottle of water, and felt miserable. The brave Frau Doctor then brought me a small glass of cognac and I became myself again.

Rosanes stayed with the patient until arranged, via Streitenfels, to have both of them taken to Sanatorium Loew. Nothing further happened that evening. The following day, that is, yesterday, Thursday, the operation was repeated with the assistance of Gersuny; [the bone was] broken wide open, the packing removed, and [the wound] curetted. There was scarcely any bleeding. Since then she has been out of danger, naturally very pale, and miserable with fresh pain and swelling. She had not lost consciousness during the massive hemorrhage; when I returned to the room somewhat shaky, she greeted me with the condescending remark, "So this is the strong sex."

I do not believe it was the blood that overwhelmed me—at that moment strong emotions were welling up in me. So we had done her an injustice; she was not at all abnormal, rather, a piece of iodoform gauze had gotten torn off as you were removing it and stayed in for fourteen days, preventing healing; at the end it tore off and provoked the bleeding. That this mishap should have happened to you; how you will react to it when you hear about it; what others could make of it; how wrong I was to urge you to operate in a foreign city where you could not follow through on the case; how my intention to do my best for this poor girl was insidiously thwarted and resulted in endangering her life—all this came over me simultaneously. I have worked it through by now. I was not sufficiently clear at that time to think of immediately reproaching Rosanes. It only occurred to me ten minutes later that he should immediately have thought, There is something inside; I shall not pull it out lest there be a hemorrhage; rather, I'll stuff it some more, take her to Loew, and there clean and widen it at the same time. But he was just as surprised as I was.[10]

In other words, Fliess had bungled the surgery badly. Freud commiserated with Fliess, was astonished "that this mishap should have happened to you," and blamed others.

Freud dreamed about this incident in July 1895. In the dream he was talking to a young woman, Irma, who had various pains and who was not doing well. At one point in the dream, he examined her nose and saw some lesions on her turbinates. He consulted with three physician friends. One of his friends had administered an injection to Irma.

Freud reviewed this dream from multiple angles. He realized that the dream was not an accurate replication of any particular event, and he wondered about the reasons for the differences between the dream and his memory. He examined all of the differences, and thought about the meanings of the words and each particular incident. By going over and over this dream—or in other words, by "analyzing" it—he had found "the royal road to the unconscious." Each difference had psychological significance. This dream became the second chapter in one of his early masterpieces, *Interpretation of Dreams*. Freud had just created psychoanalysis. A needless and slipshod operation on a young woman that had nearly killed her had led to a new way of understanding and treating psychological problems.

Quite apart from the importance of the dream in the history of psychoanalysis, Freud's discussion of the dream is interesting in the details he included or chose not to include with reference to his own history with cocaine. In his agonized discussion of the dream, he goes back to the sufferings of his friend Fleischl-Marxow and writes that his friend should not have injected cocaine. He admits that he had recommended cocaine to Fleischl-Marxow but criticizes his friend for injecting it "at once,"[11] although Freud had in fact at one point suggested that cocaine be injected.[12] He mentions the use of cocaine by one of his female patients, who might well have been Eckstein, who subsequently developed "an extensive necrosis of the nasal membrane."[13] His discussion of the dream is lengthy and convoluted but suggests that he felt uneasy about Fleischl-Marxow's addiction to cocaine and the surgical disaster, perhaps worsened by earlier cocaine use, suffered by Eckstein.

Freud continued to worry about the episode with Eckstein. In later letters to Fliess, he mentioned this incident and in an offhand way commented that, after all, it was entirely her fault. Eckstein made herself bleed.[14] Freud ended his correspondence with Fliess in 1904. We do not know when or how Freud stopped using cocaine.

Not surprisingly, Freud later requested that his vast correspondence with Fliess be destroyed. Instead, one of his acolytes, Marie Bonaparte, bought the letters from Fliess, and they were later published.

Sigmund Freud, an intelligent and sophisticated physician, thought that cocaine could be used safely. He would have been well aware of the harmfulness of most of the substances in the pharmacopoeia of the time. How could this usually cautious and pessimistic man have thought that there were shortcuts to good feelings?

Freud was young and at the beginning of his career when he fell in love with cocaine. He may not have been fully aware of the possible bias of reports of the use of cocaine in treating morphine addiction being printed in journals that were published by Parke-Davis—a company selling cocaine. And perhaps it is not reasonable to expect that Freud, who used cocaine by mouth or by application to his nose, could have predicted the risks of injected cocaine or smoked free base cocaine. Freud never became addicted to cocaine and indeed thought that the cocaine that was pasted into his nose by Fliess helped him to overcome his own "neurasthenia" and become more productive.

Freud went on to apply his theories of the unconscious to art, religion, and civilization, usually in a gloomy and qualified way. He never again wrote with the alacrity and optimism that he did about cocaine. His good cheer faded—perhaps due to a combination of maturity and being without the stimulus of cocaine.

Freud eventually developed problems related to his own nose and throat. In 1917, he noticed a painful swelling on his palate. It receded, only to recur in 1923. He told no-one at first, fearing that he would be advised to give up his beloved cigars.[15] (He smoked about 20 cigars a day.) Physicians eventually diagnosed the swelling as cancer. He suffered excruciating pain as the cancer of his jaw and palate grew. He underwent multiple operations, and so much bone was removed that he needed prostheses, which themselves were painful. His doctors, suspecting that cigars were to blame, advised him to stop smoking them, as he had feared. Freud could not give them up. He became unable to tolerate the pain of his cancer, and in 1939, at his request, his doctor administered a lethal overdose of morphine.

For Freud, cigars were more addictive and physically harmful than was coca, the gift of Manco Capac. Freud thought that cocaine had helped him to control his depression and shyness. Freud never "analyzed" his own addiction to cigars or the addiction of others to cocaine, the drug that caused exhilaration and euphoria.

Notes

1. Sigmund Freud, "Über Coca," in *White Line: Writers on Cocaine*, ed. Stephen Hyde and Geno Zanetti (New York: Avalon, 2002), 36.

2. Peter Gay, *Freud: A Life for Our Time* (New York: Norton, 1998), 44.

3. Ibid., 42. Koller's daughter described her father's discovery of cocaine anesthesia in an interesting article—Hortense Koller Becker, "Carl Koller and Cocaine," *Psychoanalytic Quarterly* 32 (July 1963): 309–73.

4. Howard Markel, *An Anatomy of Addiction: Sigmund Freud, William Halsted, and the Miracle Drug Cocaine* (New York: Pantheon, 2011), 115.

5. Gay, *Freud*, 50.

6. Markel, *An Anatomy of Addiction*, 102.

7. Jeffrey Moussaieff Masson, *Complete Letters of Sigmund Freud to Wilhelm Fliess, 1887–1904* (Cambridge, MA: Belknap Press of Harvard University Press, 1985), 106.

8. Ibid., 132.

9. Markel, *Anatomy*, 179.

10. Masson, *Letters*, 116–17.

11. Sigmund Freud and James Strachey. *The Interpretation of Dreams* (New York: Avon, 1965), 148.

12. Ernest Jones, *The Life and Work of Sigmund Freud*, ed. and abr. Lionel Trilling and Steven Marcus (New York: Basic Books, 1961), 62; Sigmund Freud, *On Cocaine*, Introduction and English trans. David Carter (London: Hesperus, 2011), 62.

13. Freud, *Dreams*, 144.

14. Masson, *Letters*, 186, 191.

15. Gay, *Freud*, 418–19.

12

Nicotine

"A custome lothsome to the eye, hatefull to the Nose, harmefull to the braine, dangerous to the Lungs."

—King James I of England, 1604

Introduction

Nicotine, the active ingredient in tobacco, is a relatively safe drug. Its effects on the mind are more subtle than those of alcohol, cocaine, or opiates. Nicotine does not generally lead to intoxicated states, behavioral problems, loss of control, or violence, and it does not dull the mind. As recently as the middle of the twentieth century, tobacco was seen as a pleasant and safe substance that lessened anxiety.

Tobacco can be ingested in many ways. In the past, tobacco was placed on the skin or tongue, or even licked. Sometimes it was used in enemas. One to two centuries ago, snuff, pipes, and cigars were common. In the twenty-first century, people trying to stop smoking chew gum, suck on nicotine lozenges, or apply nicotine patches to their skin. But all of these ways of using tobacco or nicotine are unimportant compared to smoking cigarettes.

Cigarette smoking, indulged in to get nicotine to the brain as fast as possible, is associated with more illness than the other substances reviewed in this book. It causes heart and lung diseases as well as many types of cancer. The problems are due not to nicotine itself, but to the multiple cancer-forming chemicals in burning tobacco. These substances travel with the nicotine to the lungs and then through the rest of the body to do their damage. The slim and elegant cigarette is a popular and cheap way of destroying one's health.

Tobacco companies, profitable and influential behemoths, have long been aware of the hazards of cigarette smoking. They have hidden their knowledge of the harms of tobacco from the public and continue to advertise and to market a product that destroys the health of many who use it.

The Tobacco Plant

Nicotine is found in many plants in small quantities, where it probably acts as a mild insecticide. It is present in larger quantities in the leaves of plants in the genus *Nicotiana*. The genus *Nicotiana* belongs to the large and diverse family of plants known as *Solonacae*. This family includes many plants well known to us, such as the potato, tomato, and petunia. Tobacco is a vigorous and majestic annual plant that within one growing season grows higher than a human (see Figure 12.1). It is native to the Americas. *Nicotiana tabacum* accounts for over 90 percent of the tobacco grown today.

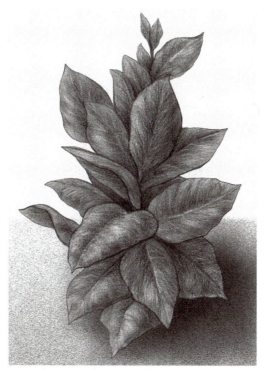

Figure 12.1 **Tobacco Plant. (© 2013 Joan M.K. Tycko)**

History

Millions of years ago, Eurasia and Africa (the Old World) split apart from North and South America and Australasia (the New World), leading to the development of different flora and fauna in the two worlds. *N. tabacum* was cultivated throughout the New World for thousands of years and was an important part of many religious rituals and ceremonies, beginning with the Mayans in what is now Mexico. The Aztecs smoked tobacco also, and many Aztec pottery engravings show priests smoking tobacco. In pre-Columbian America, the smoke was seen as mysterious and as a way of communicating with spirits. One of the most important uses of tobacco for the Northeast and Plains peoples was its inclusion in the ceremonial pipe, or calumet, used in rituals or at times of treaty making.

Native Americans recognized that tobacco led to an increase in energy and a decrease in appetite. They were eclectic in their use of it. They smoked, sniffed, snorted, and drank it, and also used it in enemas. The Aborigines in Australia rubbed tobacco leaves into their skin in some of their rituals and also chewed it for its stimulant and appetite suppressant effects.[1]

Tobacco Spreads from the Old World to the New World

The spread of tobacco from the Americas to the rest of the world is closely connected to Spanish journeys of exploration, the establishment of the English colonies in North America, and the infamous triangular trade (see figures in the alcohol chapter) in which Africans were enslaved and transported to America.

In the fifteenth century, the growing number of humans, along with their cargo, traveling back and forth across the Atlantic re-established the links between the hemispheres. Horses and cows from Europe and Asia flourished in the plains and grasslands of the Americas. Mosquitoes, honeybees, and earthworms also found new homes in the Americas. Illnesses such as influenza, malaria, and smallpox afflicted the Native Americans, who had no immunity to these illnesses. Syphilis may have traveled in the opposite direction—from the Americas to Europe.

Of particular interest here is the exchange of plants. Old World crops such as wheat, barley, and rice came to the New World. And in turn, maize, tomatoes, potatoes, and the coca leaf traveled east. Historian Alfred Crosby named this give-and-take the Columbian Exchange after the explorer Christopher Columbus. In the late fifteenth century, Ferdinand and Isabella of Spain funded Columbus to search for a westerly overseas passage to the East Indies. At this time, the trade routes used most often between Europe and Asia were long overland routes traversing deserts, mountains, and areas populated by hostile peoples. The hope was that Columbus could travel to the Indies quickly and safely and bring spices, silk, and gold back to Spain. He sailed with three small ships—the *Santa Maria*, the *Pinta*, and the *Niña*—and in 1492, he landed on the island of San Salvador, now part of the Bahamas, and encountered men of the Sarawak tribe smoking tobacco leaves. This sight was astonishing to him and his sailors, since tobacco was unknown to Europeans at that time, as was the habit of smoking any substance.

His four voyages from Spain to the Caribbean and back again established the Exchange. Subsequent transatlantic travelers brought the tobacco plant back to Europe, and it was introduced into palace gardens, where it was much admired for its beauty. Some varieties of the plant, *N. alata* and *N. sylvestris* are now grown in gardens because of their attractive appearance and scent.

In 1556, the French diplomat Jean Nicot de Villemain, who had seen tobacco plants in Portuguese gardens, introduced tobacco as a medicine to the French royal court to treat Queen Catherine de' Medici's (or her son's) migraine headaches. He is forever memorialized by having his name attached to the alkaloid, a bitter tasting chemical, responsible for some of tobacco's effects.

Two well-known Elizabethans often get the credit (or blame) for introducing tobacco into England. Sir Francis Drake may have been the traveler who first brought tobacco to England. Sir Walter Raleigh, another adventurer, made the plant popular. Raleigh was an explorer, pirate, poet, and courtier. He was one of the first people to encourage Englishmen to leave England when he arranged for Englishmen to move to Ireland, where he had established "plantations." He also was involved in some of the first European "settlements" in America. These early settlements in America failed, but he had started the process. He named the land there Virginia after his queen.

One of Raleigh's friends was Thomas Hariot. He traveled to Raleigh's settlement on Roanoke, an island in what is now North Carolina. Hariot, a skilled observer, collected and examined the Virginian flora and fauna. He was impressed by the range of plants and animals not hitherto known to the English. In the late 1500s, Hariot wrote a glowing account of the tobacco plant:

There is an herbe which is sowed a part by it selfe & is called by the inhabitants *vpp¢woc*. In the West Indies it hath diuers names, according the seur-
all places and countries where it growth and is vsed: The Spaniardes
generally call it Tobacco. The leaues thereof being dried and brought into
powder: they vse to take the fume or smoke thereof by sucking it through
pipes made of claie into their stomacke and heade; from whence it purgeth
superfluous fleame & other grosse humors.[2]

Hariot went on to become a brilliant mathematician and astronomer.
(He is little known for this work because he did not publish in this area.)
He smoked tobacco for the rest of his life. His optimistic assessment of the
benefits of smoked tobacco was of course tragically wrong.

Raleigh learned to smoke tobacco from "pipes made of claie." Because
Raleigh was a fashionable man and a favorite of Queen Elizabeth, others
followed his example. He was a trendsetter. People wanted to be like
him, so tobacco smoking became popular in the English royal court.

The introduction was not without its problems. A famous story is that
after Raleigh brought tobacco back to England, he was relaxing with a
pipe at his home in Myrtle Grove. His servant, unaccustomed to this
habit, thought that his master had caught on fire and poured a bucket of
water over him to douse the flames.

The Spanish explorers of the New World took *Nicotiana* plants to the
Ottoman Empire and to Manila in the Philippines, one of their colonies,
where it grew well. Chinese traders took the plant from Manila to Fujian
Province in China. Tobacco traveled to China via other routes. The
Portuguese took tobacco from Brazil to Macao and then to Guangdong
Province. Tobacco moved up the coast and eventually into the interior
of China, and it became very popular among soldiers. The Chinese later
smoked a combination of tobacco and opium.

Portuguese explorers brought tobacco, among other New World crops, to
Africa. The Dutch bought slaves in West Africa and sold them to the owners
of tobacco plantations in the Caribbean and Brazil. Tobacco also became
popular in India, Japan, and Korea. By the mid-seventeenth century, tobacco,
a New World plant, was smoked throughout the New and Old Worlds.

Early Doubts about Tobacco

With the increasing use of tobacco, opposition to it arose. This had less
to do with the harm that tobacco did to health, since that was not known
with certainty until the twentieth century, than it had to do with religion

and dislike of new habits. Some Spanish clergy connected tobacco smoking with what they saw as the smoke and fire of hell, and they compared smoking tobacco to satanic practices.[3]

One of the most eminent opponents of tobacco was James VI of Scotland, a man with intellectual interests and strong opinions. He was a devout Catholic and declared himself the "Devil's Greatest Enemy." In 1597, he published a treatise about demonology and was enthusiastic about prosecutions of supposed witches.

He was the closest blood relative to Elizabeth I and so succeeded her to the throne of England in 1603. James I, as he was now called, published a pamphlet, *A Counterblaste to Tobacco*, in which he showed that he was ahead of his time in noting the harm of tobacco. He mocked the belief, beginning with Hariot's observations, that tobacco was healthy. With great sarcasm, he wrote:

> ... such is the miraculous omnipotencie of our strong tasted Tobacco, as it cures all sorts of diseases (which neuer any drugge could do before) in all persons, and at all times. It cures all maner of distellations, either in the head or stomacke (if you beleeue their Axiomes) ... It cures the Gowt in the feet, and (which is miraculous) in that very instant when the smoke thereof, as light, flieus up into the head, the vertue thereof, as heauie, runs downe to the little toe. It helps all sorts of Agues. It makes a man sober that was drunke. It refreshes a weary man, and yet makes a man hungry ...[4]

But his antagonism to tobacco was primarily based on his worry for the spiritual health of his subjects. James I, like the Spanish, associated tobacco with the devil and with evil. He thought that smoke was visible hellfire.

> And surely in my opinion, there cannot be a more base, and yet hurtfull corruption in a Countrey, then is the vile use (or other abuse) of taking Tobacco in this Kingdome ... A custome lothsome to the eye, hatefull to the Nose, harmefull to the braine, dangerous to the Lungs, and in the blacke stinking fume thereof, neerest resembling the horrible Stigian smoke of the pit that is bottomelesse.[5]

The Catholic James I did not share many of the enthusiasms of his Protestant predecessor, Elizabeth I. Raleigh's Protestantism and constant raids on the Spanish Armada were unacceptable to James I, who wanted to appease his Spanish co-religionists and co-anti-tobacco crusaders.

James imprisoned Raleigh in the Tower of London for 12 years. This was not quite as brutal as it sounds, since while there he wrote a book about the history of the world and grew and smoked tobacco.

James did release Raleigh several years later so that he could search for more land and fortune for England. Raleigh sailed to South America to search for El Dorado—the golden man—but the expedition failed. Raleigh returned home with no land or gold for James I, and the king beheaded the smoking courtier. According to one story, Raleigh smoked his pipe while on the scaffold.

Other Europeans joined the English and Spanish in their concern about smoking and evil. In 1609, Henri IV of France tried to extinguish sorcery and witchcraft in rural France. A French inquisitor thought that witchcraft was often associated with tobacco smoking. But this was a brief concern as smoking also became popular among the French, including the French clergy.[6]

James I was not the most eminent Catholic to oppose smoking. Pope Urban VII had only a 13-day papacy, but during his brief time as head of the Catholic Church, he banned tobacco use inside churches on pain of excommunication.

Opposition to tobacco smoking was not just European. Authorities in China tried to prevent their subjects from smoking. Russian smokers were exiled to Siberia. In seventeenth-century Turkey, Sultan Murad IV thought that tobacco smoking was part of the decadence and corruption rife in his empire and ordered tobacco users to be executed as infidels. He would also walk in the streets of Constantinople at night, disguised as a commoner. If he came across a smoker, he would execute the person on the spot. Altogether, over 25,000 Turkish smokers are said to have been killed because of their tobacco habit.[7] The opposition of James I, Henry IV, and Murad and the specter of life in Siberia were weaker than the desires of their subjects; the spread of tobacco did not stop.

Tobacco, Colonial America, and Slavery

Tobacco was grown throughout the Americas, Asia, Africa, and Europe. Conditions were particularly suitable for its cultivation in what are now Virginia, Kentucky, and North Carolina in the southern United States. This was crucial to the health of colonial America because attempts to colonize Roanoke had failed. The next significant European effort to settle the area was made by the Virginia Company of London, a group of investors chartered by King James I in 1606. James I was carrying on the interests of Elizabeth I in counterbalancing the expansion of other European nations abroad.

The Virginia Company attempted several times to establish a viable colony in the Chesapeake Bay area. At first, they were no more successful than the Roanoke settlers. The climate was unexpectedly harsh, there was turmoil within the community, and there were few skilled workers. Clean water was not always available. The Native Americans were hostile. The English settlers could not grow food for themselves or for export. In desperation, they resorted to glassblowing and silk growing, and they failed again. Most of the English colonists died within a few years of coming to the new colony. Some were killed by the Native Americans, and others starved, died from diseases such as malaria or typhoid, or just disappeared into the wilds of America. The Virginia Company resorted to selling lottery tickets.

The settlement, known as Jamestown, grew tobacco, but the local tobacco leaf had a harsh flavor and did not sell well. A breakthrough occurred in 1612 when John Rolfe planted *N. tabacum* that he had obtained from Trinidad. This produced a much better tasting tobacco leaf and it became popular. (Rolfe later saved the colony in another way. He married the daughter of the Indian chief Powhatan, Pocahontas, which led to temporary peace with the Indians.)

Virginia gradually became a thriving colony thanks to the Trinidadian tobacco. *N. tabacum* grew well in the Virginian swampland and nurtured some of the first colonies in what is now the United States. James I would not have been pleased that a settlement named after him finally prospered because of tobacco.

Virginia was then heavily forested. The historian Steven Ambrose described the methods used to clear the land:

> Fertile land—identified by hardwood growth—was saved for tobacco. The planters had their slaves gird large trees and leave the trees to die while plowing lightly around them. Slaves created hills for tobacco with a hoe, without bothering to remove the trees. After three annual crops of tobacco, these "fields" grew wheat for a year or so before being abandoned and allowed to revert to pine forest ... The system allowed the planters to use to the maximum the two things in which they were really rich, land and slaves. Tobacco, their only cash crop, was dependent on an all-but-unlimited quantity of each.[8]

Tobacco growing took much work. Once the seeds had sprouted, they were transplanted into separate fields and then other tasks followed—weeding, worming, topping, and suckering. Harvesting involved careful selection of leaves that were then transferred to tobacco barns, where they were dried or "cured." Sometimes the tobacco was dried by exposing it to smoke from open fires.

There were not enough colonists in Jamestown to do all the work demanded by intense tobacco cultivation. Initially, indentured servants from England did much of the work in the colony. In 1619, the governor of Virginia bought 21 African slaves from Dutch ships. Tobacco, along with sugar cane and cotton, has been intimately associated with slavery ever since.

Tobacco played a part in the triangular trade as a raw product, somewhat similar to sugar. Most of the African slaves worked in the Brazilian and Caribbean sugar plantations, but they were also shipped further up the American coast, where they worked in the cotton fields and rice fields of the Carolinas. The slaves also worked on the tobacco plantations of Virginia and the Chesapeake.

By 1627, the Virginia Company was growing 500,000 pounds of tobacco a year. As the tobacco trade and profits increased, the (perceived) need for more workers grew also. As information about the harsh conditions in Virginia reached England and as the English economy improved, fewer were willing to come to Virginia as indentured servants. Thus, over the next few decades, African slaves replaced English indentured servants on the tobacco plantations.

As the number of African slaves increased, the attitudes of the plantation owners toward them hardened, which resulted in legislation known as slave codes. There were some differences between the states, but in general, in the southern slave states, it was decided that slavery was passed from mother to child and that the races should remain separate. In 1705, the Virginia General Assembly declared that slaves were "real estate" and that their "masters" could kill them without retribution.

The treatment of slaves was inhumane. Working conditions were brutal, and the slaves were often punished harshly. For example, if they associated with whites, they could be whipped, branded, or maimed. They were not allowed to learn to read. Women were raped by their "owners," and families were often broken up as members were sold to different people.

Throughout the eighteenth century, tobacco remained North America's principal export. George Washington and Thomas Jefferson were tobacco growers (and slave owners). Disagreement with England over the taxation of tobacco was another constant irritant that was one of the precipitants of the American Revolution.

Tobacco changed the American landscape. Tobacco plants deplete the soil of its nutrients so that after three crops of tobacco, the farmers had to move to new forested areas. Before the colonists arrived, the Native Americans often burnt forests, but this was done annually so that brush did not accumulate. Without the fuel of large amounts of brush, these low-intensity burns did not damage large trees. The tobacco farmers, in contrast, did kill the large trees, and this led to the loss of the forest canopy. The colonists' ploughs weakened the structure of the soil. The animals that had lived in the forests were replaced to some extent by imported cows, horses, and pigs. All of these changes degraded the land. Kirkpatrick Sale, a critic of the European settlement of America, wrote that "the first colony of what was to become the United States was saved by, and built entirely around, a product of human and environmental debilitation."[9]

People soon grew fond of tobacco in a variety of forms. Fashions about which way to use tobacco came and went; customs differed between countries and between classes within the countries. For example, chewing tobacco was popular in nineteenth-century America. This habit stimulates saliva production, and the tobacco chewer spits out large quantities of tobacco-stained saliva. Charles Dickens, himself a cigar smoker, expecting to be impressed by the new republic of America, toured the United States in 1842 and was most scathing about this American habit:

> ... the prevalence of those two odious practices of chewing and expectorating ... became most offensive and sickening. In all the public places of America this filthy custom is recognized. In the courts of law the judge has his spittoon, the crier his, the witness his, and the prisoner his; while the jurymen and the spectators are provided for, as so many men who in the course of nature must desire to spit incessantly.[10]

Dickens was also dismayed by the atrocity of slavery and noted, as many others have, the hypocrisy of those who insisted on their own freedom while owning others.

Cigar and pipe smoking, taking snuff, and tobacco chewing all have had their times of great popularity. But none of these ways of using tobacco have been as ubiquitous as the habit of smoking cigarettes.

The Cigarita *and Bright Tobacco: The Birth of the Cigarette*

The Spanish, as is befitting their prominence in the story of the European discovery and spread of tobacco, may have been the first to fashion cigarettes, as thinner cigars. They began to make cigarettes with maize wrappers and then paper, at first calling them *papelotes* and then *cigaritas*. Until the end of the nineteenth century, cigarettes were hand rolled. Even a skilled person could roll only five a minute. The most famous cigarette roller in literature was Carmen, a wild and beautiful young woman. She rolled her cigaritas in Seville, a center of tobacco preparation. The French writer Prosper Mérimée wrote his story *Carmen* about her, and then George Bizet based his opera on this story.

The cigarita moved north to France and was re-named *cigarette*. In 1845, the French state began to produce cigarettes. In a modern-sounding statement, Louis Napoleon III said, when reproached for supporting such a habit:

> This vice brings in one hundred million francs in taxes every year. I will certainly forbid it at once—as soon as you can name a virtue that brings in as much revenue.[11]

This approach to cigarettes became common. No longer would Sultan Murad roam the streets executing smokers. Governments came to rely on tobacco taxes.

Wars contributed to the slowly increasing popularity of the cigarette. The Crimean War (1853–1856) was a conflict between the Russian Empire and an alliance of Turkey, France, and Great Britain. In this war, a cross-fertilization of ideas and habits took place between the various armies. British soldiers in the Crimea encountered the Turkish soldier's hand-rolled cigarette. The Spanish had brought tobacco to the Ottoman Empire some centuries earlier, and tobacco growers in Greece, Egypt, and Turkey had learned to grow a small-leafed tobacco that was cured outside, instead of in barns. (Sultan Murad had been remarkably unsuccessful in his anti-tobacco campaign.) The cigarettes fashioned from this sun-cured tobacco were mild and aromatic and appealed to the British soldiers. The Russian soldiers also smoked cigarettes, and this too may have had some impact on soldiers from other countries.

The British officers smoked pipes and cigars, and the soldiers smoked cigarettes. The soldiers who survived the Russian artillery and scurvy, beriberi, dysentery, and fevers of the Crimea brought this habit back to England. By 1860, English tobacconists were offering hand-rolled cigarettes to their customers.[12]

Cigarettes became more common in the United States, in part as an unexpected by-product of the Civil War (1861–1865). Union and

Confederate soldiers used tobacco in different ways. Union soldiers chewed tobacco, while some of the Confederate soldiers smoked bright leaf tobacco. This tobacco, produced in the thin, poor, sandy soil of the Appalachian piedmont, was mild. Two new techniques for curing tobacco were coming into use at this time. Charcoal was used instead of wood, and flues carried the smoke from fireboxes inside the tobacco barn to the outside so that the tobacco was no longer exposed to smoke, and the risk from fires was lessened. Flue-cured tobacco, when burned, produces a mild smoke. The combination of bright leaf tobacco and flue-curing produced a cigarette that was easy to inhale.

Toward the end of the war, some Union soldiers based in Durham, North Carolina picked up the habit of smoking mild tobacco and preferred this to their earlier habit of chewing the more strongly flavored tobaccos. They brought this habit home with them and, gradually, people throughout North America began to smoke cigarettes.

In both the Crimean and American Civil Wars, diseases were rampant and indeed caused more deaths than did actual combat. One of the few comforts available to soldiers in these two wars was the cigarette, which was some compensation for the illnesses, boredom, anxiety, hunger, and pain that they suffered.

The cigarette was making a sputtering start in the United States, but it still led to some opposition. Carry Nation, the temperance crusader of the late nineteenth century, despised the "vile cigarette" and suggested that the government make tobacco illegal. She and others in the temperance movement were almost as disturbed by tobacco smoking as they were by alcohol drinking. At the beginning of the twentieth century, during the couple of decades of the Progressive Era, the cigarette was sometimes portrayed as a product used by the immoral.

The next great conflict, World War I—which brought with it the new horrors of prolonged trench warfare—was an opportunity for the cigarette to prove once again its apparent helpfulness to the soldier. Cigarettes fulfilled a number of purposes in this war. Tobacco was thought of as an "ally of virtue" in keeping soldiers away from "bad liquor and worse women."[13] Some hoped that it could be an antidote to poison gas or a prophylactic for influenza. Surgeon General William Gorgas, the U.S. Army's chief medical officer and the person responsible for controlling yellow fever during the building of the Panama Canal, reversed his earlier opposition to cigarettes and supported them as a way of leading to "contentment and morale" for the soldiers.[14]

Cigarettes were most valued by the men who were often in trenches for weeks. During this time, they slept, walked, and fought in narrow trenches that were full of mud and swarming with rats and lice. The soldiers suffered from persistent fungal infections. They were shot at by snipers and subjected to shellfire. Dead bodies could not be removed quickly, so sometimes rotting carcasses remained in the trenches with the soldiers who were still alive. Cigarettes were so important that at one point, a dog with cartons of cigarettes in a special backpack delivered cigarettes to the men in the trenches.[15]

The cigarette became a "jaunty emblem of freedom and democracy," and opposition to cigarettes seemed unpatriotic.[16] Cigarettes were included in military rations, and many soldiers became habitual smokers. The YMCA, Red Cross, and other humanitarian organizations bought cigarettes for soldiers. Cigarettes were sometimes used as currency. The *New York Sun* began a "smokes for soldiers" fund and quoted General Pershing, commander of the American Expeditionary Forces, as saying that cigarettes were as vital to the war as were food or bullets.[17]

Cigarettes were also popular in World War II, where they continued to provide soldiers a few moments of solace. Tobacco companies sent free cigarettes to the soldiers, and again they were included in their rations. Cigarettes even lent their name to army camps. The U.S. Army established camps named after American cigarettes such as Lucky Strike, Philip Morris, and Chesterfield, among others in liberated France. The American military included free cigarettes in military rations until 1975.

By the end of World War II, cigarettes were finally accepted by the public. Ashtrays were in every home, and good hosts offered cigarettes to their guests at every social occasion or meal. People smoked them in airplanes, offices, restaurants, and hospitals. One of the reasons for the availability of cigarettes in such large numbers was that cigarette production had become mechanized in the late nineteenth century.

Cigarettes were cheap. To appreciate how this happened and how the tobacco companies—despite selling such a cheap product—have become so wealthy, we will briefly review the mechanization of the cigarette and the growth of the tobacco companies.

The Tobacco Companies

Tobacco companies are immensely profitable, thanks in part to low labor costs. Until the late nineteenth century, labor costs accounted for most of the cost of the cigarette. In 1880, an American 21-year-old, James Albert Bonsack, obtained a patent for a clever machine that could roll up to 120,000 cigarettes a day. Cigarettes were soon sold in packages so that they became easier to buy and stayed "fresh" longer. For the manufacturers, inferior tobacco could be packaged into a cigarette in a way that was easier than in pipe tobacco. The cigarette paper hid the tobacco and any of its imperfections.

James Buchanan Duke, head of a small Virginia tobacco company, installed two of these machines in his factory. Within five years, he was making and selling 2 million cigarettes a day. Cigarettes were one of the first mass-produced products of the nineteenth century. Duke became so successful that he bought out his rivals. In 1890, Duke's American Tobacco Company controlled 90 percent of the cigarettes made in the United States along with about two thirds of the pipe, snuff, and chewing tobacco sales. Duke competed and then cooperated with English tobacco companies. Duke's success attracted the attention of the antitrust forces of the early twentieth century, and eventually American Tobacco was broken up. Duke remained wealthy, as he had also invested in textiles and electricity. Duke was one of the earliest tobacco magnates and a philanthropist, Duke University being the most obvious recipient of his generosity.

Tobacco companies, often following Duke's example by being international and diversified, continue to be profitable. The cigarette had been treated with some suspicion in the past but became a patriotic emblem in the two world wars. After World War II, with the discoveries of how harmful it was, the cigarette once again became an object of controversy. No longer able to rely on patriotism as way of selling their product, tobacco companies, helped by clever advertising, promoted the idea of the cigarette as a desirable object.

Cigarette Advertising, the First Amendment, and Public Health

Advertising has played a bigger part in the selling of cigarettes to the American public than in the marketing of the other substances discussed in this book. The companies have always claimed that there is no evidence that their advertising convinces people to smoke. They advertise, they say, only to encourage the already-smoking person to choose a particular brand. Common sense would suggest that advertising, on which the companies spend much money, is effective—at the very least—in establishing the normalcy of smoking. The advertising companies have shown almost limitless ingenuity, using different types of media and appealing to many interests.

The advertising has focused on *imagery*. The words in the advertisements are few and not important because the images carry the message.

For example, their advertisements suggested, by using attractive models in the right settings, that a man who smoked would be like the Marlboro man—a strong and virile cowboy who rode horses masterfully in fresh mountain air. A woman who smoked would become slim and sexually attractive.

Another focus of the tobacco companies has been children so that people would smoke for as much of their lifetime as possible. The tobacco company R. J. Reynolds developed the cartoon character Joe Camel to make smoking seem attractive to youngsters. Tobacco companies sponsored or advertised on television shows such as *I Love Lucy, I've Got a Secret*, the *Flintstones*, and the *Beverly Hillbillies*—all programs watched by children.

The Public Health Cigarette Smoking Act, passed by Congress in 1970, was one of the major bills resulting from the surgeon general's 1964 report that lung cancer and chronic bronchitis are related to cigarette smoking. This act banned cigarette advertising from radio and television in the United States. The tobacco companies turned to other venues. Indeed, advertising—by whatever means—was needed in greater amounts to counter the claims that cigarettes were harmful.

Advertising campaigns retreated from radio and television and marched into other markets. At times, almost half of the billboards in the United States have carried cigarette advertising. The sponsorship of art shows and museum events lent cigarettes an aura of sophistication. Sponsorships of athletic events, such as Virginia Slims tennis tournaments, have been advertising coups for the companies. R. J. Reynolds and its advertisements were part of race car events from 1970 to 2003. If a person drove on highways, went to a museum, or watched a tennis match or a car race, he or she would see cigarette advertisements.

Cigarettes were frequently smoked in movies. They were a boon to Hollywood because they and their rituals were evocative, symbolic, and iconic. In return, Hollywood helped the tobacco companies because the display of cigarettes in movies was free advertising.

Richard Kluger describes the thespian qualities of cigarette lighting, smoking, and extinguishing in a passage from his book about tobacco:

> To convey callow anxiety, you lit up fumblingly, whereas the powerful, controlling screen personality did so with a masterful flick—always toward the smoker himself if a male, as if manfully impervious to the flame, and away from herself with caution if a woman . . . Quick puffs and repeated tapping of the ash meant irritation or nervousness. The lovingly cupped butt, slow

draw, and billowy exhalation might signal profound contemplation or the cagey bluff. The stubbing out, depending how emphatic, might register menace or relief but announced at any rate that a decision had been reached and action was imminent.

No one smoked on screen to greater purpose than Humphrey DeForest Bogart ... (in) the 1942 film *Casablanca*, in which the hero is first encountered through a shot of his hand signing his name to a check and reaching for a half-smoked cigarette in a nearby ashtray. In that hand and in his mouth, the cigarette became endowed with a kind of ironic nobility as Bogart used it to make a moral statement about a world gone awry ... his every considered drag and expelled puff of smoke seemed to represent a mocking laugh of bitter defiance. Cool under pressure, Bogey characteristically—and *Casablanca* set the mold—wielded his smoke as a swordsman or gunslinger would his weapon in a pirate film or a Western, but instead of slaying his tormentor, he was more likely to resolve matters ambiguously by deftly discarding his still burning butt in a low, flat trajectory that ended in life's gutter. *Now Voyager* ... featured that prototypical female screen smoker Bette Davis, for whom the cigarette was laden with unspoken sexual language. She seemed to smoke with a seething intensity and, when she spoke, used the cigarette to punctuate her words ... love is perilous, and often as ephemeral and uncontainable as smoke.[18]

By 1964, more than 40 percent of the adult population in the United States smoked cigarettes. But in the next three decades, more than 40 million Americans quit smoking, and the prevalence of smoking had decreased to 25 percent.[19] What happened?

The Tobacco Companies and Their "Frank Statement to Cigarette Smokers"

By the 1950s, large studies about the harmful effects of tobacco smoking were being published in leading English and American medical journals. Public health advocates began a relentless campaign of education.

In 1954, the tobacco companies responded. They placed an advertisement in many papers, "A Frank Statement to Cigarette Smokers," acknowledging these studies but also expressing skepticism. They told the American public that they would always hold foremost the health of the smoker. The companies also announced that they would support research into the matter through the newly established Tobacco Industry Research Committee (TIRC).

The public was soothed; public health groups were not and questioned the right of the companies to advertise a substance that was harmful.

Tobacco industry spokespeople argued (in the United States) that the First Amendment supports all types of speech, even that which seems to lead to social or health problems.

The antitobacco forces countered with their own public relations campaigns and as a result, in 1966, health warnings were placed on cigarette packages. The first warnings were tentative: Caution: Cigarette Smoking May be Hazardous to Your Health. These warnings would prove to be helpful to the tobacco companies in the lawsuits that were to come. The warnings have become stronger over the years, and in some countries are accompanied by graphic pictures illustrating bodies ravaged by the toxins in cigarette smoke.

Attacks on the Cigarette Companies Lead to Release of Documents

At the same time that some antitobacco organizations were fighting tobacco company advertising, a different battle was taking place that involved attacks on the tobacco companies themselves. One of the earliest episodes in this battle was the suit of Rose Cipollone.

Cipollone was born in New York and began smoking in 1942 at the age of 16. She was enchanted by movie stars such as Bette Davis, Joan Crawford, and Norma Shearer, all of whom smoked. Cipollone felt glamorous, ladylike, and grown up when she smoked.[20] She married and moved with her husband and children to New Jersey.

She smoked for the rest of her life, averaging about a pack and a half a day. Cipollone repeatedly tried to stop and often changed cigarettes to those that were more appealing or those that were advertised to be less harmful. In 1983, at the age of 57, she was diagnosed with terminal lung cancer. She sued three tobacco companies—Philip Morris, the Liggett Group, and Lorillard. Cipollone died in 1984 from lung cancer, but her family continued the suit.

The family's move to New Jersey was an important factor in the case because New Jersey was particularly sympathetic to the plaintiff in tort suits. (Tort law governs the rights of individuals to sue others for wrongful acts that have harmed them in civil proceedings.)

In the years of legal wrangling that followed, the tobacco companies pointed out that beginning in 1966, cigarette packages contained warnings, so Cipollone had known at least since then that what she was doing was harmful. They also argued that her frequent switches indicated her knowledge of the risks. Because Cipollone had mostly smoked cigarettes made by Liggett *before* the 1966 warnings, the other tobacco companies were dropped from the suit, and the case became known as *Cipollone vs. Liggett*. The other two tobacco companies had profited from the work of their foes. The lawyers for tobacco also argued at the *same* time that cigarettes had never *decisively* been proven to be harmful.

Decisions were appealed and counterappealed. In 1988, a New Jersey jury awarded Cipollone's widowed husband $400,000. This was the first time that a tobacco company had lost such a suit, but the loss was temporary. The company appealed in 1990, won, and never paid out a penny.

The importance of the case lies in what happened during the legal arguments. During *Cipollone vs. Liggett*, Marc Edell, the attorney for the plaintiff, accused the tobacco companies of lying to the public. For many years, the companies had made public claims that their products were not addictive or harmful, so surely their own documents were fair game. Edell argued that that the conspiracy to deceive the public could be exposed only by examining the tobacco company documents. A sympathetic judge agreed, and in the process of discovery that followed, the tobacco companies were forced to disclose over 300,000 documents.

Meanwhile, some employees of other tobacco companies were becoming active in the antitobacco movement. Brown and Williamson, a large tobacco company, had hired a person with paralegal training, Merrell Williams, to review their documents in case these documents were subpoenaed. He worked for them between 1988 and 1992. However, the company made a mistake when it hired Williams because during the time that he was supposed to be working on their behalf, he copied 4,000 pages and sent them to antitobacco attorneys, who then sent them to Henry Waxman, an antitobacco Congressman, in early 1994.

In another example, Jeffrey Wigand joined Brown and Williamson as a chemist in 1989 and was fired in 1993. He subsequently served as an expert consultant for a number of attorneys and organizations. Wigand told them that Brown and Williamson manipulated the nicotine contents of cigarettes to make them addictive and knew that many of the additives were carcinogenic.

In 1994, a "Mr Butts" dropped off a box containing 4,000 pages of internal Brown and Williamson industry documents at the office of Professor Stanton Glantz at the University of California, San Francisco. The identity of "Mr Butts" has never been revealed, but it seems fair to guess that he was a tobacco company employee. Glantz made these papers available to the public at the University of California. At one point, Brown and Williamson was so alarmed that it photographed people at the University of California who were reading the documents.[21] Glantz and his colleagues then made the papers available on the Internet and wrote a book about them called *Cigarette Papers* so that anyone could read the documents without being "caught" doing so.

The Cipollone case and disenchanted employees succeeded in prying many documents from the grip of the tobacco companies. The cigarette papers were disclosed at a torrential rate and proved to be fascinating reading for antitobacco activists.

The Revelations of the Documents

The documents revealed in *Cipollone* and "liberated" by the tobacco company employees painted a very different picture from that portrayed to the public by the companies. The leaked documents showed that the tobacco companies had done much research, as they had promised in their "Frank Statement." They established facilities and hired chemists to investigate the complicated processes that happen when tobacco burns. At one point, they searched for the harmful substances in cigarettes to see if a safer cigarette could be made. But this last activity in itself highlighted the harm of cigarettes and was not publicized or supported wholeheartedly, and their research in this area was eventually halted.[22]

The tobacco companies knew more about cigarettes than did anyone else, were aware of the reports beginning in the 1950s that linked cigarette smoking and cancer, and did not doubt them. The director of research at R. J. Reynolds wrote in a 1962 memo concerning his department's work:

> Members of this [Reynolds] research department have studied in detail cigarette smoke composition. Some of the findings have been published. However, much data remain unpublished because they are concerned with carcinogenic or co-carcinogenic compounds or patentable material.[23]

The tobacco companies and their scientists, in other words, had confirmed the work of others that cigarettes were harmful, and they did not reveal this information to the public.[24] They were also well aware for many years that nicotine was addictive.[25] They were not alarmed by the addictive nature of nicotine.

One notorious television moment underlining the importance of these documents happened in 1994, when Henry Waxman was leading investigations into the tobacco companies. He arranged a televised congressional hearing at which tobacco company executives were questioned by a subcommittee. The executives said that they were not sure that cigarettes were harmful. Then the subcommittee asked the executives if they believed that their product was addictive. This question was more easily answered. Each replied that he did not. The seven tobacco executives who swore that they did not know cigarettes were addictive must have forgotten, for the moment, all of the work that their companies did to make sure that the cigarette delivered a hit of addictive nicotine. They claimed ignorance, but the documents belied their claims.

Class Action Suits and the Master Settlement Agreement: $209 Billion

There were many individual suits against tobacco companies, such as *Cipollone vs. Liggett*. The tobacco companies fought every suit as vigorously as possible to discourage others from suing. They reminded the courts that they had a legal product and that the risks of this product were well known, although not decisively proven. They also pointed out that it was impossible to prove the cause of an illness in one person. Using these arguments, the tobacco companies usually won.

As a way of more effectively combating the tobacco companies, a group of attorneys pooled their resources. They sued, not on behalf of the individual smokers, but on behalf of the entities that were paying for the smoking-related illnesses. Those entities included some health insurance companies and—overwhelmingly—Medicaid. Medicaid, funded by the federal government and the individual states, pays for medical care for the indigent. Medicaid paid for much of the health costs of the illnesses of smokers because so many people became bankrupt due to their tobacco-caused medical illnesses. The new plaintiffs were the taxpayers who funded Medicaid.

In 1994, attorneys general for most of the states joined together to sue four tobacco companies for reimbursement of costs to Medicaid associated with tobacco-caused illnesses. In 1998, the case was settled in a master settlement agreement (MSA). The tobacco industry agreed to compensate the plaintiffs $206 billion (approximately $10 billion per year over 25 years) for their Medicaid tobacco-related health care costs and to cut back on some of their advertising, particularly that directed to children. The tobacco companies promised to change their corporate culture and to release all relevant documentation involved in lawsuits to the public, which yielded yet more information about the tobacco companies. In return, the companies got some protection from future litigation from the states. They shut down their mendacious TIRC.

The MSA was a victory for the lawyers, the tobacco companies, and the states. The lawyers were paid for their work. The companies no longer had to face a steady onslaught of cases, and so had dealt with one of the situations most hated by companies—uncertainty. The companies passed along the cost of the settlement to the consumer. Medicaid did not benefit because the money was given to the states with no restrictions. Many states used the money for immediate needs not related to Medicaid costs such as debt repayment and infrastructure repair.[26]

Some states issued tobacco bonds that were backed against their future tobacco settlement payments. An unexpected result from this agreement was that many states needed tobacco companies to be solvent. It was now in the interest of the states to let the companies sell their product. In fact, 36 states filed briefs in 2003 in support of the tobacco industry in other litigation it was facing. In other words, the states were now "invested" in the tobacco companies.[27]

Cigarette Smoking in the Twenty-First Century

The MSA may not have been as effective as it could have been in weakening the tobacco companies, but even so, and despite the ongoing advertising and lobbying from the tobacco companies, smoking is less common now in the United States and most of the Western world. Some of the decrease is attributed to the increasing cost of cigarettes, due in part to the costs incurred to the tobacco companies by the MSA and to taxes. In the United States, there are federal and state excise taxes, as well as some state and municipality sales taxes. Some of the decline is presumably because of the ever-increasing evidence of the harm of smoking and the work of public health advocates.

The well educated have turned away from smoking. Smoking on television or in current movies usually signals trouble or defiance. Smoking is forbidden by most airlines, and many municipalities have banned smoking in bars, restaurants, and other public places. The smoker is now marginalized.

Smoking persists among people who get so much pleasure from smoking that they choose not to stop and others who feel that it is too difficult to stop. People with little education, low income, addictions to other drugs, and mental illnesses smoke more than do others.[28]

Cigarettes, the Third World, and the Environment

As the pressures against cigarette smoking continue to erode the market in the developed world, American tobacco companies have turned to the huge markets of the developing world. Most of the world's 1 billion smokers live in low- and middle-income countries. Although cigarette smoking is decreasing in wealthy countries, it is increasing worldwide.[29]

The tobacco companies have the muscle of the U.S. State Department behind them and are fortified by righteous claims of free trade. The United States has forced Japan, South Korea, and Taiwan to open their markets to U.S. tobacco products.

Thailand, however, fought back. It wanted to keep the U.S. tobacco companies out of their country, both to protect its own tobacco companies and also (perhaps) to protect its population from the smoother and more slickly advertised and hence more appealing American cigarettes. This was blocked by the World Trade Organization (WTO). The attempts of the United States and WTO to force American tobacco into Thailand are reminiscent of the Opium Wars, in which the English and other Western countries forced opium into China.

The tobacco companies are helped, as ever, by clever advertising. A description of advertisements and smoking in Burkina Faso, one of the poorest countries in the world, illustrates many of the points already made:

> Cigarette advertising in Burkina Faso is ubiquitous: Indeed it is one of the only products advertised there and certainly no other advertising comes near it in scale ... But who are the smoking public in Burkina? Well, for the time being, it is predominantly masculine, urban and young. Cigarettes can be bought on almost any street corner, but the association between smoking and alcohol is strong. Cigarettes are always on sale at the entrances to Ouagadougou's many bars. They are within the price range of almost anybody since they can be bought singly. Cigarette smoking, though, is a luxury people in Burkina Faso can ill afford ... the habit shows no signs of abating in Burkina Faso at the moment. New recruits, in the form of young boys, are joining the ranks of the smokers every day. The only two pictorial advertisers, Marlboro and Ormond, sum it up between them: Marlboro smokers are cool and cowboy; Ormond smokers are connected with the jet set. (There is an airplane in their stickers.) Smoking is seen as classy and Western.[30]

The largest cigarette market is the most populous country in the world—China. In the past, tobacco in China was mixed with opium and smoked as madak. Tobacco smoked in the form of cigarettes became more popular with the advent of the Communists and after opium use was eliminated by Mao Zedong in the mid-twentieth century. Cigarettes were part of life in Communist China. In the past, China began to grow her own opium to weaken the English opium importers; China now grows her own tobacco for similar reasons. In 2010, more than a quarter of adults in China smoked. Most of these smokers are men. China is now both the world's largest tobacco producer and its largest consumer.

Most of the world's tobacco is now grown in the developing world. Forests are cleared so that tobacco can be planted. (This is similar to the deforestation of the Caribbean so that sugar cane can be grown.) Trees are also used for fuel to dry, or cure, the tobacco leaves. The tobacco plant is prone to many diseases, so tobacco growers use large amounts of pesticides and herbicides. Tobacco depletes soil nutrients at higher rates than do food crops and most cash crops (such as coffee, tea, and cotton). The loss of soil fertility associated with tobacco growing was known to George Washington, who stopped growing tobacco because of this. Tobacco is harmful to the smoker and also to the environment.

The Cigarette and Smoking

Smoking burning tobacco is quite different from any other activity that we have described in this book. It used to be somewhat cumbersome because smoking cigars and pipes requires some manipulation and frequent relighting. The development of mild tobacco, cigarettes, matches, and lighters has made smoking tobacco easier. The cigarette itself is a brilliantly designed nicotine delivery device. To understand why cigarette smoking is so powerful, we will describe the structure of the cigarette and then the mechanics and physiology of breathing.

The Cigarette

The cigarette fits easily between our fingers and is a good match for our lips. We kiss and smile with our lips, and we use them to help us eat and drink efficiently and neatly. Our lips articulate some consonants and vowels, and they are so pliable and well supplied with nerves and muscles that they can form an airtight seal around the cigarette; this allows a good draw on the cigarette and inhalation of the smoke deep into the lungs.

This ability to draw on a cigarette distinguishes us from other animals. Some chimpanzees and birds use tools, but no other animals have the coordination of the lips or the motivation to be able to smoke. In the infamous smoking experiments described elsewhere, beagles smoke, but only through tracheal tubes, and even then it is only an approximation of

smoking. There is one exception. Dr. Murray Jarvik, developer of the nicotine patch, was able to teach monkeys to smoke through tubes.[31]
Smoking machines have been constructed, but they too are not quite the
same as human lips, fingers, and lungs.

The cigarette is cleverly constructed in all of its other aspects. Cigarette
paper burns at the same rate and temperature as tobacco. Good cigarette
paper has no odor or taste and burns to an ash.

The cigarette burns well. It lights easily when a match or light is applied
to it and as the person draws or puffs on it. It smolders when the smoker is
not puffing and then burns when the person draws on the cigarette. The
cigarette does not "go out" when the smoker is not smoking, and it does
not burst into open flame when pulled on. (Cigarette burning is not
entirely problem free, as unattended or dropped lit cigarettes lead to fires.)

The tobacco inside the cigarette consists of leaves and mashed tobacco
stems. Some of the tobacco is puffed or expanded, with the help of dry
ice. Tobacco itself is a mixture of cellulose-like compounds, proteins, sugars, phenols, fatty acids, and minerals. Tobacco contains many alkaloids,
one of which is nicotine. Compounds are added to the tobacco to make
it moist and flavorful and to make the smoke easier to inhale. Additives
include sugars, cocoa, licorice, and almost 600 other substances.

One additive is ammonia. Tobacco companies had known since the
early 1950s that adding ammonia to the tobacco gave smoke a richer flavor. It is also used to prepare "reconstituted tobacco" so that the otherwise
discarded bits and pieces could hold together in the cigarette.

Ammonia also allows nicotine to be "free based," so that nicotine is no
longer bound to other compounds. When companies lowered tar and nicotine levels in cigarettes, they had to make sure that the act of smoking
still got the nicotine into the lungs, which was done by adding ammonia
to "free" the nicotine. This form of nicotine gets into the brain much
more easily.[32] Smokers of low-nicotine cigarettes could still get a "kick."
The tobacco companies discouraged their scientists from using the words
free base because of the similarity to the term *free base cocaine.*[33]

Some cigarettes have filters at the "puffing" end of the cigarette that
trap some of the particulate matter in the smoke. Most cigarettes with filters have ventilation holes around the circumference of the filter. These
holes admit air that then dilutes the smoke. Many smokers cover these
holes with their lips or fingers.

When the cigarette is lit, combustion takes place at the tip, where the
temperature quickly becomes over 800 degrees Celsius. The cigarette
burns about 50 degrees hotter when air is being drawn through the

cigarette. The tobacco and additives are burned and change into smoke. The smoke contains many compounds resulting from the burning of the tobacco and chemical additives, including carbon monoxide, nitrosamines, polycyclic aromatic hydrocarbons, and about 4,000 other compounds.

The smoke travels from the burning tip through the body of the cigarette and cools down as it moves through the cigarette. The composition of the smoke is complex and varies according to the vigor and frequency of the puffing, the position of the person's fingers on the filter, the temperature of the burning, and the amount of unsmoked cigarette that the smoke is pulled through. The smoke travels from the mouth cavity to the bronchi and then into the alveoli of the lungs.

Smokers of filtered cigarettes can use various methods to increase the nicotine that gets into their brain. They can cover the ventilation holes in the filter, pull very hard on the cigarette, hold the cigarette longer in their mouth, inhale more frequently and deeply, and smoke the cigarette down to the butt. The cigarette companies have always known this. Filters and lower amounts of nicotine and tar in cigarettes have not resulted in safer or less addictive cigarettes.[34]

Milder smoke can be pulled deeper into the lungs to increase the power of nicotine. This may explain why soldiers in the Crimean and American Civil Wars became so fond of the mild Oriental tobacco and flue-cured bright leaf tobacco.

Smoking

The person who smokes burning cigarettes does this by using one of our most basic activities—breathing. The healthy person breathes effortlessly and without thinking about it. The chest wall muscles and diaphragm work together smoothly so that air travels in and out easily through the airways, or bronchi. Inhaling brings air to the small elastic pockets of lung tissue known as alveoli, where oxygen and carbon dioxide are exchanged. The surface area of the alveoli is huge—as big as a tennis court—so the exchange of the gases is rapid. Cells need oxygen to burn along with carbohydrates, protein, or fats to produce energy for the body's various functions. The end products of the burning of carbohydrates are water, carbon dioxide, and energy. A simple chemical formula for the burning of carbohydrate, a major fuel source, that takes place in all body cells, is the following:

carbohydrate (CH_2O) + oxygen (O_2) → water (H_2O) + carbon dioxide (CO_2) + energy

The carbon dioxide is the waste product of the burning of the carbohydrate. It is dissolved in the blood and then carried back to the alveoli of the lungs to be exhaled.

Just as we can choose to change the frequency and volume of our breaths, we can also choose to breathe, instead of air, smoke from the convenient and easy-to-use cigarette. Inhaling smoke is so peculiar, and such a perversion of the purpose of breathing, that it was not understood when first observed by Europeans. Thomas Hariot, an intelligent man, was baffled by the tobacco smoking of the Native Americans. He described the smoking as "sucking it . . . into their stomacke and head." Many early observers described smoking as "drinking smoke."[35]

The smoker draws the smoke into his or her lungs, where there are no enzymes to metabolize the nicotine or any other substances. (We usually ingest foreign substances through our gut. Enzymes there and in the liver metabolize unfamiliar or unwanted molecules.) The lack of metabolizing enzymes means that inhalation is a way of ingesting substances without any interference from the body's usual defenses. The nicotine in the smoke is absorbed by millions of innocent, helpful alveoli directly into the bloodstream and, unchanged, speeds to the brain.

Effects on the Mind and the Body

Tobacco is used in many ways, but here we will concentrate on the effects of smoking tobacco in cigarettes.

Effects on the Mind

Relief of Anxiety

Tapping the cigarette package (or cigarette) to pack the loose tobacco, flipping open the package and taking the cigarette out, lighting the cigarette, deliberately drawing in the smoke and slowly exhaling it, knocking off the ash, and then stubbing it out—all are enjoyable, ritualistic activities. From the first tap, the cigarette smoker feels calmer and distracted from his problems. The nicotine rush to the brain decreases anxiety and boredom, and leads to mild euphoria.

The person most afflicted by boredom and terror—the soldier—has used tobacco for centuries to alleviate the miseries of war. Benjamin Rush wrote that

Fear creates a desire for tobacco. Hence it is used in greater quantities by soldiers and sailors than by other classes of people.[36]

The relief is amplified when the tobacco is ingested via a cigarette. The cigarette might have been designed for soldiers. It is quickly lit, smoked, and finished. It is easy to transport and store, and it is helpful to smoke when rations are low because it suppresses the appetite. Chewing tobacco is even easier to use, since there is no light or smoke that could alert the enemy, but it does not get the nicotine to the brain so quickly and with such satisfaction.

Cigarettes are a cheap source of relief. To the nonsmoker, the price still seems too high given the risks of illness, but to some smokers, this risk is outweighed by the distraction from boredom and anxiety.

Addiction

Smoking burning tobacco is more addictive than other ways of ingesting tobacco because of the speed with which inhaled nicotine gets to the brain. Nicotine levels peak in the brain within 10 seconds of inhalation. The immediate effects of nicotine fade in a few minutes, causing the smoker to smoke frequently to maintain the drug's pleasurable effects and prevent withdrawal. Smokers will take about 10 puffs on a cigarette over the period of five minutes that the cigarette is lit. Chewing tobacco or nicotine gum, or applying nicotine patches to the skin, gets nicotine to the brain but not with the addicting rush that comes with smoking a cigarette.

Repeated exposure to nicotine results in tolerance, meaning that higher "doses" are required to produce the same initial stimulation. Nicotine is broken down fairly rapidly and disappears from the body in a few hours. Therefore, some tolerance is lost overnight, and smokers often report that the first cigarettes of the day are the strongest or the "best." As the day progresses tolerance develops, and later cigarettes have less effect. Oscar Wilde described this well: "A cigarette is the perfect type of a perfect pleasure. It is exquisite, and it leaves one unsatisfied. What more can one want?"[37]

Withdrawal

The person who stops smoking usually suffers from withdrawal symptoms such as irritability, difficulty thinking and concentrating, sleep disturbances, and increased appetite. Frequent mild weight gain dissuades some people from quitting. These unpleasant symptoms peak within the first few days but may last for several weeks.

An important but poorly understood part of the nicotine withdrawal syndrome is craving, which may persist for six months or longer. While the withdrawal syndrome is related to the pharmacological effects of nicotine, many behavioral factors also can affect the severity of craving. The feel, smell, and sight of a cigarette—and the rituals of handling, lighting, and smoking the cigarette—are pleasurable and difficult to relinquish. While nicotine gum and patches may ease the pharmacological aspects of withdrawal, they do not replace the rituals.

Many people can stop smoking, and most do so without treatment, but it may take multiple attempts. The presence of psychiatric illnesses such as depression or schizophrenia makes quitting more difficult, as is discussed in the following section.

Smoking and Psychiatric Disorders

People with psychiatric problems are more likely to smoke than others. The clearest example is schizophrenia. There is a high rate of smoking among people with schizophrenia that may in part be due to the ability of cigarette smoking to reduce side effects caused by medications. Also, nicotine may be associated with improvement in some types of memory and thinking ability in schizophrenia.

People with attention deficit hyperactivity disorder start smoking earlier and smoke more than others. One reason may be that nicotine addresses the problem of poor attention. Researchers have found that nicotine may be associated with improvement in the ability to pay attention. For example, airplane pilots performed better when given nicotine in the form of chewing gum.[38]

Nicotine has a complicated relationship with depression. Although smoking itself does not seem to treat depression, smoking cessation is associated with a return of depression in smokers with a history of depression.[39] Consistent with this is the finding that bupropion, an unusual antidepressant that enhances the effects of dopamine, may help people to give up cigarettes. Bupropion is now marketed in the United States under the name Zyban to help people stop smoking.

There is a high rate of co-substance abuse. In other words, people who use the three other substances of this book are more likely to smoke tobacco than are abstemious people.[40] In programs dealing with alcohol, cocaine, or opiate addiction, the addiction to tobacco is not always taken seriously. Alcoholics Anonymous meetings are famously redolent with the smell of coffee and cigarettes. (Some meetings now are designated as nonsmoking.) Tobacco smoking is not always addressed because tobacco addiction does not involve illegal activities and does not lead to out-of-control behavior. There is also some sense that people can give up only one addiction at a time. But many experts report that giving up tobacco does not make giving up other substances any more difficult.[41]

Effects on the Body

Cigarette smoking damages the body, and thus the cigarette smoker chooses momentary pleasure over future health problems. The person who smokes burning tobacco inhales thousands of toxic compounds. Nitrosamines and polycyclic aromatic hydrocarbons are among the compounds that cause much of the illness associated with smoking. Although the lungs are the organs most commonly thought of with respect to harm from cigarettes, cigarette smoking actually causes more deaths by damaging blood vessels and the heart. In the United States, tobacco smoking is responsible for more deaths than HIV, car crashes, suicides and murders, alcohol, and illegal drug use combined.[42]

Heart and Blood Vessels

Cigarettes interfere with the circulation of blood throughout the body in a number of ways. Tobacco smoke toxins enhance the stickiness of platelets, blood cell fragments that form clots, so that the cigarette smoker is more likely to have clots that can interfere with blood flow in their blood vessels. Smoking is also associated with large-vessel atherosclerosis, meaning that plaque, consisting of cholesterol and other substances, deposits on the walls of large arteries. The artery walls become thicker and harder, so blood vessels become narrower and less flexible, and blood flow to organs decreases. If a plaque ruptures, it can lead to a blood clot blocking blood flow. If a blood clot prevents flow in the brain, a stroke results; a blood clot in a blood vessel in the heart can cause a heart attack.

Smoking also damages smaller arteries, which in turn damages the heart and other organs. Cigarette smoking worsens the problems caused by high blood pressure, high levels of cholesterol, or other fats in the blood. The leading cause of death in the United States is coronary heart disease, and cigarette smoking is a major and preventable risk factor for this disorder. Cigarette smoking can cause peripheral arterial disease, leading to poor circulation and pain in the legs.

Lungs

The lungs are of course sorely battered by the toxins in cigarette smoke. Most people with lung cancer have been, or are, cigarette smokers.

The risk of lung cancer increases with the length of time one has smoked and the number of cigarettes smoked. Lung cancer is the leading cause of cancer deaths in the United States. Exposure to the several thousand toxic chemicals in cigarette smoke, particularly nitrosamines and polycyclic aromatic hydrocarbons, is probably the culprit, although the exact mechanism by which cigarette smoking causes lung cancer remains unknown.

Cigarette smoking causes other types of damage to the lungs as well. Smokers develop chronic obstructive pulmonary (lung) disease (COPD), either chronic bronchitis or emphysema. Chronic bronchitis is a long-lasting infection or inflammation of the bronchi. The person with bronchitis produces too much mucus and develops a persistent cough as well as repeated lung infections. In the person with emphysema, the small airways and alveoli of the lungs are damaged, so gas exchange, usually a rapid and easy process, is hindered.

Once again, it is not known exactly how cigarette smoking does so much damage, but it is not surprising that constant inhalation of so many foreign substances harms the delicate tissues of the bronchi and alveoli.

Once the airways become plugged with mucus or the alveoli and small airways lose their elasticity, breathing becomes painfully effortful. In both chronic bronchitis and emphysema, it is difficult for the person to bring in oxygen or get rid of carbon dioxide. At the end stage of chronic obstructive pulmonary disease, the person sits bolt upright and breathes with the help of accessory muscles because the chest wall muscles and diaphragm are no longer capable of doing the work by themselves. The person feels short of breath all the time. The work of moving air—practically a weightless substance—overwhelms all other tasks.

One of the testaments to the strength of the addictive powers of nicotine is the sight of a thin person sitting in a wheelchair with a nasal cannula delivering oxygen to her. Warning signs attached to the oxygen tank declare: "No smoking when oxygen is in use!" She hunches forward, using all of her strength to smoke a cigarette.

Pregnancy

Pregnant women who smoke have smaller babies and an increased risk of pregnancy complications. The toxins in the cigarette smoke damage the blood supply of the placenta as well as the organs of the embryo or fetus.

Cancers

Cigarette smokers have higher rates of cancer throughout the body. The higher rates of lung and head and neck cancers are well known. But rates of cancer are also higher in parts of the body not so obviously connected with breathing, such as the esophagus, stomach, pancreas, liver, kidney, ureter, urinary bladder, and uterine cervix. Smokers also have higher rates of some types of leukemia.

The other nicotine habits (not so common now), such as chewing tobacco, using snuff, or smoking cigars and pipes, are less harmful than cigarette smoking. Chewing tobacco, as was so clearly described by Dickens, is not an attractive habit. But spitting at least saves the chewer from quite so much exposure to the poisons of tobacco. Pipe and cigar smokers do not inhale the smoke. But these are still not safe habits. For example, Ulysses Grant, Sigmund Freud, and perhaps Thomas Hariot all died from head and neck cancers possibly related to smoking pipes or cigars. Grant's years of alcohol consumption might have played a role also in his final illness.

Appetite

Nicotine suppresses the appetite. It is sometimes used for this reason in times of inadequate food. For example, aboriginal people in Australia used tobacco when food was scarce, as did soldiers. Now, of course, advertising companies use this property to make cigarettes appealing to women who are more interested in being thin than in being well.

The Good Effects of Nicotine

People who smoke have lower rates of ulcerative colitis, preeclampsia during pregnancy, Parkinson's disease, and aphthous ulcers, perhaps due to their intake of nicotine. As is discussed in the brain chapter, the increase of neurotransmitters such as dopamine and acetylcholine due to nicotine has inevitably led some scientists to wonder if nicotine could be used in a therapeutic manner.

Conclusion

The Mayans and Aztecs, terrified soldiers in the trench, and women wanting to look like Bette Davis have smoked tobacco. In the past, it was connected with spirituality and peaceful negotiation. Now that we have made it more efficient by developing the cigarette, tobacco smoking has become the cause of one of the largest public health epidemics. Cigarettes are cheap and easily consumed. Nearly half of the 1 billion smokers in the world will die sooner than they have to because of a disease caused by their smoking.[43] While the tobacco companies and those who invest in them are able to tolerate this, public health advocates would like the long relationship between humanity and tobacco to end.

Notes

1. Iain Gately, *Tobacco: A Cultural History of How an Exotic Plant Seduced Civilization* (New York: Grove, 2001), 130.

2. Thomas Hariot, *A Briefe and True Report of the New Found Land of Virginia*, 1590, Project Gutenberg, eBook Collection, EBook #4247, released July 2003 (last updated August 6, 2012).

3. Gately, *Tobacco*, 38.

4. James I. *A Counter-Blaste to Tobacco, 1604*, ed. Edmund Goldsmid 1884, Project Gutenberg, eBook Collection, #17008, released November 5, 2005.

5. Ibid.

6. Timothy Brook, *Vermeer's Hat: The Seventeenth Century and the Dawn of the Global World* (New York: Bloomsbury, 2008), 126–27.

7. Gately, *Tobacco*, 86.

8. Stephen E. Ambrose, *Undaunted Courage: Meriwether Lewis, Thomas Jefferson, and the Opening of the American West* (New York: Simon & Schuster, 1996), 32.

9. Kirkpatrick Sale, *Christopher Columbus and the Conquest of Paradise* (London: Tauris Parke, 2006), 283.

10. Charles Dickens, *American Notes*, 1842. (New York: Fawcett, 1961), 134–35.

11. Gately, *Tobacco*, 181.

12. Gately, *Tobacco*, 185–86.

13. Cassandra Tate, *Cigarette Wars: The Triumph of "The Little White Slaver"* (New York: Oxford University Press, 1999), 66.

14. Ibid., 88.

15. Ibid., 79.

16. Ibid., 65.

17. Ibid., 71.

18. Richard Kluger, *Ashes to Ashes: America's Hundred-Year Cigarette War, the Public Health, and the Unabashed Triumph of Philip Morris* (New York: Vintage, 1996), 114–15.

19. Allan M. Brandt, *The Cigarette Century: The Rise, Fall, and Deadly Persistence of the Product That Defined America.* (New York: Basic Books, 2009), 337.

20. Kluger, *Ashes to Ashes*, 645.

21. Stanton A. Glantz et al., *The Cigarette Papers* (Berkeley: University of California Press, 1996), 10.

22. David Kessler, *A Question of Intent: A Great American Battle with a Deadly Industry* (New York: Public Affairs, 2001), 252.

23. K. Michael Cummings, Christopher P. Morley, and Andrew Hyland, "Failed Promises of the Cigarette Industry and Its Effect on Consumer Misperceptions about the Health Risks of Smoking," *Tobacco Control* 11, suppl. 1, (March 2002): i114.

24. Robert N. Proctor, *Golden Holocaust: Origins of the Cigarette Catastrophe and the Case for Abolition* (Berkeley: University of California Press, 2011), 340–41; Kessler, *Intent*, 252.

25. Much of the argument in Kessler, *Intent*, has to do with the tobacco companies knowing for decades about the addictive nature of nicotine.

26. Steven A. Schroeder, "Tobacco Control in the Wake of the 1998 Master Settlement Agreement," *New England Journal of Medicine* 350, no. 3 (2004): 296.

27. Ibid.

28. Ibid., 293.

29. World Health Organization (WHO), "Tobacco Fact Sheet No. 339," updated July 2013, http://www.who.int/mediacentre/factsheets/fs339/en/ (accessed August 3, 2013).

30. Simon Chapman, *Great Expectorations: Advertising and the Tobacco Industry* (London: Comedia, 1986), 127–28.

31. Murray Jarvik, "Tobacco Smoking in Monkeys," *Annals of the New York Academy of Sciences* 142 (December 1967): 280–94.

32. G. Ferris Wayne, Gregory N. Connolly, and Jack E. Henningfield, "Brand Differences of Free-Base Nicotine Delivery in Cigarette Smoke: The View of the Tobacco Industry Documents," *Tobacco Control* 15 (June 2006): 189–98.

33. Terrell Stevenson and Robert N. Proctor, "The Secret and Soul of Marlboro: Philip Morris and the Origins, Spread, and Denial of Nicotine Freebasing," *American Journal of Public Health* 98, no. 7 (2008): 181–94.

34. Michael J. Thun et al., "50-Year Trends in Smoking-Related Mortality in the United States," *New England Journal of Medicine* 368, no. 4 (2013): 363.

35. Wolfgang Schivelbusch, *Tastes of Paradise: A Social History of Spices, Stimulants, and Intoxicants*, trans. David Jacobson (New York: Vintage, 1992), 96.

36. David T. Courtwright, *Forces of Habit: Drugs and the Making of the Modern World* (Cambridge, MA: Harvard University Press, 2001), 141.

37. Oscar Wilde, *The Picture of Dorian Gray*, 1891. (New York: Dover, 1993), 58.

38. Martin Mumenthaler at al., "Psychoactive Drugs and Pilot Performance: A Comparison of Nicotine, Donepezil, and Alcohol Effects," *Neuropsychopharmacology* 28, no. 7 (2003): 1366–73.

39. Alexander Glassman, "Cigarette Smoking: Implications for Psychiatric Illness," *American Journal of Psychiatry* 150, no. 4 (1993): 546–53.

40. Schroeder, "Tobacco Control," 293.

41. Catherine Theresa Baca and Carolina E. Yahne, "Smoking Cessation during Substance Abuse Treatment: What You Need to Know," *Journal of Substance Abuse* 36 (2009): 207.

42. Centers for Disease Control and Prevention (CDC), "Fact Sheet: Tobacco-Related Mortality; Smoking and Tobacco Use," http://www.cdc.gov/tobacco/data_statistics/fact_sheets/health_effects/tobacco_related_mortality/ (accessed July 12, 2013).

43. WHO, "Tobacco Fact Sheet."

13

Tobacco and Illness: The Discovery

The discovery of the damage done to our health by inhaling burning tobacco is one of the great accomplishments of modern medicine. Scientists demonstrated a relationship between smoking and a variety of illnesses, beginning with lung cancer, by counting and tabulating. Yet the century's greatest statisticians and many physicians were unconvinced by these numbers for some years.

For the first half of the twentieth century, cigarette smoking seemed benign, since cigarette smoking does not cause immediate damage. People smoked and felt well. In fact, many people feel *better* after smoking a cigarette, especially after the first cigarette of the day. It was difficult to perceive damage in something as evanescent and soothing as cigarette smoke.

Nonetheless, some noticed the problem. In 1938, Dr. Raymond Pearl of Johns Hopkins wrote a report in *Science*, a preeminent journal, that heavy cigarette smoking led to premature deaths.[1] Angel Roffo, an Argentinian physician, produced a large body of work over several decades in the early twentieth century about the dangers of smoking tobacco. One of his most striking observations was that lung cancer seemed to affect just men. Because Argentinian men smoked while women did not, he thought that cigarettes could be the cause. He also made the connection between tars from coal burning and tars from tobacco burning. This had been a century and a half in the making. In 1779, Percivall Pott suggested that young boys who climbed up and swept clean the smoky chimneys of London developed scrotal cancer because of their exposure to soot. Roffo knew that tar, whether from coal or from cigarette burning, contained polycyclic aromatic hydrocarbons, such as benzopyrene, which he suspected could lead to cancer.[2]

Roffo also worked in the laboratory. He painted tar from cigarette smoke on rabbit ears; cancers resulted. He published prolifically about his research, mostly in German. German scientists and American tobacco companies, but few others, were aware of his work. In Germany, Franz Müller showed in 1939 that smokers were more likely to develop lung cancer than nonsmokers. It seems to have been widely accepted in Germany that smoking was the leading cause of lung cancer. Physicians in Germany also believed, correctly, that there was a link between smoking and heart disease. Yet Müller's work, and that of other German scientists, is not known to many today. Perhaps there is a reluctance to acknowledge the scientific work done by doctors who collaborated with the Nazi regime, or who published in the German language, as did Roffo. Müller himself was a member of the Nazi Party, and Adolf Hitler had a personal dislike of smoking, and this too makes the German research of the time uncomfortable to acknowledge.[3]

Cigarette smoking was common throughout much of the Western world in the middle of the twentieth century, and it was accepted as a normal and safe habit. For example, in mid-twentieth-century England, four-fifths of men smoked.[4] Rates of smoking were high in part because cigarettes were so avidly smoked by soldiers of the wars of the nineteenth and twentieth centuries. Cigarettes were omnipresent among young men in the British Army in World War I so by the 1950s, many older British men had been smoking heavily for at least 30 years.

This increase in the number of people smoking tobacco happened at the same time that much of the world's population, at least in the developed world, was becoming healthier. Sanitation, nutrition, and safety at work had improved. The discoveries of the infectious causes of illnesses such as typhoid, cholera, and tuberculosis and then the amazing effects of insulin, penicillin, and the sulfa drugs made medicine, for the first time, a scientific and helpful discipline. Because of asepsis and anesthesia, surgery was safe and tolerable. Life expectancy was increasing in the Western world. Chronic disorders and the illnesses of the elderly were not much worried about. Optimism prevailed.

Lung cancer was rare. A few physicians had reported that smoking cigarettes was linked with lung cancer, but these reports usually involved small numbers of people or were not published in leading or English-language journals. Pearl's article in *Science* was ignored. However, by the middle of the twentieth century, pathologists performing autopsies in the United States, Australia, New Zealand, and Switzerland noticed an increase in lung cancers. Suspicion about cigarettes grew, even outside Argentina and Germany.

In the United States, medical student Ernest Wynder, after seeing a heavy smoker die of lung cancer, became interested in the possible connection with cigarettes. He persuaded one of his instructors, Dr. Evarts Graham, a thoracic surgeon, to investigate this with him. They compared smoking habits of over 600 hospital patients with lung cancer to those of a roughly equal number of hospital patients with other diseases, and in 1949 concluded that long-term cigarette smoking can cause lung cancer. Graham and Wynder noted the greater incidence of lung cancer in men than in women and commented on the long lag time between smoking and the development of lung cancer that made studies very difficult.[5]

More studies were done by Richard Doll and Austin Bradford Hill in the United Kingdom at the behest of the British Medical Research Council. The suspected culprits with respect to the increase in lung cancer were environmental. In mid-twentieth-century England, automobiles were becoming common, and roads were being paved at a rapid rate. The two researchers thought that the culprit could be related to road coal tar or coal burning.

The researchers questioned people with and without lung cancer. Doll and Hill recorded background information such as age, sex, urban or rural place of residence, and social class. They asked questions about what they suspected to be important: exposure to air pollution and domestic coal fires. The two researchers also recorded data related to the length of time the patients smoked and whether they smoked cigarettes or pipes.

To the surprise of Doll and Hill, all of the patients with lung cancer—but not the comparison patients—turned out to be cigarette smokers. The other factors that they inquired about were not implicated.[6]

Doll and Hill went on to do a second study. This time, they worked forward and used nonpatients. In 1951, they recruited 34,000 English physicians, mostly male. The choice of doctors was clever. They thought that doctors would report their health accurately, get good medical care, cooperate with studies to do with health, and be easier to follow, since they always had to let the medical authorities know where they were working. Over 80 percent of the doctors were lifelong smokers. Within three years, Doll and Hill found an association between high rates of lung cancer and smoking.[7]

Many physicians and statisticians were skeptical of these findings. Edward Cuyler Hammond, a Yale statistician, had not been convinced by the work of Graham and Wynder or by that of Doll and Hill. He began another prospective study that was four times as large as the British study. Together with Daniel Horn, a psychologist with expertise in statistics, he mailed questionnaires to nearly 188,000 white U.S. males of all levels of income and education between the ages of 50 and 69 in 1952. This was a larger and more representative sample than the British one. They found that cigarette smokers were more likely to get lung cancer than non-smokers. They also found an increase in heart disease among the cigarette smokers that had not been suspected. This would turn out to be of great importance.[8]

Doll and Hill published their findings in the prestigious *British Medical Journal* and Hammond and Horn in the equally well-respected *Journal of the American Medical Association*. Other research groups had similar findings. The quality of these reports, the similarity of findings from groups in different countries, and the imprimatur of the journals in which these articles were published began to change the way in which smoking was perceived.

However, these findings were all large population studies and subject to all of the weaknesses therein. Were people's reports and memories accurate? The tobacco companies rejected the findings and were supported by the century's most respected statisticians.

Ronald Fisher, perhaps the greatest statistician of the time, argued that the studies showed, at the most, only an *association* between smoking and lung cancer. The studies were not designed to show *causation*. Perhaps there was another condition that led to both cigarette smoking and lung cancer. Perhaps men who smoked were the same people who had the genotype that put them at risk for lung cancer.[9]

Another statistician, Joseph Berkson, pointed out the surprising number of diseases associated with smoking. This weakened the findings. At that point, the concern was primarily with lung cancer. To him and many others, particularly those who smoked and enjoyed it, the connection between cigarettes and lung cancer was not obvious, and it was made less so by what seemed to be a spurious link with too many other illnesses. The anticigarette scientists were weakening their case by claiming too much. Berkson wrote that "we have here a great deal more than was bargained for, and most of it without relation to what it was intended to explain, the observed risk in death rate from cancer of the lung."[10]

Another problem in the smoking-illness theory was that it lacked the clarity of the work done with infectious diseases. Louis Pasteur and Robert Koch had done brilliant laboratory work in the late nineteenth century showing that microorganisms caused specific illnesses, such as cholera and tuberculosis, and did so quickly. Smoking, in contrast, was associated with many illnesses and with a long lag time. The lack of specificity, slowness, as well as a lack of obvious mechanism worried medical scientists.

Was there any other kind of evidence that could prove or disprove the link? Since numbers and tables did not convince everyone, more animal experiments were started. The advantage of animals is that they can be exposed to cigarettes and then killed so that the effects of the cigarettes can be studied on actual tissue. In the mid-1950s, Wynder (by now a physician) and his colleagues applied chemicals from cigarette smoke to the skin of mice and found that the mice developed skin cancers. (This was similar to Roffo's work.) But this was not cigarette smoking.

The American scientists who took another step in studying cigarette smoking in animals were Hammond, the statistician, and Oscar Auerbach, a pathologist. Auerbach had a background that prepared him well—his work with tuberculosis.

Tuberculosis was common in the early twentieth century.[11] The discovery of effective antituberculosis medications was one of the reasons for the widespread belief of the time that medicine was leading to greater health for everyone. Few people thought that there would be other causes of lung disease once tuberculosis was treatable.[12]

Auerbach, who worked at a public tuberculosis sanatorium, documented the success of streptomycin in treating tuberculosis. He had worked himself out of a job once the value of streptomycin became clear. He kept his interest in lung diseases but moved from tuberculosis to smoking. He joined the Veterans Administration in 1952 and led a team of researchers in examining lung tissue samples from people with a variety of illnesses. They examined more than 100,000 lung tissue samples. By 1957, he was fairly certain that smoking was associated with lung cancer. His group also saw changes associated with emphysema, a progressive disease that destroys tissue in the lungs of smokers.[13]

He joined forces with Hammond to do work with animals. Hammond understood numbers, and Auerbach understood lungs. The experiments were difficult because no animals apart from humans smoke cigarettes.

They tackled this problem by what many would consider to be cruel techniques.

In 1967, Auerbach and Hammond began to work with beagles, a species often used in animal studies, and particularly useful in these studies because of the similarity between beagle and human lungs. The two researchers trained 86 beagles to smoke cigarettes through a tube inserted into the trachea. Animal rights activists became aware of the use of beagles. The problem was not so much the smoking, since the dogs seemed to enjoy it, but the fact that the beagles had to be killed so that their lung tissue could be examined. The activists made death threats against the researchers themselves and organized protest marches. But the researchers continued and showed that the dogs who became heavy smokers of non-filter cigarettes were the most likely to develop lung cancer and emphysema. The beagle lung cancers resembled human lung cancers.[14]

Berkson had thought it improbable that cigarettes could be linked with so many different types of illnesses and in so many parts of the body. Research has confirmed the findings that Berkson thought to be suspicious. Cigarette smoking leads to head, neck, and lung cancer but also to other lung diseases such as chronic bronchitis and emphysema. Cigarette smoking also is a risk factor for other cancers and for cardiovascular illnesses. Some of these illnesses develop only in people with relatively long lives. As the general health of the population improved and people lived longer, the problem of chronic illnesses has emerged, as has the connection with cigarettes. It bears repeating that in the United States, tobacco smoking is now responsible for more deaths than HIV, car crashes, suicides and murders, alcohol, and illegal drug use combined.[15]

In 1996 benzopyrene, a polycyclic aromatic hydrocarbon, was identified as a carcinogen. Angel Roffo's suspicion that there was a link between chimney sweeps' cancer and lung cancer was supported. Benzopyrenes can damage DNA and are responsible for at least some of the cancers in both chimney sweeps and cigarette smokers.

Of the researchers described earlier in this chapter, Doll is perhaps the best known. He went on to do much other epidemiological work and was responsible for several advances in public health. He never abandoned his interest in cigarettes. He followed his group of doctors for 50 years, publishing his last survey of their smoking practices in 2004. He showed that persistent smoking will lead to the deaths of about half of those with that habit, that smoking was the cause of most lung cancer, but that lung cancer accounted for less than half of the excess mortality caused by cigarette smoking. Much of the mortality is due to other lung diseases and cardiovascular illness.[16]

The work of Auerbach, Doll, Graham, Hammond, Hill, Horn, Müller, Pearl, Roffo, and Wynder (and others not mentioned here), has been replicated and thus confirmed in later studies. The work of these early scientists runs the risk of not being appreciated because it seems so obvious now that cigarettes are bad for our health.

Notes

1. Raymond Pearl, "Tobacco Smoking and Longevity," *Science* 87 (1938): 216–17.

2. Robert N. Proctor, "Angel H. Roffo: The Forgotten Father of Experimental Tobacco Carcinogenesis," *Bulletin of the World Health Organization* 84, no. 6 (2006): 494–96.

3. Robert N. Proctor, *The Nazi War on Cancer* (Princeton, NJ: Princeton University Press, 1999), 194–97.

4. Iain Gately, *Tobacco: A Cultural History of How an Exotic Plant Seduced Civilization* (New York: Grove, 2001), 278.

5. Ernest L. Wynder and Evarts A. Graham, "Tobacco Smoking as a Possible Etiologic Factor in Bronchiogenic Carcinoma: A Study of Six Hundred and Eighty-Four Proved Cases," *Journal of the American Medical Association* 143 (1950): 329–36.

6. Richard Doll and Austin Hill, "Smoking and Carcinoma of the Lung: Preliminary Report," *British Medical Journal* 221(ii) (1950): 739–48.

7. Richard Doll and Austin Hill, "The Mortality of Doctors in Relation to Their Smoking Habits: a Preliminary Report," *British Medical Journal* 228(i) (1954): 1451–55.

8. Edward Cuyler Hammond and Daniel Horn, "Smoking and Death Rates: Report on 44 Months of Follow-Up of 187,783 Men; I. Total Mortality," *Journal of the American Medical Association* 166 (1958): 1159–72.

9. Robert N. Proctor, *Golden Holocaust: Origins of the Cigarette Catastrophe and the Case for Abolition* (Berkeley: University of California Press, 2011), 280.

10. Quoted in Colin White, "Research on Smoking and Lung Cancer: A Landmark in the History of Chronic Disease Epidemiology," *Yale Journal of Biology and Medicine* 63 (1990): 37.

11. Hill contracted tuberculosis at the age of 17 and was ill for four years. He had intended to study medicine, but his long illness made this impossible, so he got a degree in economics instead. He retained his earlier interest in medicine and turned to medical statistics. Doll, a medical doctor, also had been ill with tuberculosis that had affected one of his kidneys but was well enough to practice medicine. In 1946, Hill was the statistician for the British Medical Research Council's

successful trial of streptomycin in the treatment of tuberculosis, probably the first randomized clinical trial ever performed.

12. Tuberculosis is still a significant cause of illness and death in Asia and Africa and is becoming more common due to the HIV/AIDS epidemic and the emergence of drug-resistant strains of the tuberculosis bacterium. It may be a risk factor in the development of lung cancer in smokers, and tobacco may be a risk factor for becoming ill with tuberculosis.

13. Oscar Auerbach et al., "Changes in Bronchial Epithelium in Relation to Cigarette Smoking and in Relation to Lung Cancer," *New England Journal of Medicine* 265 (1961): 253–67.

14. Oscar Auerbach et al., "Effects of Cigarette Smoking on Dogs: II. Pulmonary Neoplasms," *Archives of Environmental Health* 21 no. 6 (1970): 754–68.

15. Centers for Disease Control and Prevention (CDC), "Fact Sheet: Tobacco-Related Mortality; Smoking & Tobacco Use," http://www.cdc.gov/tobacco/data_statistics/fact_sheets/health_effects/tobacco_related_mortality/ (accessed July 12, 2013).

16. Richard Doll et al., "Mortality in Relation to Smoking: 50 Years' Observations on Male British Doctors," *British Medical Journal* 328 (2004): 1519.

14

Women and Cigarettes

Women have never used tobacco as much as have men. Women who did smoke, and particularly those who dared to do this in public, were often ridiculed in the past. In a German newspaper article from the 1840s, the sight of women daring to smoke on the street was greeted with sarcasm:

> Women's emancipation takes remarkable strides forward in Germany, especially in Berlin, Germany's most discerning city, with the most startling results. In the brilliant circles of that city, girls aged nineteen or twenty speak confidently about Guizot, Thiers, and search laws—it all verges on the incredible! At this point many of these miniature George Sands don't even disdain the cigar; recently an elegant lady stopped a gentleman on the street who was smoking to ask him to light *hers*. Charming prospects, these! How long before they put on trousers, force men into the kitchen with riding whips, and nurse their babies on horseback! Easy for the emancipated woman! A public coffeehouse is already being opened for women ...[1]

George Sand, born Aurore Dupin, mentioned so derisively in the preceding quotation, was a renowned French novelist who shocked people in many ways. She had multiple love affairs, took on the name and the habits of males, and often wore men's clothing. In her novels, she attacked the ideas of arranged marriage and class discrimination. She defied social convention by smoking in public.

Another example of a woman who dared to smoke in public is Lola Montez, a famous courtesan and dance hall star of the mid-nineteenth century. She sang and danced throughout Europe and America, and she too had many lovers, including Franz Liszt and Alexandre Dumas père.

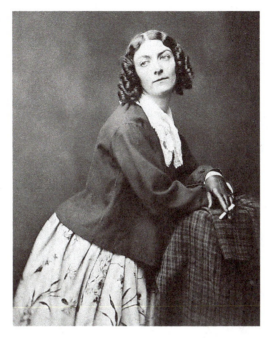

Figure 14.1   **British Dancer Lola Montez in America.**
(© **Corbis**)

Her most notorious liaison, lasting five years, was with King Ludwig I of Bavaria. A photograph of her, taken in Boston in 1851, shows her dressed formally, wearing black gloves, looking brazenly at the camera, and holding a cigarette. As Figure 14.1 shows, she is calm, sure of herself, sophisticated, and theatrical. Montez chain smoked and used her cigarette as a prop and provocation.

In the United States at the beginning of the twentieth century, women who smoked still raised eyebrows. Paula Fass, in her description of the United States in the 1920s, writes that smoking cigarettes was "sexually suggestive and associated with disreputable women or with bohemian types"[2]—in other words, with women like George Sand and Lola Montez. Fass goes on to write that "undoubtedly, many women in the twenties began to smoke because it was a glamorous affectation and somewhat naughty."[3]

Tobacco Smoking and Women: "A New Standard of Female Loveliness"

The difference between the genders in smoking rates is now smaller. This may be due to the greater independence of women, but another reason may be advertising, and particularly that done by Edward Bernays, the "father of public relations." Bernays was a nephew of Sigmund Freud —twice over. His mother was Freud's sister, and his father's sister was Freud's wife, Martha. Bernays was born in Vienna in 1891 and was raised in New York. He pioneered the use of "product placement" and the creation of mass events for marketing purposes. He encouraged the public to eat bananas on behalf of the United Fruit Company, which owned banana plantations in Guatemala.

Some of his cleverest work was for the American Tobacco Company, which manufactured Lucky Strike cigarettes. By the mid-1920s, cigarette smoking had become popular. But the company knew that its sales could be larger if it could convince more women to smoke, and in 1928 it hired Bernays to do just this.

Bernays had many approaches. He first exploited the well-known appetite-suppressant properties of nicotine and explicitly connected cigarette smoking with thinness and elegance. He recruited "experts" to argue that "the slender woman who, combining suppleness and grace with slenderness, who instead of overeating sweets and desserts, lights a cigarette . . . has created a new standard of female loveliness."[4] Bernays cajoled a letter from Arthur Murray, the famous dance instructor, in which he wrote:

> On the dance floor, results of over-indulgence are quickly revealed—causing embarrassment not only to one's dancing partner but also to other dancers by encroaching on more than a fair share of space on a crowded or, as is often the case, on a dance floor of limited proportions. Dancers today, when tempted to overindulge at the punch bowl or the buffet, reach for a cigarette instead.[5]

Bernays understood the importance of ritual, and he popularized the habit of ending a meal with a cigarette. He enlisted the British Association of Medical Officers of Health to suggest that "the correct way to finish a meal is with fruit, coffee, and a cigarette" to prevent gum decay and soothe the nerves. He even intruded into home design. He suggested to kitchen cabinet makers that they build special cigarette drawers in new kitchens. Bernays had brought cigarettes into the domain of the domestic.[6]

There was more. The American Tobacco Company noted that women were "allowed" to smoke only in their own homes. George Washington Hill, president of the company, wanted to increase market share by encouraging women to smoke in public. Hill and Bernays seized on the women's rights movement. Bernays persuaded women's rights marchers in New York City to hold up Lucky Strike cigarettes as symbolic "torches of freedom." In 1929, he arranged for attractive and slim women to walk up and down 5th Avenue while smoking during the New York Easter Day Parade. Supposedly this effort was to support the concept of freedom for women, but Bernays's goal was to make smoking outdoors by women socially acceptable. Feminism had been suborned by a tobacco company.

Sigmund Freud had promoted cocaine; his nephew promoted cigarettes. Bernays, who had convinced women that smoking would make them slim, never smoked himself. He tried to discourage his wife from smoking. Perhaps influenced more by her husband's professional advertising than by his personal advice, she smoked a pack a day for many years. Sigmund Freud, famously, had been perplexed by half of the human race: "What do women want?" His nephew knew the answer: "to be thin."

Bernays died in 1995 at the age of 103. He was active and healthy for most of his 100 plus years. Perhaps his lifelong habit of not smoking had kept him healthy—in contrast to his famous uncle who smoked cigars and suffered terribly from cancer of the jaw and palate.

Another advertising expert, Albert Lasker, also was involved with the tobacco companies. He had been astonished when his first wife, told by her physician to take up smoking in order to lose weight, was forbidden to smoke in a restaurant.[7] Lasker created the slogan "Reach for a Lucky instead of a Sweet" and variations thereof for the American Tobacco Company (see Figure 14.2).

Albert Lasker, also a nonsmoker, died in 1952 at the age of 72, leaving behind his second wife, Mary, a philanthropist. She was instrumental in the formation of the American Cancer Society and in the massive increase of federal funding for medical research. On her husband's fiftieth birthday, she gave him a gift, the Albert Lasker Medical Research Awards Program. The Lasker award is now one of the most respected prizes in medical research. She funneled the money that her husband had made from advertising tobacco into science.

In 1968, the tobacco company Philip Morris continued this appeal to women's interest in slimness by introducing a new brand, Virginia Slims, and trumpeting "You've come a long way, baby." This slogan, offensive to many, was effective. Rose Cipollone, the New Jersey housewife discussed in the nicotine chapter, found the advertising and packaging of these cigarettes appealing and switched to Virginia Slims.

Some women, such as Sand and Montez, smoked to assert their independence from or equality with men. That now seems old-fashioned, since

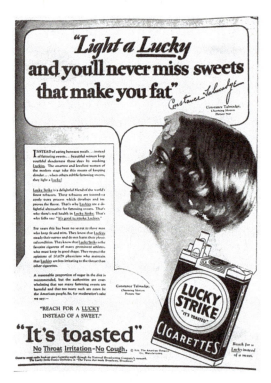

Figure 14.2   Lucky Cigarette Advertisement.
(© Corbis)

women are no longer mocked if they smoke. Women in the Western world smoke today not to assert their equality with men but because they have succumbed to the promises of the advertisers—that they will be independent and adventurous, and, even better, thin and sexually alluring if they smoke cigarettes.

Effects on Health

Women suffer all of the ill effects of smoking that men do. Lung cancer kills more women in the United States than breast, uterine, and ovarian cancer combined. Most women who develop lung cancer smoke or have smoked tobacco. Women also face some risks that men do not. The use of oral contraceptives increases the risk of stroke connected with smoking. The pregnant woman and the fetus are both harmed by cigarette smoking. Women may find it more difficult than men do to stop smoking. Rose Cipollone is a sad, well-publicized, and litigated example of some of these issues.

Women in the Third World

Smoking is becoming less common now in the developed world. Tobacco companies have responded to this loss of market by promoting smoking in less developed countries, and their particular targets are girls. Their advertisements link smoking with the Western lifestyle of pleasure, wealth, and consumption. For women, an added implicit message is emancipation or freedom. The message seems to be getting through, as the World Health Organization estimates that the biggest rise in female smoking will be in less-developed countries.[8] The health consequences of tobacco smoking can be overshadowed by the many other problems in Third World countries. Nonetheless, women who smoke, no matter how poor and oppressed they are, are increasing their risk of illness. The cigarette companies once again have suborned the message of women's rights.

Conclusion

The image of Montez smoking is striking, but Bernays and Lasker created images that were designed to make smoking even more appealing to women. Women want to be free, but even more they want to be slim. Tobacco companies suggest that women who smoke will look more attractive and become more independent. In reality, they will develop cardiovascular disease, chronic obstructive pulmonary disease, lung cancer, and a variety of other cancers, and they will put their pregnancies and babies at risk.

Notes

1. Wolfgang Schivelbusch, *Tastes of Paradise: A Social History of Spices, Stimulants, and Intoxicants*, trans. David Jacobson (New York: Vintage, 1992), 120.

2. Paula Fass, *The Damned and the Beautiful: American Youth in the 1920s* (New York: Oxford University Press, 1977), 293.

3. Ibid., 300.

4. Larry Tye, *Father of Spin* (New York: Henry Holt, 1998), 24.

5. Ibid., 25.

6. Ibid.

7. Jeffrey L. Cruickshank and Arthur Schultz, *The Man Who Sold America: The Amazing (but True!) Story of Albert D. Lasker and the Creation of the Advertising Century* (Boston: Harvard Business Review Press, 2010), 252.

8. Amanda Amos and Margaretha Haglund, "From Social Taboo to 'Torch of Freedom': The Marketing of Cigarettes to Women," *Tobacco Control* 9, no. 1 (2000): 3–8.

15

Opiates

Introduction

Opium and related drugs, such as heroin and morphine, are celebrated as the strongest treatments for pain. For most of recorded time, they have been the only useful medication available to humanity. Just one century ago, on his deathbed, William Osler, one of the most distinguished physicians of his time, wrote to his sister-in-law about his exhausting and painful bouts of coughing,

> ... There is nothing I do not know of the varieties & vagaries of coughs & coughing—the outcome is far away. Shunt the whole pharmacopoeia, except opium. It alone in some form does the job. What a comfort it has been![1]

Yet in the twenty-first century, people who become addicted to any of the opiates are shunned or looked at with a frisson of horror. The opiate addict is dismissed as a "junkie."

Opium comes from the lovely poppy (see Figure 15.1). These annual flowers grow in many climates and soils but thrive in hot, dry conditions and in mountainous regions with poor soil. Areas in Asia, Colombia, and Mexico are particularly hospitable to this flower.

Opium is the dried and concentrated juice of the unripe poppy seed capsule. Morphine ($C_{17}H_{19}NO_3$) is the alkaloid in this juice that is responsible for the effects of opium. The species of poppy with the highest proportion of morphine in this juice is known colloquially as the opium poppy and scientifically as *Papaver somniferum*. It has been known for

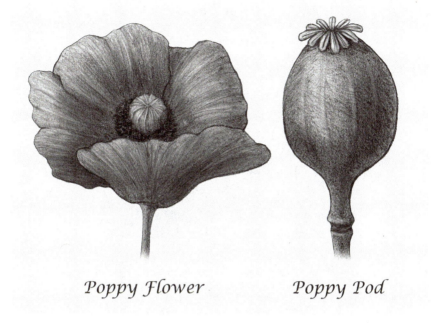

Poppy Flower   *Poppy Pod*

Figure 15.1   **Opium Poppy. (© 2013 Joan M.K. Tycko)**

many centuries that the juice that drips out of this poppy seedpod, or cap-sule, causes sleepiness. Other alkaloids contained in the resin of the opium poppy include codeine and thebaine.

Harvesting opium is simple. The seed capsule of the poppy produces a milky liquid during a two-week period. The harvester cuts the ripening seed pods and collects the white liquid that oozes out. The liquid hardens into a gum, which is then dissolved in boiling water and simmered. The result is prepared or cooked opium (see Figure 15.2).

Opium and related drugs do not lead directly to the out-of-control behavior associated with alcohol and cocaine. Nicotine and alcohol both cause much more medical harm than do opiates. Yet opiates, apart from those used in medicine, are illegal in many parts of the world because of their powerfully addictive nature and their ability to suppress breathing, which can lead to lethal overdoses.

The strong addictive power of opium and its derivatives means that people will purchase them even if they are unregulated and illegal. Trafficking involves individuals, gangs, multinational cartels, and coun-tries themselves. In some regions, including present-day Afghanistan, opium poppies are a leading agricultural cash crop. The profits associated with opiates led to the Opium Wars in China in the nineteenth century,

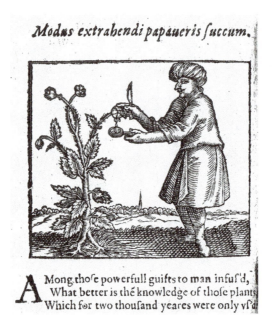

Modus extrahendi papaueris succum.

A Mong thofe powerfull guifts to man infuf'd,
   What better is the knowledge of thofe plants
   Which for two thoufand yeares were only vf'd

Figure 15.2 **Method of Extracting Juice from Poppy. (Wellcome Library, London)**

and poppies grown in the Golden Triangle and Golden Crescent are now associated with much international conflict.

History

Mesopotamia, Egypt, Greece, and the Middle and Far East

The first people to use opium were probably, once again, the clever Sumerians who settled in Mesopotamia in about 5000 BCE. Not much is known about how they used opium, but their name for it was the "joy plant," suggesting that they had some experience with its effects on the mind.

Later, the ancient Egyptians, Greeks, and Romans became familiar with the poppy and its products. Poppies were grown in the Middle and Far East, and opium was used in Arab medicine. Although the addictive nature of opium was known from early times, and Diagoras of Melos, in about 400 or 500 BCE, warned about the possibility of dependence,[2] opium was not then as reviled or feared as it would be much later.

Laudanum

In sixteenth-century Europe, the use of opium dissolved in alcohol was advocated by one of the great physicians of that time, Philippus Aureolus

Theophrastus Bombastus von Hohenheim, who chose to be called Paracelsus. He named this beverage laudanum—after the Latin word *laudare*, "to praise."

Thomas Sydenham, a renowned English physician, further developed this powerful and appealing drink in the seventeenth century. He concocted a compound of opium, sherry wine, and herbs that became popular in England. The wine enhanced the effects of the opium, and, along with the herbs, would have masked the bitter taste of the opium. Laudanum was considered a useful medicine and sedative. One of its uses was to calm discomfort associated with fevers such as the aches of malaria.

Opium, Malaria, and "Jesuits' Bark"

Although we now think of malaria as a tropical disease, it also afflicted temperate climes until as recently as the mid-twentieth century. Malaria was common in the Fens, a lowland area in the east of England, and other marshlands of coastal southern England, and may have led to the death of King James I of England in 1625. Until the mid-nineteenth century, the only remedy for malaria was the bark from *Cinchona calisaya* trees, which grew in the mountains of South America. The first Europeans to use cinchona bark were Jesuit missionaries working in South America. They were familiar with malaria because it was endemic to the Italian swamps and marshes, and had caused the deaths of popes and cardinals. The active ingredient of the bark was later discovered to be the alkaloid quinine.

Beginning in the 1600s, this botanical cure spread throughout Europe and was known as "Jesuits' bark." Oliver Cromwell, Lord Protector of England, became ill with malaria but, suspicious of anything to do with the Catholics, died of the illness in 1658 after refusing to use the Jesuits' bark.

Other treatments were available for those not wanting to benefit from the Jesuits. In England, Robert Talbor made a mysterious potion for use by Protestants. In 1672, Talbor, who described himself as a "feverologist," warned others: "Beware of all palliative Cures and especially of that known by the name of Jesuit's Powder . . . for I have seen most dangerous effects follow the taking of that medicine."[3]

Talbor was, of course, using the Jesuits' bark or powder. He "improved" on this by adding wine and opium. Charles II of England was convinced that Talbor saved his life in 1678. He knighted Talbor and sent him to France to save French royalty. Was there enough cinchona bark or quinine in Talbor's remedy to be effective? Or was it the opium and alcohol that made the patient feel better? Or feel less? Whatever the answer, it is clear that the addition of certain drugs such as alcohol, cocaine, or opiates to herbal potions will make a better-selling product. Talbor's cure was clever. The quinine might have treated the malaria, and if the person did not have malaria but another illness, the alcohol and opium would have made him or her feel temporarily better no matter what the illness.

Opiates in the Nineteenth Century

Mrs. Winslow's Soothing Syrup

The use of opium slowly increased, and by the nineteenth century, opium and its derivatives were widely used in America and England. The English who lived near the marshes used opiates in prodigious amounts to treat their discomforts. For example, in 1858, journalists reported that in one town in the Fens district, laudanum "is sold in immense quantities, not only by our druggists, but by almost every little country shopkeeper and general dealer."[4] Laudanum would not have treated any illnesses (some of which might have been malaria) but, as with Talbor's potion, the alcohol and opium would have lessened aches and pains. Until the twentieth century, there was no effective or specific medicine for any illnesses. Opiates at least provided symptomatic relief, so it is not surprising that laudanum was popular.

Opiates, possessing strong sedative properties, were used in preparations sold to calm fretful babies. Laudanum soothed the baby and allowed the baby and the rest of the family and neighbors to sleep. A popular medicine in the United States and England was Mrs. Winslow's Soothing Syrup, an improved form of laudanum (see Figure 15.3). This was sold as a teething elixir for babies and contained fennel, anise, and caraway dissolved in syrup. But the important ingredients were alcohol and morphine. The people who made this syrup "issued a series of chromolithographs featuring loving mothers soaking their babies in alcohol and morphine sulfate."[5] This soothing syrup was labeled by the American Medical Association as a "baby killer."

Opiates were used by the ill for other reasons. As well as relieving pain and anxiety, the opiates have a concrete action—they slow down the bowels. If opiates are being used to treat pain, this action can cause unrelenting constipation. On the other hand, for people with severe diarrhea, slow bowels are a godsend.

This might seem a trivial point, but in the past (and still today in the underdeveloped world), clean water was not always available, and cholera

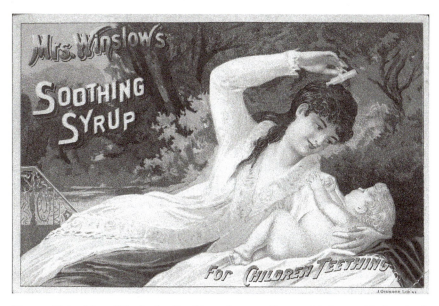

Figure 15.3 Mrs. Winslow's Soothing Syrup. (Patent Medicine Trade Cards [12.1.60.3], History Collections, Laupus Library, East Carolina University)

and dysenteric illnesses were common. (This was one of the reasons for the appeal of alcoholic beverages.) Without sewers to carry waste away from sources of drinking water and without chlorination, fecal contamination of drinking water was common—as were diarrheal illnesses. Without reliable clean water, diarrheal diseases caused severe illness and often death because of dehydration. Substances that could calm overactive bowels were valuable.

Laudanum was used in all classes of society. One historian writes that "most people in early nineteenth-century Britain dosed themselves with opium at some point in their lives."[6] William Wilberforce, the English abolitionist, began to use opium in 1788 when his physician prescribed it for a diarrheal illness and he used opiates for the next several decades.[7]

Women were particularly prone to use laudanum because of menstrual discomfort and pains associated with childbirth. (This would be seen again with morphine.) In the United States, one of the most famous people suspected of laudanum addiction was Mary Todd Lincoln, the president's wife. Some biographers think that she started to use laudanum to treat migraines and that it gradually took over her life.[8]

Although opium poppies were actually cultivated for a brief period in England and various parts of the United States, most of the opium in the nineteenth century came from India and Turkey. Mrs. Winslow's

Soothing Syrup probably owed its calming powers to poppies grown in one of those two countries.

Opiates and Writers

Many writers of the nineteenth century used laudanum and wrote about their experiences with it. The essayist Thomas De Quincey, for example, wrote *Confessions of an Opium Eater* about his use of laudanum. He said that he used so much that he might as well have bathed or swum in it.[9] Samuel Taylor Coleridge, the poet and critic, used laudanum for many years. He may have written the exotic and otherworldly poem *Kublai Khan* as well as the *Rime of the Ancient Mariner* under the influence of opium.

Coleridge and De Quincey initially used opiates to treat illnesses or pain. But they noticed that the laudanum also made them feel less anxious and more cheerful. They began to use laudanum even when not ill and they eventually became addicted. Coleridge and De Quincey had complicated attitudes toward the use of this substance. They disapproved of the other's laudanum use, and they criticized each other for using laudanum, for exaggerating their use of it, for not stopping, and for letting it interfere with their work.

Wilkie Collins, another great English writer of the time and a friend of Charles Dickens and Coleridge, wrote one of the first detective novels, *The Moonstone*. In this book, one of the narrators is withdrawing from tobacco, cannot sleep, and is given laudanum to help him sleep. Collins was writing, in part, from his own experience. He used laudanum to control arthritic pain. He, too, tried to withdraw from laudanum and followed custom by substituting one dangerous drug for another. He was treated with morphine, and in 1869 he explained to a friend why he had to decline a dinner invitation:

> One line (written most unwillingly) to ask you to forgive me if I am absent tomorrow night. My doctor is trying to break me of the habit of drinking laudanum. I am stabbed every night at ten with a sharp-pointed syringe which injects morphia under my skin—and gets me a night's rest without any of the drawbacks of taking opium internally. If I only persevere with this, I am told I shall be able, before long, gradually to diminish the quantity of morphia and the number of nightly stabbings—and so emancipate myself from opium altogether.[10]

In this brief note, Collins refers to his drinking laudanum as a habit and also notes that it helps him to sleep. It is clear that he thinks that injections are safer than taking a drug by mouth. He used the word *emancipate*; he was one of many who have compared addiction to slavery. Substituting morphine for the laudanum did not work, and he continued to drink large quantities of laudanum for the rest of his life. Walter Scott is said to have written *The Bride of Lammermoor* under the influence of opium and then not to have remembered a word of it. Other English-speaking writers of the time who may have used opium or its derivatives include Elizabeth Barrett Browning and Edgar Allan Poe.

Whether opium enhances or hinders the abilities of these writers has been debated.[11] It certainly provided some writers with good subject material. Did writers use opium more than others did? Perhaps there was no difference between the writers and the general population; the writers were just more skilled at describing their habits. The writers may also have thought that others would share their fascination with their own habits.

The addictive properties of opium were known. However, since opium was not illegal, addicts were able to get what they needed fairly simply and without breaking any laws. As noted in the alcohol chapter, opium was seen as a lesser evil than alcohol, and no less an authority than Benjamin Rush recommended opium as a safer alternative to distilled spirits.

Concern about Opiates Grows

Toward the end of the nineteenth century, unease about the use of opiates developed, due, in part, to the increasing use of patent medicines. Many of these medicines contained opiates, but, in a fraudulent manner, were sold to people who wanted to *stop* using opium. An exposé in the United States in 1886 revealed that 19 of 20 advertised opium cures contained opium (and that patent medicines sold to cure alcoholism contained alcohol). The sellers of these cures charged more than it would have cost the consumer just to buy opium. To make matters worse, these cures sometimes contained more opiates than the person was originally taking.[12] The cure worsened the problem and guaranteed that the customer would keep returning. This was a business with faithful customers.

By the early twentieth century, it was clear that opiates were being overused and oversold. Laudanum and patent medicines became disreputable, and their sellers seemed like charlatans. (The unsavory business of patent medicines and its demise are discussed at greater length in the chapter about Lydia Pinkham.) Regulation of medicines sold in the United States and England increased, and the use of laudanum and narcotics in patent medicines decreased.

In contrast to later opiate users, laudanum drinkers and patent medicine takers never seemed degenerate or criminal. They seemed innocent rather than wicked and aroused concern and pity.

Morphine Is Isolated

Opium is drunk (if dissolved in alcohol), or smoked. The discovery of morphine and then the manufacture of the syringe changed the ways in which opiates were used. After these advances, people began to inject morphine or heroin with more powerful effects.

In 1804, Friedrich Wilhelm Adam Sertürner, a 20-year-old German chemist, isolated the active ingredient of opium—the molecule within opium that is responsible for the pain-relieving and euphoriant effects. He named the substance *morphium* after Morpheus, the Greek god of dreams or sleep. Opium varies in the amount of morphine that it contains, depending on a number of factors. For example, some varieties of poppies produce opium with more morphine than do others. The growing conditions and ways in which poppies are cultivated and processed also change the amount of morphine in the opium. Raw opium has a morphine content that ranges from 3 to 30 percent, but each milligram of morphine has the same strength as the next milligram. The effects of morphine, therefore, are more predictable than those of opium and make it easier to use as medicine.

The development of the syringe was also important in the story of opium. In mid-seventeenth-century London, 24-year-old Christopher Wren had made a syringe-like device consisting of a bladder and quill, and he used this to inject a solution of opium and dry wine into a dog's hind leg vein. In other words, Wren injected laudanum into a dog. This was the first intravenous use of opiates.[13]

Much later, in the mid-1800s, Sir Alexander Wood in Scotland perfected the syringe and hollow needle. Medicine could now be given to people who were too ill to swallow or who were vomiting. Morphine injected under the skin or into veins has other advantages. It is stronger and works faster than morphine taken by mouth because so much of swallowed morphine is broken down in the liver. During the Crimean War (1853–1856) and the American Civil War (1861–1865), morphine was used as an analgesic and calming agent. Giving patients morphine was one of the few helpful medical activities of those wars.

At first, injectable morphine was thought to be safer than opium taken by mouth. Physicians thought that the smaller quantity of morphine compared to opium would make addiction less likely. In 1869, Wilkie Collins thought that an injection, or "stabbing" with "morphia," was less dangerous than drinking laudanum. Addiction was thought to be related to hunger, or the need for oral ingestion of a substance. People did not realize that one could come to crave an injection *more* than something taken by mouth.

In 1870, Sir Thomas Clifford Allbutt, an eminent British physician and professor of medicine at the University of Cambridge, wrote about the changing medical perception of morphine:

> Is [the physician] to withhold that means which relieves pain, which restores appetite, which encourages activity and promotes ease and cheerfulness? I honestly confess that, during a long period, I could not see my way to forbidding the repetitions of the morphia. Injected morphia seemed so different to swallowed morphia, no one had experience of any ill effects from it, and we all had the daily experience of it as a means of peace and comfort, while pain on the other hand was as certainly the forerunner of wretchedness and exhaustion. Gradually, however, the conviction began to force itself upon my notice, that injections of morphia, though free from the ordinary evils of opium-eating, might, nevertheless, create the same artificial want and gain credit for assuaging a restlessness and depression of which it was itself the cause ...[14]

Many observers noted that more women than men abused morphine. William Osler wrote about what he called the "morphia habit:"

> The habit is particularly prevalent among women and physicians who use the hypodermic syringe for the alleviation of pain ... physicians should exercise the utmost caution in prescribing morphia, particularly to female patients. Under no circumstances whatever should a patient with neuralgia or sciatica be allowed to use the hypodermic syringe, and it is even safer not to intrust this dangerous instrument to the hands of the nurse.[15]

Perhaps some of his pessimism was due to his contact with Dr. William Stewart Halsted. Osler knew that Halsted continued to use morphine throughout his life. Halsted's story illustrates the strong hold of opiate addiction, the ability of people to work despite the addiction, and the ease of deceiving physicians. (Halsted's story is recounted in a separate chapter.) Osler had a description, but no solution, for the problem of the "morphia habit," since we cannot trust the patient, especially if a female, nurse, or physician.

In the late 1800s and early 1900s, doctors prescribed morphine liberally. As noted by Osler, women were particularly likely to be prescribed morphine, presumably because of gynecological complaints. Gradually, the problem of morphine addiction, also known as morphinism, became apparent. Physicians frequently caused the problem with their generous use of the drug and, not immune to stress or disease, often themselves became addicted. Prescribing morphine began to be seen with disfavor and to become less common.

Gradually, a shift in the population of morphine users occurred. Young men from disadvantaged social backgrounds in urban locales began to use opiates to treat their anomie and to flaunt middle-class values. The situation would worsen with the synthesis of heroin.[16]

Bayer Laboratories in Germany Makes Heroin

The synthesis of heroin was worked out twice. In 1874, C. Alder Wright synthesized it in England. A later, but more consequential, synthesis belongs to Bayer Laboratories in Germany. Bayer, initially a dye factory, was about to become a pharmaceutical giant. In 1897, Felix Hoffmann at Bayer had made aspirin by adding an acetyl group to salicylic acid. Heinrich Dreser suggested that he do the same to morphine. Hoffmann added two acetyl groups to morphine and made diacetylmorphine ($C_{21}H_{23}NO_5$).

Bayer named this substance heroin either after the German word *heroisch* or the Greek work *heros*, both of which refer to the heroic effects of the drug. Bayer thought that it had found a safe substitute for opium or morphine and marketed it as an effective and nonaddictive oral sedative and cough suppressant (see Figure 15.4). As we now know, the marketers were too enthusiastic and oversold their product. The hope for a safe commercial product overwhelmed any caution.

The addition of two acetyl groups turned morphine, an addictive analgesic medication, into a more powerful substance. Heroin is fat soluble and therefore easily passes through the blood-brain barrier. This protective arrangement of cells around small blood vessels in the brain lets in, or transports in, only a small number of substances with the correct balance of fat and water solubility. Morphine does not pass through easily; heroin does. Once through the blood-brain barrier, the acetyl groups are removed and heroin is converted back into the active drug, morphine. As with the preparation of cocaine from coca and the distillation of alcohol from fermented brews, the more potent and quick-acting the substance, the more damaging it can be.

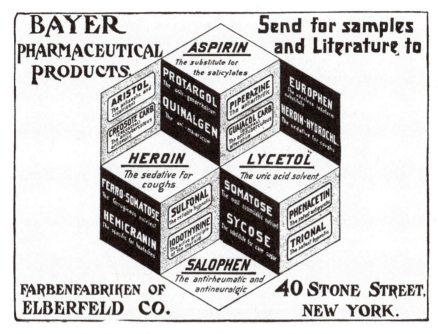

Figure 15.4   **Early Bayer Pharmaceutical Advertisement.** (© Corbis)

Opiates in the Twentieth Century

In the twentieth century, the use of opiates changed once again. The development of heroin made opiates more addictive and more easily transported. Unlike morphine, heroin never became a significant drug within medicine. It did become a drug that was abused.

Harrison Narcotics Tax Act of 1914

The Harrison Narcotics Tax Act of 1914 is often credited as the legislation that changed the way in which opiates were treated in the United States. It thrust the federal government into issues of health and commerce previously left to the states. The act was the beginning of the American criminalization of opiates.

The history of the Harrison Act is as complex as its legacy. It involves racism, a federal power-grab from the states, and a concession to China. It was a product of the Progressive Era and a precursor to Prohibition. The word *narcotic* in the name of the act is confusing. To physicians, narcotic means an opiate. But to others, including those who wrote the Harrison Act, it refers to any addictive drug, including cocaine.

In the 1800s in America and Europe, doctors, pharmacists, and mail order companies had few restrictions with respect to drugs. Sigmund Freud encountered no problems, other than expense, when he ordered cocaine from a pharmaceutical company. John Pemberton added coca leaf to beverages with no governmental interference. Cocaine-laced beverages were sold to help alcoholics, and patent medicines contained a panoply of substances, many addictive. In short, entrepreneurs marketed whatever they wanted.

As the use of cocaine and morphine increased toward the end of the nineteenth century, there was uncertainty about what to do. Many states and municipalities required cocaine and morphine to be available only with a physician's prescription, with a few loopholes for patent medicines.

At the same time, the American Medical Association (AMA) was attempting to increase the prestige and income of physicians. They claimed that physicians, in contrast to Lydia Pinkham and her colleagues, used "ethical drugs." Ethical drugs were those that were prescribed by a physician during an office visit and dispensed by a pharmacist. Unlike patent medicines, they were not advertised to patients (until recently). The AMA argued that only physicians could be trusted to decide what patients needed, and that they would never be influenced by thoughts of profit. The AMA supported more regulation, which fit with their interest in promoting their professionalism and high fees.

Meanwhile, racism and fears of immigration were also playing a role. Newspapers published sensational and spurious stories of cocaine exacerbating violent crimes committed by black Americans and of opium being used by Chinese men to seduce white women.

There were also international reasons for increased regulation. China deeply resented the Indian opium smuggled in by the English, and the United States was eager to appease the Chinese, important trading partners, by banning opiate trade at international conferences. There was pressure for the United States to be consistent by banning opiates within its own shores. In 1909, Congress passed the Smoking Opium Exclusion Act. This act banned the importation of opium for the purpose of smoking, but this was not enough. Indeed, in some ways this act worsened the situation, in that some opium smokers switched to other opiates such as morphine or heroin.

In 1913, Representative Francis Burton Harrison was in charge of convincing Congress to pass more antinarcotic legislation, against the wishes of the patent-medicine makers and some politicians, especially those from the South, who feared that states' rights were being compromised. States were responsible for health issues within their borders, and they were not eager to relinquish any control to the federal government.

The Federal Harrison Narcotics Tax Act of 1914 was eventually introduced, after many compromises, as a revenue and control measure. The goal was to stop nonmedical use of opiates and cocaine. All people who handled opiates or cocaine were required to register with the government, pay a "special tax," and maintain records of the drugs that they dispensed. The act contained no penalties for actual use of these drugs and was to be enforced by the Bureau of Internal Revenue. Purchasers of narcotics were to complete paperwork and give copies to district internal revenue offices. Patent medicines containing small amounts of cocaine, morphine, opium, or heroin could still be sold by mail order. Cocaine could not be used in any over-the-counter remedies. Persons violating the requirements of the act could be fined up to $2,000 or imprisoned for up to five years.

The Harrison Act allowed small quantities of opiates to be prescribed to people dependent on them. But the act was not clearly written, perhaps because of all the compromises that had been needed to get it passed. What exactly was appropriate medical use of opiates? Many people had become dependent on opiates because their physicians had prescribed them. Was it reasonable for those people no longer to be able to receive them? Whether the act involved police powers or allowed addicts still to obtain narcotics was not clear. The act was interpreted by subsequent Supreme Court decisions as forbidding the prescription of opiates to prevent withdrawal. The punitive and criminalizing approach of the American legal system toward drug abuse began with passage and interpretations of this revenue act.

Morphine clinics that had legally treated addicts with steady doses of opiates closed. Some had a difficult time withdrawing from opiates, and therefore some physicians continued to prescribe opiates for these people. Between 1914 and 1938, more than 25,000 physicians were indicted for prescribing opiates for addicts. Twenty thousand paid fines, and 3,000 went to jail.[17]

The Harrison Act and the way it has been interpreted ended easy and legal access to opiates. The days when respectable people, usually women, became addicted to laudanum or morphine were over. The Harrison Act, however, did not deter young thrill seekers from using opiates. Opiate addiction became an expensive, illegal, and possibly far more dangerous problem than it otherwise might have been. The Harrison Act decreased opiate and cocaine use but did not stop it, and the subsequent imprisonments of addicts who were now breaking the law led to overcrowding in the nation's jails and prisons.

Lexington Narcotic Farm

Because of a need for more drug abuse treatment programs, the federal Public Health Service (PHS) established two facilities to treat addicts and to conduct research. The PHS was dedicated to investigating illnesses affecting large parts of the community, such as the infectious diseases smallpox, yellow fever, tuberculosis, hookworm, malaria, and leprosy.

In 1935, the PHS United States Narcotic Farm was opened in Lexington, Kentucky, under the leadership of Dr. Lawrence Kolb Sr., one of the country's experts in drug addiction. The Farm occupied a thousand acres in a rural setting and had a dairy and chicken coop. It was an amalgam of rural prison, hospital, and rehabilitation facility. The idea of quarantining people came naturally to the PHS, given its history of involvement with contagious diseases. Perhaps people who started using opiates because of the stress, overcrowding, and filth of inner cities would find it easier to give up this habit in bucolic surroundings where they could work with animals and crops and be removed from their usual haunts.

Some residents of the Farm were federal prisoners who were opiate addicts, and some came voluntarily. The residents/inhabitants/patients/inmates also included artists, physicians, and street hustlers. One of the most famous residents was William S. Burroughs. He wrote about the Farm in his 1953 semiautobiographical novel *Junky*. Others who stayed at the Farm included jazz musicians such as Chet Baker, Sonny Rollins, and other entertainment figures such as Peter Lorre and Sammy Davis Jr.

Training of future physicians was an important part of the Farm. Physicians who trained there included Marie Nyswander and Jerome Jaffe, who will be discussed later.

Research was carried out at a part of the Farm known as the Addiction Research Center (ARC). The director from 1945 to 1963 was Dr. Harris Isbell, a highly respected medical scientist. Opiate withdrawal was studied and described. Methadone was used first in the United States at the Lexington Narcotic Farm. The nature of alcohol withdrawal was established here. Inmates were exposed to new drugs to see if they had addictive potential. Other drugs were studied also, including lysergic acid diethylamide (LSD) and other hallucinogens.

Another type of research was being carried out at the Farm. At the time of the Farm's existence, the U.S. government was concerned about the use of "brain washing drugs" possibly being used by other countries such as China and the Soviet Union. MK-Ultra was a secret program run by the

Central Intelligence Agency (CIA) in the 1950s that attempted to discover ways of behavioral modification that could be used by, or against, the enemy. The program involved about 80 institutions, including universities and prisons. MK-Ultra enrolled many people, including psychologists and psychiatrists, who experimented on the Farm's residents. Isbell worked for MK-Ultra and was described as a "gung-ho research scientist who remained on the CIA payroll for over a decade."[18] The connection with the CIA—which was fanatically interested in beating the Communists in mastering drugs to control either enemy agents or populations—was not publicized. However, some knew about parts of the program:

> It became an open secret among street junkies that if the supply got tight, you could always commit yourself to Lexington, where heroin and morphine were doled out as payment if you volunteered for Isbell's wacky drug experiments.[19]

Many of the Farm inmates participating in these experiments were prisoners. This was not particularly unusual at that time. Indeed, one of the greatest triumphs of the PHS had been accomplished using prisoners. Dr. Joseph Goldberger had used prisoners at Mississippi's Rankin State Prison farm to discover the cause of pellagra.[20] Much research involving drugs and infectious diseases in the twentieth century was performed on prisoners, who would be considered, in the twenty-first century, a vulnerable population. The idea of giving prisoners who were heroin addicts heroin for their participation in experiments now could be considered a form of coercion.

Despite the rural surroundings and the talent of many of the patients and clinician-investigators, most of the residents who left Lexington seemed unable, at least at the time of follow up, to maintain sobriety. The relapse rate was between 80 and 90 percent.[21] The idea that addiction was a chronic relapsing disorder was developed. Indeed, the PHS had more success in treating pellagra than it did in treating addiction.

In the 1970s, the climate surrounding research involving governmental agencies changed. There was increasing unease about the use of prisoners and embarrassment about another PHS project, the Tuskegee study. In that study, black men with syphilis were not told about their illness and were not treated. In 1975, a U.S. Senate committee investigated intelligence gathering by the CIA and Federal Bureau of Investigation (FBI), and discovered Project MK-Ultra. The project was ended as a result of this investigation. The ARC itself had been subsumed in 1948 by the newly established National Institutes of Mental Health. All of these factors, combined with the dismal recovery rate, led to the end of the Lexington Narcotic Farm in 1974 and its conversion back into a federal prison.

Trafficking Heroin: "The French Connection"

Heroin is potent, and its effects are short lived. These properties make it powerfully addictive and, therefore, a profitable commodity. The distribution of illegal drugs such as heroin is known as trafficking and involves chemistry and capital. Heroin traffickers have to be able to fund the purchase of large volumes of opium, laboratories, and protection from law-enforcement agencies.

One group of criminals that became involved in narcotics in the 1900s was the Italian American Mafia, and one of their infamous schemes was the "French Connection." This arrangement dated back to the 1930s, when Corsican gangs organized heroin labs in France. Opium from French Indochina or Turkey was shipped to Lebanon, where it was converted to morphine and then shipped to the French port city of Marseille, processed into high quality heroin, and smuggled into the United States.

Heroin abuse and smuggling increased after World War II. This development was related to the repeal of Prohibition, the invasion of Sicily in World War II, and the fear of Communism. The American Mafia had done well during Prohibition. After Prohibition was repealed and smuggling alcohol was no longer profitable, the American Mafia moved into narcotics. Charles "Lucky" Luciano was one of the new leaders (or dons) of the Mafia. He strengthened the organization, but he was successfully prosecuted after a police raid on 200 brothels that he was accused of running. He was sentenced to prison for 30 to 50 years. Nonetheless, there must have been a grudging sense of respect for him because he was approached by the U.S. government to help in the war effort. Authorities asked him to use his influence to make sure that dockworkers in New York did not go on strike and then they asked him for help in planning the Allied invasion of Sicily. Mussolini had persecuted the Mafia in Sicily, so Luciano, the Italian Mafia, and the U.S. government shared a common enemy.

Luciano was released from prison and deported to Italy in 1946 as a reward for assisting the war effort. Once in Italy, he established one of the world's most successful narcotics syndicates and continued the

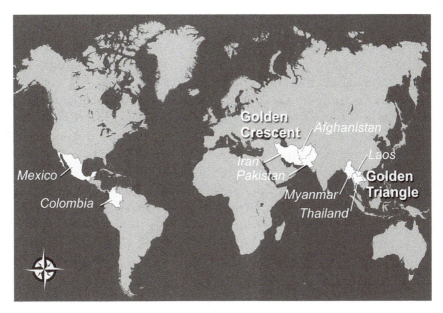

Figure 15.5 **Opium Growing Areas.** (© 2013 Joan M.K. Tycko)

French Connection, which supplied increasingly large quantities of heroin to the United States. The connection was weakened when, under pressure from the United States, illegal opium production was greatly diminished in Turkey. The Corsican syndicates of Marseille found another source of heroin in the jungles of Southeast Asia. This area—a roughly triangular zone in the highlands of Laos, Thailand, and Burma (now Myanmar) known as the Golden Triangle—supplied heroin to American soldiers during the war in Vietnam (see Figure 15.5).

Opiates and Vietnam

Soldiers have often used cigarettes and/or alcohol to help them deal with the horrors of war. American soldiers smoked cigarettes during the Vietnam conflict, but they used other drugs as well, including opiates. Their opiate use had a surprising result: it changed the way in which heroin addiction was treated.

American soldiers in Vietnam had trained in conventional warfare but became embroiled in a jungle-based guerilla conflict. It was difficult to know who was enemy and who was ally. Public support declined as the war went on. Alcohol was available but was not sold to soldiers under the age of 21 on army bases in Vietnam, and many soldiers were under this age. (The average age of the American soldier in Vietnam was 19.)

They were old enough to use a gun but not to drink beer. Marijuana was forbidden, but it grows well in Vietnam. It was easy to buy but difficult to transport, store, and hide because of its bulk and persistent and distinctive odor. Some soldiers thus turned to opiates.

Heroin and opium were available, potent, and cheap because opiate production in the Golden Triangle was flourishing. The connections between this area and the U.S. soldiers fighting in Vietnam were forged, some argue, by the United States itself. The theory is that in its efforts to contain Communism, the United States allied itself with the local enemies of the Communists, who were often involved in drug production. For example, when the French, also concerned about Communism, left Indochina in the 1950s, they turned over their own connections with the Laotian opium producers to the CIA. Opiates were flown from the Golden Triangle to South Vietnam and American soldiers. Drug trafficking in Saigon involved people in the South Vietnamese government and Corsican drug traffickers.[22] Young girls sold heroin at roadside stands along the highway from Saigon to American army bases.[23] Soldiers mixed opium with tobacco or marijuana and smoked it. They had unknowingly re-created the old Chinese custom of smoking *madak*.

In May 1971, two U.S. congressmen went to Vietnam on an official visit and reported that 15 percent of American servicemen were actively addicted to heroin. Journalists and army officials agreed that 10 to 25 percent of American soldiers in Vietnam were addicted to heroin.[24]

President Richard Nixon was criticized because of the war in Vietnam and also because of increasing domestic crime. The news of opiate use among the soldiers was therefore particularly unwelcome. His administration feared that opiate-using soldiers in Vietnam returning to the United States would continue to use heroin and that this would exacerbate tensions and crime in the cities, since much inner-city violence was perceived to be fueled by heroin addiction. Nixon declared heroin addiction to be the nation's "No. 1 Public Health problem" and declared an "all-out war on drugs" in the summer of 1971.

Nixon's administration was helped by American medicine. Dr. Jerome Jaffe, a psychiatrist, had trained at the Lexington Narcotic Farm and in 1971 was director of the Illinois State Rehabilitation Program. He organized drug treatment programs in Chicago and told President Nixon that his programs led to a 40 percent reduction in crime.[25] Nixon appointed him director of the newly established Special Action Office for Drug Abuse Prevention, and he became the first "drug czar."

One of Jaffe's first steps was to address the issue of soldiers returning from Vietnam. Rather than considering heroin use to be a crime that deserved punishment, he exploited the soldier's desire to leave Vietnam. He arranged to screen the urine of all military personnel who were leaving Vietnam to return to the United States. If a soldier's urine was positive for opiates, he could not go home for several weeks. This mandate meant that soldiers would not return to America while actively using opiates and was intended to stop the spread of the virus of opiate abuse. In other words, this process was a version of quarantine. The number of positive urine tests dropped from 10 percent of soldiers at the beginning of testing to less than 2 percent six months later.[26]

These results raised questions about opiate abuse in Vietnam. Was it indeed so common in soldiers? Had the press and the army overestimated its prevalence or severity? How was it possible that the soldiers could stop it so easily? Jaffe recruited an expert in the epidemiology of drug abuse, Dr. Lee N. Robins, to study opiate abuse in these veterans.

Robins, a sociologist familiar with drug abuse, interviewed over 800 veterans returning from Vietnam, almost all of whom had been exposed to opiates. She had access to a large amount of information about her subjects and cooperation from many agencies. This was an extraordinary opportunity, since most studies—to obtain large enough numbers of drug users—recruit from treatment centers. (As we shall see later, drug users in treatment centers are different from drug users in the general population.)

She and her co-investigators found that opiate use in Vietnam was indeed common. Almost half of the enlisted men used opiates in one form or another; about one third used heroin and one third opium. About 20 percent reported that they were addicted, meaning that they used opiates heavily and had withdrawal symptoms when they tried to stop. Use of alcohol and marijuana, despite the difficulties in obtaining them, was more common than the use of opiates.[27]

Robins re-interviewed these men three years after their return from Vietnam, and her findings became even more interesting. About half of the men addicted to opiates during their time in Vietnam did go on to use heroin when back in the United States. However, of this group, only about 12 percent of those addicted in Vietnam became re-addicted, and often only for a short period. In other words, many soldiers addicted to heroin in Vietnam used heroin on their return to the United States, but only briefly. Most who stopped had not been in treatment.[28]

The findings were reassuring. The problem was not as severe as Nixon feared. About half of the soldiers fighting in the jungles of Vietnam used opiates, but most were able to stop when they returned stateside. This was the opposite of what had been observed at the Lexington Narcotic Farm. It seemed that the gloom about heroin addiction was not deserved and that heroin would not become as common as the cigarette. We will return to these findings in the chapter about addiction.

Nixon and Methadone Clinics

Concern about heroin use in Vietnam had led to urine testing and research into the use of heroin in Vietnam. Another result was a new form of treatment that arose from Nixon wanting effective anticrime policies. In the United States, crime is a local—not federal—issue, but Nixon had promised to be a law-and-order president and in preparation for the 1972 election, he wanted a decrease in urban crime. Heroin was thought to drive urban crime, and Nixon saw the chance to fight crime by fighting heroin addiction. Methadone clinics were seen as a way of lowering urban crime.

Methadone was developed in Germany by I. G. Farben during World War II. The Allies controlled the supply of opium, and German scientists, in the absence of secure supplies of opiates and looking for ways to treat wounded soldiers, synthesized methadone as an analgesic.

In 1947, Eli Lilly and Company, a large American pharmaceutical corporation, began to manufacture methadone. Methadone is usually taken by mouth, and its effects last for at least 24 hours. The onset of action is slow and, partly because of that property, it does not lead to euphoria. Methadone is a useful addition to the opiate-like drugs that can be used to treat pain. However, it is not the long-sought-after synthetic substitute for opiates, since it is itself addictive. Methadone is still used for pain relief but also for another quite different purpose.

The story of methadone clinics begins at the Lexington Narcotic Farm. Marie Nyswander had worked there as a public health physician, switched specialties to psychiatry, and then trained in psychoanalysis. She also treated heroin addicts for four years in East Harlem, and wrote a book about this experience called *The Drug Addict as a Patient*. Vincent Dole, an endocrinologist, was impressed by her work and recruited her to work with him at Rockefeller University in devising new treatments for opiate addiction. (They eventually married.)

In early 1964, they tried to treat their opiate-addicted patients by hospitalizing them and giving them regular doses of morphine. The hope was that if the addict had a steady supply of opiates, the importance of the drug would diminish. This did not happen because the patients were either heavily sedated, in withdrawal, or focused only on their next morphine dose. It seemed that drug withdrawal did not work, nor did a steady drug supply.

Later, the two physicians treated two young men, both with long histories of heroin addiction and prison time, with high doses of methadone. Over a couple of months, their cravings for heroin faded. A generous daily dose of methadone broke their focus on the next dose. They also received much psychosocial rehabilitation. The two men became interested in normal activities of life and gave up their antisocial ways.

Dole and Nyswander established a methadone maintenance treatment program, or clinic, at the Beth Israel Medical Center in New York City. They argued that heroin had changed the brain chemistry of the addict and that methadone in high enough doses treated these changes, much as insulin treated diabetes. They emphasized that methadone controlled the problem but did not cure it and could be required indefinitely, just as a diabetic must take insulin for life. Dole's background in endocrinology perhaps helped them to see addiction in this way.

Other addiction experts noted that the heroin addiction itself had not been cured; the addiction had just moved to a legal drug that was easier to take. Was methadone that different from the fraudulent patent medicine addiction cures? Many experts believed that abstinence from drugs was the goal of treatment, but Dole and Nyswander disagreed.

Six years after they began to treat addicts with methadone, these clinics received an infusion of funding from Nixon's administration. This new funding was due to the efforts of Jaffe, Richard Nixon's drug czar. In the 1960s, he had worked for six months with Dole and then returned to Chicago in 1967, where he established methadone clinics as a treatment option. Jaffe changed the idea of the methadone clinic as an *experiment* to the methadone clinic as *treatment*. (His success with this is what had led to his appointment as drug czar.) He convinced the federal authorities that crime decreased with the introduction of methadone clinics, and Nixon's administration funded methadone clinics as part of the crusade against crime. By the end of 1972, over 60,000 people were being treated at methadone clinics in the United States. The Nixon administration actually allocated more federal funds for treatment than for law enforcement.[29]

Methadone clinics continue into the twenty-first century. Methadone maintenance is safe and effective. It is, for example, the treatment recommended for pregnant women addicted to heroin. Participation in methadone clinics also has the potential to reduce the transmission of infectious diseases, such as hepatitis and human immunodeficiency virus (HIV; the cause of acquired immunodeficiency syndrome [AIDS]), that is related to the intravenous use of heroin.

But methadone clinics are associated with some problems. For example, the clinics tend to be depressing and regimented facilities where regulations, paperwork, and rigid guidelines abound. Many patients have multiple problems, including addiction to other substances and unemployment. Diversion of methadone and deaths due to overdose are not uncommon. The air of optimism and excitement that surrounded the first methadone clinics has become stale.

Opiates in the Twenty-First Century

It is not difficult to grow poppies, and they continue to be grown around the world where conditions are suitable. Because they are annuals, the investment in them is minimal. That may explain why *P. somniferum* is mostly grown in parts of the world where there is much poverty and conflict, and few other ways of making a living. One area of great interest to the United States in the twenty-first century is the Golden Crescent, an area comprised of parts of Iran, Pakistan, and Afghanistan (see Figure 15.5). Poppies grown in Afghanistan are the principal cash crop of this poor country, but they also support crime and groups working against Western governments.

Poppies are low-cost plants, but once their opium is changed into heroin, large profits can be made. Because heroin is so potent, small quantities are valuable, and smuggling is easy. People known as mules sometimes carry it on them (e.g., in padded bras) or swallow it in packages (e.g., balloons or condoms). It is smuggled across borders in coffins, diapers, and children's toys. The mules travel from poppy-growing countries in Asia or South America to heroin-hungry countries such as the United States at great risk to themselves. The farmers and mules are not well paid for their work; the drug lords are some of the wealthiest people in the world.

Heroin

Heroin is perhaps the prototype of addictive drugs. It is associated with many problems, all of which are exacerbated by its illegal status. Heroin's effects are short lived, so frequent use is necessary. This explains why heroin use is often inimical to regular employment. A person addicted to heroin needs a regular supply of the drug, and this need can interfere with work. As he or she becomes more tolerant of heroin, he or she will have to consume higher doses to get the desired effect. Addicts may be driven to illegal activities to support their habit. Women may resort to prostitution, thus exposing themselves to sexually transmitted diseases and violence.

One of the problems of Prohibition was that alcohol was not always safely prepared, and that is one of the problems with heroin as well. There is little quality control over illicit substances, and the person buying heroin can never be sure of the potency or purity of the product. Heroin available on U.S. streets varies in quality and often is contaminated or adulterated. It is commonly diluted by a variety of substances, including lactulose or other sugars, powdered milk, quinine, caffeine, and strychnine.

Pure heroin can be sniffed or snorted, but heroin of poorer quality is more often injected. People sometimes progress from snorting or smoking heroin to injecting it (most commonly into veins) because tolerance to heroin grows rapidly.

Buprenorphine

Buprenorphine is a semisynthetic opiate derived from thebaine, one of the alkaloids found in the opium poppy. It binds tightly to the *mu* opiate receptor in the brain, but it is only a partial agonist. This means that it does not lead to the usual opiate effects of euphoria and relief from anxiety if taken by mouth. It does have enough opiate activity so that people dependent on, for example, heroin, can stop using heroin, take buprenorphine, and not suffer withdrawal or craving. However, there is a way around this for people intent on misusing the drug. If a person crushes the buprenorphine pill and then injects the buprenorphine, it can indeed lead to a "high."

To avoid this misuse, buprenorphine is often prescribed in combination with a full opioid antagonist, naloxone. Naloxone opposes the effects of opiates but is active only when injected. This stops people from "abusing" the combination of buprenorphine-naloxone because if the person injects the combination hoping for a high from the buprenorphine, the naloxone—now active—will block any effects of the buprenorphine.

Control of Pain in the Twenty-First Century and Oxycodone

Scientists have created several semisynthetic and synthetic opiates to treat pain. The hope is to create a medication as effective as morphine, without the problems of addiction and suppression of respiration. Instead, a new problem has arisen—prescription drug abuse. In the late 1800s, morphine and laudanum were commonly used to treat pain; in the twenty-first century, opiates in the form of pills such as oxycodone or Oxycontin have become popular. Oxycodone was developed in Germany in 1916. Like buprenorphine, it is derived from thebaine, one of the ingredients of opium. Researchers developed a time-release version of oxycodone and introduced this as Oxycontin in 1995. The time-release mechanism ensured that the drug would be delivered slowly to the body, thus making abuse difficult.

As so often happens with opiates, it turned out that this drug, too, could be abused. If the Oxycontin was ground up, the time-release mechanism was broken, and the powder could be snorted. Oxycontin abuse began in the Appalachians, Ohio, and Maine, and the drug became known as "hillbilly heroin." Oxycontin has also been involved in the phenomenon of "doctor shopping," or going from doctor to doctor to get prescriptions for Oxycontin or other opioids.

One measure of the magnitude of this problem is death by overdose. Deaths from accidental overdose of prescription opioids are increasing and, in 2010, overtook the number of deaths from heroin. Most of the people who died from these overdoses had a background of substance abuse and were taking Oxycontin in combination with other drugs and/or alcohol.[30] In other words, some people are re-creating laudanum but in a more potent form.

Effects on the Mind and the Body

How Opiates Get into the Body

Opiates are consumed in a number of ways. Opium itself can be dissolved in alcohol and drunk as laudanum. Morphine, heroin, and many of the synthetic or semisynthetic opioids can also be consumed by mouth. Morphine, heroin, and fentanyl, a synthetic opioid, can be injected just under the skin (skin popping), into muscle, or into veins. Pure heroin can be sniffed or snorted. Fentanyl patches applied to the skin are often used for patients with severe and chronic pain. Sometimes opium is combined with tobacco and smoked as madak, or it can be smoked alone. Some people smoke heroin; this is sometimes known as "chasing the dragon."

Effects on the Mind

Immediate

One of the most welcome effects of opiates is the relief from anxiety that has been compared to a "warm cocoon." Hallucinations and vivid fantasies may occur. Intravenous heroin is reported to be associated with intense pleasure often described as a whole body orgasm. The pleasure associated with the first use of opiates becomes more difficult to achieve over time as the person develops tolerance to the euphoriant effects.

Dependence, Withdrawal, and Addiction

With repeated use, opioids lead to physical dependence, meaning that the person develops withdrawal symptoms when he or she stops using them. Most people report that they continue using the drug mainly to relieve the discomfort that arises as the effects of the drug wear off. Moreover, the addict has to increase the dose of the drug just to prevent symptoms of withdrawal. Drug-seeking and drug-taking activities take over the person's life, interfering with other activities or interests.

Opiate withdrawal is marked by rebound exacerbation of anxiety. The withdrawing person is physically uncomfortable, with a runny nose, sweating, yawning, insomnia, loss of appetite, gooseflesh, back and abdominal pain, and tremor. The gooseflesh may be responsible for the phrase *cold turkey*. Sometimes, there are kicking movements, which may have led to the phrase *kicking the habit*. These symptoms peak between 48 and 72 hours after the last dose and can last for about a week. Although unpleasant, withdrawal from heroin is not as life threatening as withdrawal from alcohol can be.

People may crave opiates long after withdrawal has ceased, a phenomenon difficult for those without addiction to understand. This craving is easily exploited, and to great monetary advantage, by drug dealers. A few people use opioids infrequently, a pattern that is known as "chipping" and that can easily change into dependency.

Effects on the Body

Pain Relief

Opiates are powerful analgesics, or pain relievers. They also decrease the unpleasant arousal and fear often associated with pain. Over time, however, they can sometimes lead to hyperalgesia, or increased sensitivity to pain.

Gut

Opiates are constipating due to their activity at nerves controlling activity in the gastrointestinal tract.[31] The ability to slow the bowels was one of the reasons for the popularity of opium and laudanum. The muscles of the bowel that move waste through the gut slow down, so feces stay in the intestine for a longer time, which allows water to be absorbed from the feces and back into the circulation. People with diarrhea who are becoming exhausted and dehydrated may welcome slower bowels, but constipation can be problematic for ill people who use an opiate for pain relief.

Endocrine

Opiates affect the endocrine, or hormone, system. Serum concentrations of cortisol (a stress hormone) are lowered, and there is also a decrease in sex hormones. Opiate users often have decreased libidos.

The Nervous System

Opiates cause the pupils to constrict, leading to the well-known sign of pinpoint pupils. They can cause nausea and vomiting because of their effects on the chemoreceptor trigger zone in the medulla oblongata. This zone is the area that reacts to noxious substances that may be dangerous and should be expelled from the body by vomiting. Opiates also suppress the impulse to cough, which was why Bayer initially developed and marketed heroin.

In high doses, opiates are sedating and slow down breathing through their effects on the reticular activating system of the brain stem, where arousal occurs. This is the only part of the brain that is crucial to life, and opiates can cause death due to their ability to effect this system. Lethal heroin overdoses may occur accidentally when a user is unaware that his or her heroin is particularly pure and potent—that is, without the usual diluents.

Other Effects

If a person spends most of his or her money on heroin, he or she is prone to malnutrition and then more likely to develop infectious diseases such as pneumonia and tuberculosis. In addition, contaminants or additives present in injected heroin can damage blood vessels and lungs. A complication of heroin abuse that developed in the late twentieth century and persists is the problem of infections passed from person to person by the use of shared needles. Intravenous needle users became one of the first groups of people to become ill with HIV/AIDS. Heroin users are susceptible to other infections as well, including hepatitis B and C (serious liver infections). They are also susceptible to bacterial endocarditis, a serious infection of the inner lining of the heart.

Conclusion

Opium and its derivatives have eased pain and diarrheal diseases for many centuries but have also led to treatment refractory and complicated addictions. William Osler was aware of the terrible hold that opiates had on his Johns Hopkins colleague Halsted, and he warned that they must be used with great care. Yet he used opiates for his own patients, and as he was dying, he noted that opiates were the only remedy for his cough and agonal pain.

Notes

1. Quoted in Michael Bliss, *William Osler: A Life in Medicine* (New York: Oxford University Press, 1999), 469.

2. Martin Booth, *Opium: A History* (New York: St Martin's Griffin, 1996), 17.

3. Fiammetta Rocco, *The Miraculous Fever-Tree: Malaria and the Quest for a Cure That Changed the World* (New York: HarperCollins, 2004), 101.

4. Barbara Hodgson, *In the Arms of Morpheus: The Tragic History of Laudanum, Morphine, and Patent Medicines* (Buffalo, NY: Firefly, 2001), 48.

5. Ibid., 113.

6. Paul Johnson, *The Birth of the Modern* (New York: HarperCollins, 1991), 763.

7. Hodgson, *Morpheus*, 52.

8. Anne E. Beidler, *The Addiction of Mary Todd Lincoln* (Seattle: Coffeetown Press, 2009), 150–56.

9. Hodgson, *Morpheus*, 60.

10. Andrew Gasson, *Wilkie Collins: An Illustrated Guide* (Oxford: Oxford University Press, 1998), 119. The first part of the letter only is in the book; the second part of the letter can be found in a website, Wilkie Collins Information Pages, in the section titled Wilkie Collins and laudanum, last updated October 2013, ©Andrew Gasson 1998–2013, accessed November 9, 2013.

11. Alethea Hayter, *Opium and the Romantic Imagination* (London: Faber and Faber, 1968), 331–41.

12. William L White, *Slaying the Dragon: The History of Addiction Treatment and Recovery in America* (Normal, IL: Chestnut Health Systems/Lighthouse Institute, 1998), 67–68.

13. Dean Latimer and Jeff Goldberg, *Flowers in the Blood: The Story of Opium* (New York: Franklin Watts, 1981), 50–51. Wren is better known for his later and different achievements. He worked with Thomas Willis in describing brain anatomy and later still, he designed St. Paul's Cathedral.

14. David F. Musto, *Drugs in America: A Documentary History* (New York: New York University Press, 2002), 230–31.

15. William Osler, *The Principles and Practice of Medicine* (New York: D. Appleton, 1892). Facsimile reprinted by the Classics of Medicine Library, 1978; Gryphon Editions, 1005–7.

16. David Courtwright, *Dark Paradise: A History of Opiate Addiction in America* (Cambridge, MA: Harvard University Press, 2001), 85–88.

17. White, *History*, 114.

18. Martin A. Lee and Bruce Shlain, *Acid Dreams: The Complete Social History of LSD; The CIA, The Sixties, and Beyond* (New York: Grove, 1985), 24.

19. Ibid.

20. Frances Frankenburg, *Vitamin Discoveries and Disasters* (Santa Barbara, CA: Praeger, 2009), 41.

21. Michael Massing, *The Fix: Under the Nixon Administration, America Had an Effective Drug Policy; We Should Restore It (Nixon was Right)* (New York: Simon & Schuster, 1998), 85; Lee and Schlain, *Acid Dreams*, 24.

22. Alfred W. McCoy, *The Politics of Heroin: CIA Complicity in the Global Drug Trade*, 2nd rev. ed. (Chicago: Lawrence Hill, 2003), x–xi.

23. Ibid., 223

24. Ibid.

25. Edward J. Epstein, *Agency of Fear* (New York: Putnam, 1977), 147.

26. Jill Jonnes, *Hep-Cats, Narcs, and Pipe Dreams: A History of America's Romance with Illegal Drugs* (New York: Scribner, 1996), 276.

27. Lee N. Robins, "Vietnam Veterans' Rapid Recovery from Heroin Addiction: A Fluke or Normal Expectation?" *Addiction* 88 (1993): 1041–54.

28. Ibid.

29. Massing, *The Fix*, 119–20.

30. Centers for Disease Control and Prevention (CDC), "Vital Signs: Overdoses of Prescription Opioid Pain Relievers; United States, 1999–2008," *Morbidity and Mortality Weekly Report* 60, no. 43 (2011): 1487–92.

31. This property was used by Hans Kosterlitz in his Aberdonian guinea-pig studies described in the chapter about the discovery of the opiate receptor.

16

Discovery of the Opiate Receptor

The poppy is connected with some astonishing discoveries in neurochemistry, the science of the chemical makeup of the brain. In the 1970s, scientists discovered that there were opiate receptors in the brain, meaning that some molecules in the brain are poised to "recognize" opiates that come from poppies and react to them. The chain of discoveries leading to opiate receptors began with electric fish.

We usually think of electricity as an inanimate force connected with lightning or human-made generators, but small-brained and non-tool-building animals also generate electricity. The two most widely studied are the electric ray (found throughout the Atlantic, Pacific, and Mediterranean) and the electric eel of South America. The electric ray, also known as the torpedo fish, lurks in sand at the bottom of the ocean and uses an electric organ in its head to stun and capture prey with over 200 volts of electricity.[1]

David Nachmansohn was a scientist interested in the link between nerve and muscle. He saw that the fish's electric organ is composed of a series of electrocytes, or electric cells, in the same way that muscle is composed of a series of muscle cells. Nachmansohn realized that studying the large single-purposed electric organs of fish could help in understanding the nerve-muscle connection.

In 1937, Nachmansohn, then working in France, attended the World's Fair in Paris, saw some electric rays, and acquired some specimens. When describing this fish and its usefulness, he often quoted the words of a Nobel Prize–winning German chemist August Krogh: "Nature has created quite a few animals with the special purpose to help biologists to solve their problems."[2] Later, he moved to the United States and began to work with the electric eel.

Three decades later, Jean-Pierre Changeux, a French neuroscientist working at the Pasteur Institute in Paris, was studying transmission between nerves and looking for the long-wondered-about *receptor*. The receptor was then a *theoretical* structure on the cell membrane that received or recognized specific chemicals and that was involved in transmitting messages from nerve to organ. Acetylcholine was involved—were there acetylcholine receptors? Changeux joined Nachmansohn's lab at Columbia University in the 1960s and studied the synapses between the eel's nerve cells and electrocytes. Changeux wrote:

> As all these microscopic synapses have the same chemical composition, working with a kilogram of electric organ becomes practically the same as working with a single giant synapse of the same weight! The quantities of acetylcholine receptor available attain several grams. One need only separate it from the other components of the electric organ to identify its chemical nature.[3]

To find the acetylcholine receptor, one more animal was needed. In 1970, a Taiwanese psychopharmacologist, Chen-Yan Lee, gave Changeux some venom from the krait, a snake in his country. We fear snakes and their poisons, but their venom has scientific value. The Taiwanese krait paralyzes its prey using a protein, alpha-bungarotoxin. This protein binds to the acetylcholine receptor and stops the acetylcholine from activating muscle. This leads to the snake victim's paralysis and then death. Changeux wrote about the usefulness of toxins:

> [I]t is, in some ways, a wrong key that fits the right lock; once in the lock, it can no longer be removed, blocking the action of the receptor and paralyzing it. With radioactive tagging, it can serve as a very selective indicator of the receptor lock . . .[4]

Radioactive tagging, or radiolabeling, is a method of tracking substances by replacing certain atoms with radioactive isotopes. The structure can be "followed" by detecting the radioactivity to see where it sticks, or binds. Changeux and Lee used tagged alpha-bungarotoxin and the electric eel to find the actual acetylcholine receptor. They showed that acetylcholine latches onto a receptor that recognizes it and that this leads to a cascade of effects resulting in an electric discharge or a muscle twitch. The receptor was no longer theoretical and is now a cornerstone of our understanding of how the body works.[5]

Researchers then set to work to find receptors in the brain. Studying the electric organ or muscle is relatively easy: one can measure electric output or muscle activity. But the brain is a quiet organ. No sparks are emitted, and no muscles contract. Finding receptors, or binding sites, in the human brain was bound to be more difficult.

The search was arduous, but the potential rewards were large. There was particular interest in finding the opiate receptor (if it existed) because of opiates' powerful effects. The idea that opiates from poppies were attaching to something ready to accept them in the brain was intriguing. The search was also helped by the hope that money could be made. The market is large for safe ways to treat pain. If the opiate receptor existed and could be located and described, this might lead to effective and non-addicting pain-controlling drugs.

The acetylcholine receptor was an easier target than a possible opiate receptor. Researchers estimated that putative opiate receptors, in comparison to the abundant electric fish acetylcholine receptors, made up only a millionth of the brain's weight. The fish electric organ is a kilogram of one type of synapse; the brain in comparison is 1.5 kilograms of many different types of synapses. Researchers in Scotland, California, New York, Sweden, and Maryland looked for the receptor.

The researcher in Scotland was a German refugee. Hans Kosterlitz had fled from Nazi Germany in 1933 to England and then moved north to Aberdeen in Scotland. He did research on insulin and glucose but in the mid-1950s became interested in opiates. He developed techniques for finding opiate sensitivity in surprising body parts of the guinea pig, including nervous tissue surrounding smooth muscle in the intestines and the muscle in the vas deferens that propels sperm from the testicles to the urethra. Kosterlitz applied an electrical current to the bowel or vas deferens to make them twitch. Opiates such as morphine in the solution in which the bowel or vas deferens was suspended blocked muscular activity.

He used this preparation to study opiate antagonists, substances that block opiate activity. If he applied opiate antagonists to the solution containing opiates and then applied an electric current, the muscle fibers twitched.

Kosterlitz worked on these preparations for a couple of decades. He wondered why these tissues responded to morphine and came up with an idea that was so strange that he was hesitant to talk about it. Did the body produce its own morphine-like chemicals that the morphine mimicked?

Avram Goldstein, a physician and pharmacologist in Stanford, California, used radiolabeling to try to find the receptor. Goldstein used rat brains and because the brains were ground, his activity was called grind and bind. He labeled opiates with radioactive isotopes. Eric Simon at New York University Medical School and Lars Terenius at the University of Uppsala in Sweden were also working in this area.

The final steps were provided by Richard Nixon. His war on drugs involved more than incarceration and military intervention. The war also included (some) money for research and for treatment. In 1971, Dr. Jerome Jaffe, the first "drug czar," was given $2 million to spend on laboratory research. Grants were quickly prepared, and money was awarded to Kosterlitz, Goldstein, and also to one of Jaffe's colleagues, Solomon Snyder. Snyder and his group at the Johns Hopkins Medical School in Baltimore were newcomers to the opiate receptor brotherhood. In describing his relative ignorance, Snyder later said that he "hardly knew horseradish from heroin."[6]

In California, Goldstein was labeling opiate *agonists*, molecules that are like opiates and will bind to the receptor in the tissue to activate it. But Snyder's group refined this technique by tagging opiate *antagonists*. Snyder and his graduate student Candace Pert used radiolabeled naloxone, an opiate antagonist. This was an effective way of finding the receptor and tagging it. The antagonists bound more strongly than Goldstein's Californian agonists. This is another example of Changeux's "wrong key" that sticks in the lock better than does the correct key.

Snyder's group used some of the techniques developed by Kosterlitz and worked with strips of muscle from guinea pig intestines. In 1973, they discovered that radiolabeled naloxone attached specifically to the nervous tissue attached to guinea pig intestines—they had found the opiate receptor. Front pages of newspapers across the United States trumpeted the news. Journalists announced that the cure for opiate addiction would surely follow. Nixon's war on drugs had a victory.

Snyder and his students worked with other animals. They dissected rat and monkey brains and found opiate receptors in parts of the brain that process deep pain, emotions, breathing, and pupillary size—all areas that fit with the actions of opiates. Their discovery inevitably led to the question of the purpose of the opiate receptor. Why are there opiate receptors in intestine and brain?

Kosterlitz, meanwhile, was continuing his work with a young colleague, John Hughes, in gloomy Aberdeen. Every other day, Hughes would bicycle to an abattoir with bottles of whiskey. He would give whiskey to the butchers and in return was given pig heads. He dug out the pig brains and bicycled back to his lab, this time laden down by pig brains but no whiskey. He mashed up the brains with acetone into "soup" and then, laboriously, screened different pig brain extracts by applying them to Kosterlitz's bowel and vas deferens preparations. This work led to a "reek of rendered fat and airplane glue."[7] In 1975, when Kosterlitz was 72 and had officially retired and after many bicycle carriers of whiskey and pig brains, the Scottish team isolated two short peptides and worked out the amino acid sequence. This was a simple stretch of five amino acids. They named these peptides enkephalins. Later the name was switched to endorphins, short for endogenous morphines.

The Aberdonians had shown that Kosterlitz's strange idea had been correct. The juice from the seed capsule of *Papaver somniferum* has substances in it that mimic the brain's own peptides, which have their own receptors. These receptors recognize the peptides, now well characterized as five amino acid endorphins, but are also ready and willing to recognize and respond to opiates from poppies. The similarity between our own endorphins and the poppy's opiates explains some of the powers of these drugs.

Strenuous exercise, sexual activity, laughter, and eating foods such as chocolate and hot pepper cause the release of endorphins. The "purpose" of endorphins remains somewhat mysterious. Presumably they are involved in the body's capacity to deal with pain.

The laboratory work that led to the discovery of the opiate receptor involved electric fish, Taiwanese snakes, guinea-pig bowels, and pig brains. Nachmansohn highlighted the importance of acetylcholine in the delivery of messages by nerves, Changeux discovered the acetylcholine receptor, Snyder and Pert found the opiate receptor, and Kosterlitz and Hughes found endorphins. But these brilliant accomplishments have not yet led to safe opioids. Scientists have been unable to synthesize endorphin-like molecules that treat pain without leading to addiction.

Notes

1. Early Roman physicians used rays to shock their patients to cure their headaches and gout. The torpedo fish's name comes from the Latin *torpere*, "to be stiff or numb," which is what happens to prey when shocked by the fish.

Torpedo also refers to a self-propelled missile, which destroys its target on contact. The missile was named after the fish.

2. David Nachmansohn, "Biochemistry as Part of My Life," *Annual Review of Biochemistry* 41 (July 1972): 12.

3. Jean-Pierre Changeux, *Neuronal Man: The Biology of Mind* (Princeton, NJ: Princeton University Press, 1985), 91.

4. Ibid., 91–93.

5. This particular receptor turns out to also be a *nicotinic* acetylcholine receptor.

6. Solomon Snyder, *Brainstorming: The Science and Politics of Opiate Research* (Cambridge, MA: Harvard University Press, 1989), 10.

7. Jeff Goldberg, *Anatomy of a Scientific Discovery* (Toronto: Bantam, 1988), 19.

17

Pain and Anesthesia: The Role of Cocaine and Opiates

Introduction

Pain is an unpleasant sensation, easy to recognize and remember but difficult to define. We fear that our body is damaged. We use the same words—*hurt, suffering, pain, agony,* and *anguish*—to refer to both physical and mental distress. Indeed, physical and emotional pain may be processed in the same part of the brain, the anterior cingulate cortex.

Three of the substances of this book—alcohol, cocaine, and opiates—have been used to control pain. Alcohol is not a subtle or reliable pain reliever. It mutes the perception of pain but also dulls consciousness and leads to unpredictable behavior. Cocaine and opiates, in contrast, have specific effects on pain itself. Cocaine was the first local anesthetic, and opiates are our best pain-relieving drugs.

We will briefly describe pain by dividing it into three types. Then we will review the invention of local anesthesia using cocaine and the undignified discoveries of general anesthesia. Finally, we will review the use of opiates in controlling pain.

Acute Pain

Acute pain gets our attention and alerts us to do something. For example, if our finger touches a hot stovetop, we jerk our finger away quickly. We do not consciously control this response, yet we note the event, remember how unpleasant the experience was, and decide not to touch the hot stovetop again. This process begins when a pain receptor on a sensory neuron detects the extreme heat and sends a signal to motor nerves in the spinal cord. The motor nerves then direct the muscles of the arm to pull the finger away from the hot object. This automatic reflex happens without any input from our brain. At the same time, information travels up the spinal cord to the lateral thalamus, a relay station in the brain, which sends messages to the sensory cortex so that we know where the pain is. The lateral thalamus also sends messages to the cerebral cortex so that we can think about the pain, know which part of our body hurts, and tend to it. Finally, information also goes to the medial thalamus and from there to the anterior cingulate cortex in the limbic system, where we "feel" the pain. Some of the most vivid attributes of pain are the fear and suffering generated in this part of the brain.

Chronic Pain

Some pain is not as well understood or as useful as finger-on-the-stove pain. Pain receptors located on deep internal surfaces such as heart, lungs, or bowels send messages of vague and chronic aches. This kind of pain is difficult to localize or describe. Some pain occurs with no corresponding detectable physical problem and is known as idiopathic pain. Neuropathic pain due to a variety of neurological conditions can be long-lasting and severe. Ernst von Fleischl-Marxow, a friend of Sigmund Freud, suffered from severe neuropathic pain, as is discussed elsewhere. Diseases of the joints, such as osteoarthritis and rheumatoid arthritis, can lead to chronic pain. Finally, many types of cancer are associated with pain.

The purpose of these types of pain is not clear. The pain may encourage us to slow down and take care of ourselves, but moving less is not helpful for a person with arthritis or indeed for anyone. Severe and long-lasting pain can lead to insomnia, irritability, isolation, dependence on others, and depression.

With many types of chronic pain, there may be no outward sign of the problem. Those lucky enough not to have chronic pain often have trouble understanding this condition. Jon Kabat-Zinn, a molecular biologist who studies mindfulness, describes with empathy what it is like to have one of the most common of all pain syndromes, chronic low back pain:

> Just bending over the sink when brushing your teeth, or picking up a pencil, or getting into the bathtub or out of a car can trigger days or even weeks

of intense pain that may force you onto your back in bed just to bear it. Not only pain but also the threat of pain if you make a wrong move constantly affect your ability to lead a normal life. Thousands of things have to be done slowly and carefully, taking nothing for granted. Lifting heavy objects may be out of the question. Even lifting very light objects can cause major problems. And at those times when you are not in pain, the strange feeling of instability and vulnerability in that central region of your body can still lead you to feel insecure and precarious. You may not be able to stand up straight or turn or walk in a way that feels normal. You may feel a need to brace yourself or guard yourself from people or circumstances that might throw your body off balance. It is very hard to have your body feel "right" when its central fulcrum feels unstable and vulnerable.[1]

Surgical Pain

Rotten teeth, kidney stones, cavitating tumors, broken or gangrenous limbs, and the like have plagued humankind for millennia. There have always been surgeons who would fix or remove the offending organ or problem. But people trying to help others sometimes cause pain.

There were many ways of temporarily numbing a body part to eliminate the pain of a surgical procedure. Ice or restricting blood supply, for example, can limit inflammation and swelling, and decrease bodily sensations. But these techniques cannot be used for long periods of time without damaging the body. Also, it is difficult to restrict blood supply to some parts of the body. Tourniquets can restrict blood supply to a limb but not to a tooth or an eye. Perhaps this was why the great discoveries in pain relief came from dentists and ophthalmologists.

In the past, there were a number of ways of making a person unconscious so that surgery could take place. People were sometimes partially suffocated. A procedure might be helped by two bottles of whiskey—one for the patient and one for the surgeon so that he could tolerate the screams of the patient. In the 1800s, mesmerism or hypnosis was used. These methods were ineffective or lethal, or both.

Until a century and a half ago, surgical procedures were done without the aid of local or general anesthetics. Patients were held down by strong men or by straps. The best surgeons were the fastest. These gifted men were able to amputate limbs or remove kidney stones in less than a minute. For example, Robert Liston was a legendary nineteenth-century British surgeon. This six-foot two-inch man was a knowledgeable anatomist and skilled knife wielder. Sometimes, like a pirate in the Caribbean, he would hold a knife in his teeth. He sawed off limbs—asking medical students to time him—in 30 seconds. However, working in a slippery, bloody field and distracted by the patient's screams and writhing, his attention could wander or a knife could slip. During one operation, in a terrible moment, he amputated the finger of one his assistants. The patient and assistant both died of infections, and an observer collapsed and died. Even in those times, it was unusual for an operation to have a 300 percent mortality rate.[2] In another incident, a patient changed his mind before Liston could start cutting, fled the operating theater, and locked himself into a bathroom. Liston charged after him, broke down the door, hauled out the terrified man, dragged him back to the theater, tied him down to the table, and proceeded with the operation.

There was little people could do to control any of these three types of pain until the nineteenth century, when scientists began to take advantage of some unusual characteristics of the coca leaf.

Cocaine and Local Anesthesia

People chewing coca leaf or ingesting cocaine by mouth noticed a numb tongue and lips. Many suggested the use of coca and then cocaine as a local anesthetic. Carl Koller, an ophthalmologist, usually gets the credit for developing this idea and introducing it into medical practice to allow for pain-free surgery.

Cocaine was the first safe and effective local anesthetic. It causes numbness with no tissue damage and can be applied to any area of the skin or to membranes. The effect lasts long enough for brief surgery and then ends, so the body part can retain its useful sensitivity. Cocaine also constricts, or tightens, blood vessels so that there is less bleeding. Cocaine was useful in the removal of teeth, the treatment of toothache, and surgery on the eye, such as cataract removal. However, if cocaine was applied generously, some was absorbed into the body, made its way to the brain, and led to addiction.

William Stewart Halsted developed regional anesthesia in which cocaine was injected into the vicinity of large nerve trunks so that large areas of the body could be anesthetized. The person retained full consciousness. Halsted also became addicted to cocaine, as is discussed elsewhere.

Biochemists altered the cocaine molecule to make local anesthetics such as novocaine and xylocaine. These drugs work well as local anesthetics and have none of the stimulant, euphoriant, or addicting properties of the parent molecule, cocaine. Cocaine and its derivatives block the functioning of ion channels in the cell membranes of some nerves and thus interfere with transmission of the pain message to the brain. The person stays awake. Cocaine is still used in some operations involving the ear, nose, or throat.

Laughing Gas, Ether Frolics, and General Anesthesia

The most powerful way of preventing pain is to eliminate the conscious perception of it. General anesthesia is a deliberately induced unconsciousness in which the person is not aware of his or her surroundings. During general anesthesia, the person feels no pain and remembers nothing. The person cannot be woken and does not dream.

One of the agents that leads to general anesthesia is nitrous oxide—the famous laughing gas. This colorless gas, with the formula N_2O, was first synthesized by the English chemist Joseph Priestley in the late eighteenth century. Humphrey Davy experimented with the gas in 1799 and noted its analgesic properties, but the main use of nitrous oxide for the next four decades was for amusement. For example, nitrous oxide was used in traveling medicine shows and carnivals where people would be intoxicated for a few minutes and act foolishly.

Diethyl ether, also known simply as ether, was used for similar purposes. Ether is a colorless and volatile liquid that is highly flammable. Paracelsus, the chemist who named laudanum, noted that ether put chickens to sleep harmlessly. It was known in the past as "sweet oil of vitriol." College students and others used ether to intoxicate themselves at parties that became known as "ether frolics."

The discovery that these substances could lead to general anesthesia was one of the greatest events in medicine. The main impetus came from laughing gas parties and ether frolics rather than from laboratories or hospital clinics. The people who made the jump from medicine show to medicine were four Americans: Crawford Long, Horace Wells, William Morton, and Charles Jackson. Long was a physician; Wells was a dentist, Morton was a medical student and dentist, and Jackson was a chemist, physician, geologist, and polymath.

Long, the only practicing physician of the four, stole kisses from young women during ether frolics. He recognized that ether lowered consciousness and could be used for more serious purposes. In 1842, he used it to render a patient unconscious while he removed a tumor from the person's neck. He received little credit for this achievement, perhaps because he himself did not publicize what he had done for six years and played no part in the melodramatic events of the discovery of general anesthesia.

Wells was a young dentist who was troubled by the pain he caused his patients. In 1844, he thought of using nitrous oxide after attending a traveling nitrous oxide exhibition and seeing a man, while under the influence of this gas, injure his leg. Wells asked the man if he was in pain, and the man replied that he was not. Wells decided to try this gas on himself and under its influence, he had one of his own molars painlessly removed. He went on to use nitrous oxide in his dentistry practice. In 1845, Wells demonstrated the use of nitrous oxide in a tooth removal at the Massachusetts General Hospital (MGH) in Boston. This did not go well. The patient howled, the doctors jeered, Wells was humiliated, and he stopped his work in this area.

But Wells had a partner, Morton, who was not so easily discouraged. Morton was restless and entrepreneurial, a dentist, and a medical student. Morton worked with one of his medical school instructors, Jackson, a skilled chemist, to devise an efficient way of delivering Long's agent—ether—to the patient. Morton used Jackson's technique and ether to render a patient with a rotten tooth unconscious. Morton pulled the tooth and the man woke up, not even realizing that the tooth had gone. Patient and dentist were thrilled.

A short two weeks after this, Morton followed in the steps of his earlier partner and convinced MGH physicians to try his new substance. In mid-October 1846, John Collins Warren, an eminent surgeon, allowed Morton to etherize a young man who had a large vascular tumor on his jaw. Morton applied ether, and the man lost consciousness. Warren removed the tumor and the man woke up, having suffered no pain. Warren famously announced, "Gentlemen, this is no humbug." This event became widely publicized, and general anesthesia was born. October 16 is now celebrated as Ether Day and the operating theater where it was first used at MGH in Boston is still known as the Ether Dome.

Morton tried to keep the nature of his substance secret so that he could be the sole and wealthy provider. However, the characteristic smell of ether could not be hidden, and his attempts at secrecy and interest in personal reward did not endear him to those desperate for pain relief. The quarrels among the last three men and their supporters about who deserves the most credit were bitter. Morton claimed credit for the introduction of ether and was not shy about his claims. He appealed to Congress for recognition and tried to sue the government when it was not forthcoming. Jackson, who had assisted Morton, turned against him, claiming that he was the person responsible for the discovery. In the summer of 1868, Morton was in New York, still pursuing his dispute with

Jackson, when he became ill, possibly due to a severe heat wave, and died at the age of 48.

Jackson had been a fierce adversary. He never backed down from a fight over discoveries. He had a long running dispute, for example, with Samuel Morse over who invented the telegraph. Jackson recruited supporters, including his brother-in-law Ralph Waldo Emerson. Jackson was convinced that his work with the delivery of ether was the key. Despite support from Emerson, one of the most respected men of the day, Jackson did not succeed. He also felt, as did Morton, unappreciated for his work with anesthesia. In 1873, he suffered a neurological event, lost his power to speak, and was hospitalized at McLean Hospital, a psychiatric hospital outside of Boston, and remained there as a patient for seven years until his death at the age of 75.

Wells, meanwhile, fared no better. From his point of view, he had the courage to experiment on himself and then take his idea to MGH. And he had tutored Morton. He heard about Morton's success at MGH and became enraged at his exclusion. He developed an interest in the newly popular liquid chloroform. One evening, possibly under the influence of chloroform, he assaulted prostitutes by throwing sulfuric acid on them. He was jailed. He anesthetized himself with chloroform, cut open an artery in his thigh, and bled to death at the age of 33.

Despite the tragic and sordid background to this discovery, general anesthesia changed medical practice. It made operations tolerable. One more achievement was necessary for the science of surgery to develop: control of infection. Influenced by the discovery of Louis Pasteur that there were airborne bacteria, the Scottish surgeon Joseph Lister had introduced asepsis into surgery by using carbolic acid sprays. The rate of infections dropped. The Hungarian physician Ignaz Semmelweis and the American physician Oliver Wendell Holmes Sr. showed that transferring cadaveric germs to pregnant or postpartum women often led to fatal infections and that washing between examining corpses and delivering babies led to fewer maternal deaths. After much foot-dragging, physicians accepted these findings, and surgery became a safe and effective discipline. Surgeons could operate with some thoughtfulness and deliberation, without the reckless speed of Liston and without infecting their patients.

Nitrous oxide and ether were not without their problems. They were unpredictable in their anesthetic effects and could lead to coughing and vomiting. Ether was more effective than nitrous oxide but quite dangerous because it was easily ignited. General anaesthesia was achievable, but needed better agents.

The invention of liquid chloroform, another agent that led to general anesthesia, is also a debated event. Justus von Liebig, one of the rivals of Louis Pasteur, claimed the honor. In 1872, he published a paper claiming that in 1831 he had been experimenting with chlorine and alcohol, and thus formed chloroform. An American, Samuel Guthrie, claimed that he had first made it in that same year. Finally a French pharmacist, Eugene Soubeiran, argued that he had invented it.

The discovery of this liquid as a useful anesthetic agent is less debated. James Simpson, a renowned Scottish obstetrician who had studied with Robert Liston, met with a group of friends weekly to experiment with different chemicals. In 1847, they discovered that chloroform led to brief unconsciousness. It became the preferred anesthetic agent in Edinburgh and then the United Kingdom. Chloroform was not flammable and in some respects easier to use than ether. But chloroform led to liver damage and unpredictable deaths.

Chloroform was an element of many patent medicines. Chlorodyne, for example, was a famous English patent medicine. In one formulation, it was made of treacle, opium, capsicum, chloroform, ether, and peppermint. Other formulations included cannabis, laudanum, or chloroform. Kimball White Pine and Tar Cough Syrup was a popular American product containing alcohol and chloroform.

Chloroform also developed an unpleasant reputation in a different field of endeavors. Liquid chloroform was easily obtained by people with no medical interests. It was a useful tool for criminals. A person could soak a sponge in it and then hold it over someone else's face. The victim would quickly succumb to the chloroform vapors. In the nineteenth century, chloroform was used as an aid to burglary and murder.[3]

Although most welcomed the idea of freedom from pain, there was some opposition to the use of anesthetics. One physician claimed, "Pain is the wise provision of nature and patients ought to suffer pain while their surgeon is operating; they are all the better for it, and recover better!"[4]

The opposition was fiercer with respect to the use of anesthesia in labor. Some of this was founded on the reasonable fear that it might interfere with the natural process of birth or injure the mother or baby. Some resistance was founded on the belief that pain in childbirth was mandated by Genesis 3:16: "I will greatly increase your pains in childbearing; with pain will you give birth to children."

The dispute was settled by Queen Victoria in 1853. The queen knew a considerable amount about labor and childbirth, since she had had seven children with no anesthesia. For her eighth child, she chose to use chloroform, the agent recommended by Simpson. Her anesthetist was John Snow.

Snow was a good choice because he was one of the most careful physicians of the time. By mapping the outbreaks of cholera in London, he proved that a particular water supply was contaminated. He persuaded the local council to remove the Broad Street pump handle, which was delivering contaminated water to the inhabitants of some parts of London. This action is associated with ending a cholera outbreak in London (although the cholera outbreak was already ending). Snow was also interested in the delivery of anesthetic agents and worked out ways of calculating correct dosages of these drugs. He devised an apparatus to ensure that the correct dose was administered. Anesthesia was becoming more scientific.

The royal anesthesia and delivery went well. The queen was pleased, and Dr. James Simpson became Sir James Simpson. Victoria's eighth child was Leopold, who subsequently became Duke of Albany. He suffered from hemophilia and died at the age of 30 after a fall, but as far as we know, he suffered no complications from being the first royal baby to be born while his mother was free of pain. Snow later administered chloroform to the queen when she delivered Beatrice, her ninth child, in 1857.

Scientists have devised new drugs that are safer than the early anesthetic agents. General anesthesia now involves induction or initiation, often with propofol or a barbiturate, and maintenance with sevoflurane or desflurane. These improvements, although important, lack the game-changing nature of the discoveries made by the unhappy and quarrelsome quartet of Long, Wells, Morton, and Jackson.

Opiates as Analgesic Drugs

None of the four substances discussed in this book are used as general anesthesia agents. Opiates come the closest but cannot be used as general anesthetics because in doses sufficient to stop the perception of pain, they depress the brain center that controls breathing and can cause death. However, opiates are sometimes used along with other general anesthesia drugs to allow smaller doses of the general anesthetic to be used.

The body has its own system of analgesia. This is odd, since pain protects the body. Yet there are some circumstances where pain, if only briefly, should be ignored. For example, the person fleeing from a predator should not be slowed down by a painful twisted ankle or broken toe. Stories of soldiers in battle who sustain horrific wounds yet do not complain of pain at the time are legion. We do not experience pain if we are concentrating on an important task or are swept away by emotion. The body's own opiates, the endorphins, suppress incoming pain signals.

This may be the clue to the riddle of the effectiveness of opiates. To the opiate receptors, the opiates look like our own endorphins. Opiates mimic our endorphins and let us bear pain with equanimity. They block nerve transmission in sensory pathways of the spinal cord and brain that signal pain. Opiates also act in the anterior cingulate cortex. They differ from local anesthetics, such as cocaine, in that they work in the body as a whole, not locally.

Chemists have altered molecules found in the poppy to modify their effects. Some pain-killing drugs are made from substances in opium and are therefore called semisynthetic. Hydrocodone, which is often combined with acetaminophen, is made from codeine or thebaine, both of which are found in opium. Oxycodone and buprenorphine are both made from thebaine. Methadone, fentanyl, and meperidine are synthetic opiates, meaning that they are made in the laboratory. Fentanyl is sometimes used intravenously or in a patch that delivers the drug over several days. Buprenorphine and methadone are used primarily to treat opiate addiction. The gold standard of pain medications continues to be morphine, the active ingredient of opium.

Patients in pain generally do not become addicted to opiates, and they stop using them once the pain has gone. However, some people may claim to be in pain and get opiates to maintain their addiction or to sell to others. This latter activity is known as diversion, and it causes problems to the prescribing physician, who can be investigated for the patient's misuse of the drugs. The people who suffer most from diversion are those in chronic pain who may find physicians reluctant to prescribe adequate doses of pain-relieving medicine. Patients who divert opiates cause turmoil (mostly to themselves) out of proportion to their number and may create the false impression that opiates used to treat pain are often addicting.

Opiates are also used in hospice and palliative care. Patients at the end of their lives can, if necessary, take doses high enough to eradicate pain without unduly worrying about addiction or the medication's effects on breathing.

Control of Pain in the Twentieth and Twenty-First Centuries

Salicylic acid, a bitter extract of willow bark, had long been used to treat aches and pains, but its use was limited by its irritant effects on the stomach. In the 1890s, Felix Hoffmann of Bayer Laboratories in Germany replaced the hydrogen of salicylic acid's phenolic –OH group with an acetyl group (CH_3CO) and formed acetylsalicylic acid. Hoffmann tested this on his father, who had arthritis, and then Bayer then tried it on many of its own employees. It was successful and was patented in 1900 as aspirin, one of the most successful medications ever made. (During the same time period, Hoffmann added two acetyl groups to morphine to form heroin.)

Other pain medications include other nonsteroidal anti-inflammatory medications, such as ibuprofen, and acetaminophen. Corticosteroid creams and lotions ease the pain of skin irritations. Tricyclic antidepressants or selective serotonin reuptake inhibitors sometimes alleviate pain. Anticonvulsants such as carbamazepine, gabapentin, and pregabalin can lessen pain in some neurological disorders. These medications have few or no effects on the pleasure centers of the brain and are not taken for pleasure or abused in the way that cocaine and opiates are. They all have their own side effects and are not as effective as the opiates.

There are other nonpharmacological approaches to managing pain such as hypnosis, massage, electrical stimulation, and acupuncture. Even with the use of these therapies and medications, opiates continue to be considered the most effective treatment for pain.

Conclusion

In the twenty-first century, we are lucky that we no longer have to be tied down or made drunk to withstand surgery. The first useful pain relievers—nitrous oxide, ether, and chloroform—seemed miraculous. They were all used at times recreationally as intoxicants or as drugs of abuse. They never became popular because of their unpleasant side effects and the difficulty involved in either making or transporting them. Cocaine, opiates, and their derivatives are more useful pain-relieving substances but have powerfully addicting properties that also make them dangerous.

One-and-a-half centuries after the remarkable events of Ether Day, patients and surgeons no longer have to dread operations. General, local, and obstetrical anesthesia are common, safe, and effective. However, for people with chronic pain, problem-free relief remains elusive.

Notes

1. Jon Kabat-Zinn, *Full Catastrophe Living* (New York: Delta, 2009), 300–301.

    2. Richard Hollingham, *Blood and Guts: A History of Surgery* (New York: Thomas Dunne, 2008), 42.

    3. Linda Stratmann, *Chloroform: The Quest for Oblivion* (Stroud, UK: Sutton, 2005), 116–33.

    4. Julie M. Fenster, *Ether Day* (New York: HarperCollins, 2001), 164.

18

The Gladstones and Opium

The Gladstones were a prominent family in eighteenth-century England whose experiences with opium and laudanum illuminate the complex and contradictory role of these drugs in England. William Gladstone, the best-known member of the family, spoke out passionately against the Opium Wars. He and his sister, Helen, both used laudanum, and Helen became addicted to it. The family was also involved with slavery and sugar cane plantations in the West Indies.

John Gladstone (1764–1851), a Scottish businessman, was the patriarch of the family. He had six children and is remembered today chiefly as the father of William, who was prime minister of England four times (see Figure 18.1.) But John Gladstone had many achievements of his own. He was a religious man with unrealized political ambitions and was successful in business due to his skill in international commerce, trading in grain from England and in cotton from America.

He made a good part of his fortune in sugar plantations in the West Indies. He "owned" over a thousand slaves in British Guiana (now known as Guyana). Although it was well known that the treatment of the slaves there was cruel, John thought that on his plantations, the slaves were treated well. How is it that he could have thought this? The answer is simple—he never set foot on the plantations and was convinced (or chose to be convinced) by his overseers that slaves on his plantations were well treated and content. Olaudah Equiano (ca. 1745–1797), a slave in the West Indies in the eighteenth century, wrote this about absentee landlords:

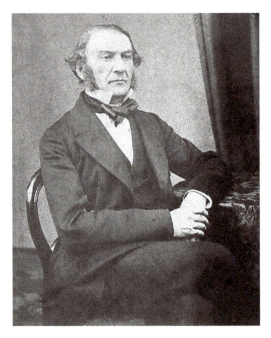

Figure 18.1 **William Ewart Gladstone. (Wellcome Library, London)**

Another negro man was half hanged, and then burnt, for attempting to poison a cruel overseer. Thus by repeated cruelties are the wretched first urged to despair, and then murdered, because they still retain so much of human nature about them as to wish to put an end to their misery, and retaliate on their tyrants! These overseers are indeed for the most part persons of the worst character of any denomination of men in the West Indies. Unfortunately, many humane gentlemen, by not residing on their estates, are obliged to leave the management of them in the hands of these human butchers, who cut and mangle the slaves in a shocking manner on the most trifling occasions, and altogether treat them in every respect like brutes.[1]

Because John Gladstone was the owner, some of the slaves on his plantations took his name. One slave, Quamina, named his son Jack Gladstone. In 1823, these two men organized an uprising among the slaves on the coast in Demerara (now a name of sugar) in British Guiana. The uprising was quelled. Quamina was hung at the entrance to Gladstone's plantation, and Jack Gladstone was deported. Accounts of this revolt strengthened the growing abolition movement in England.

In the early 1800s, William Wilberforce, a friend of the Gladstone family, spearheaded the English abolition movement. John's wife and eldest daughter, Anne, were distraught about their family's involvement in slavery. But John and his sons, profiting handsomely from their sugar estates, were incredulous of Wilberforce's belief that slaves should be freed. John insisted that abolition would be disastrous for the sugar plantations and also for the slaves themselves. Nevertheless, slavery was abolished in the British Empire in 1834.

William Gladstone (1809–1898), John's youngest son, inherited his father's interest in religion and politics. He was an intelligent and prodigiously energetic man who struggled all his life to do what he thought was demanded by his Anglo-Catholic beliefs. He had considered a career in the Church before he went into politics. John's wealth allowed his son to pursue a political career, and William became known for his thundering speeches.

Some of William's first political activities had to do with protection of his father's commercial interests. He protested against the abolitionists, and when he saw that his family was on the losing side of the argument, he helped arrange generous compensation for his father (and indirectly for himself) and other English planters for the loss of "their" slaves. Since William's political career was funded by the work of his father's slaves—growing and processing sugar cane in the deforested West Indies, he might have felt that he owed it to his father to argue for compensation. The Gladstones won this argument. The British government paid £20 million, a large amount of money at the time, as compensation to the slave owners for the loss of their slaves.

Helen Gladstone (1814–1880) was the youngest of John's six children. Helen and William were close as children and had intense discussions about religious matters, with William instructing and haranguing. At the age of 14, she began to be seen as a "difficult" child and to be treated by a doctor who was also treating her invalid mother. She and her mother were both treated with galvanism, the application of electricity to the body, which was a popular treatment at that time for "nervous" complaints. By the age of 21, Helen was being treated with laudanum.

In 1838, at the age of 24, her use of laudanum became out of control, and the family looked for a cure in Europe. (Faith in geographic cures, as we saw with William Halsted, is not rare.) She was sent with William to a health resort in Ems, a small town in Germany with hot springs. Here she met a Russian Polish count, Leon Sollohub. A romance developed, and they planned marriage. Back in London, Helen was told that Sollohub's family in Russia would not allow the marriage, and this possible escape route from England, laudanum, and her overbearing brother was blocked. She never married.

At the age of 26, Helen began to correspond with Dr. Wiseman, a leading member of the English Roman Catholic clergy. A couple of years later, she went to a convent in Birmingham and converted to Roman Catholicism. This was anathema to William, a stout opponent of this religion, who suggested that she be expelled from the family. John, a calmer man in matters of religion, refused to do this.

In 1845, at the age of 31, Helen and a companion went to a spa in Baden-Baden, Germany. When the companion tried to stop Helen from using laudanum, Helen dismissed her. While there, Helen's laudanum use continued and worsened. The family sent William to Germany to bring her back to England. Once William arrived at the spa, terrible scenes ensued. Helen locked herself in her room for several days at a time. Sometimes she stopped speaking and seemed paralyzed. She refused to talk to William or to eat for 12 days. She was force fed liquids. The drama eventually ceased, and her doctors returned her to England with a doctor, a priest, and William.

Back in London, she stayed in one room. This time it was not at her request but at the insistence of her family. "She attempted to send messages by dropping them from the window to a street musician and tried to sell jewelry to raise money. Tom [another brother] caught one of the maids with a parcel of things Helen had given her to sell."[2] Her efforts to get laudanum continued.

In 1847, at the age of 33, Helen went to a spa in Leamington, England. The stay was again unsuccessful, and her use of laudanum continued. A year later, she was sent Edinburgh to be under the care of a "nerve specialist." While there, she was in a particularly agitated state: "her jaw was locked, both hands were clenched, and she was calling loudly for chloroform."[3] Her doctor in Edinburgh, with some disapproval, reported to William that she was visited by Dr. Wiseman and that the following happened:

> The party assembled. The folding doors were thrown open between the drawing-room and Miss G.'s bedroom. Paraphernalia were brought from the nunnery. A book-case was converted into an altar ... High Mass was performed. Dr. Wiseman, advancing with a relic (the knuckle bone of some female saint) touched with this relic the jaw! It flew open. The hand! The fingers sprang open. The other hand! it, too, unclosed. Then "Te Deum" was sung by the whole assemblage! A miracle was, of course, declared![4]

Clearly this physician did not appreciate the involvement of Dr. Wiseman and described the event in an unpleasant and mocking way. The physician was writing to someone who shared his prejudices against Roman Catholicism, and perhaps this sharpened his pen.

The miraculous cure was not permanent, and, for the rest of her life, Helen had relapses. In 1855, at the age of 41, she was once again using opium heavily. A religious community in Rome cared for her. She remained eccentric until her death at the age of 66.

Helen's addiction to laudanum deeply upset her family. Despite his interest in global trade, John argued against England's opium trade with China, based in part on his observations of the effects of laudanum on his daughter. John, the absentee landlord, could not understand what slaves in the West Indies suffered. But close contact with his daughter taught him about the agonies of opium addiction. William was equally blind to the horrors of slavery in the West Indies and also had an easier time understanding the painful bonds of opiate addiction. He wrote, with respect to his sister, "The ruin brought by opium on the moral as well as the physical constitution of human beings is one of the saddest sights this world can offer."[5] Father and son had been as one on the subject of slaves and were just as allied in their feelings about the opium trade in China.

When the first Opium War began in 1839, William was 30 years old and had been in Parliament for eight years. He defied the powerful Palmerston who was then prime minister and denounced the war. He spoke eloquently:

> a war more unjust in its origin, a war more calculated in its progress to cover this country with permanent disgrace, I do not know, and I have not read of . . . under the auspices of the noble Lord [our] flag is hoisted to protect an infamous contraband traffic . . .[6]

He even suggested that the Chinese were justified in poisoning British wells.[7] His opposition to his country's warfare continued and in 1857, his condemnation of the second Opium War led in part to the dissolution of Parliament. But in a wave of patriotic fervor, Palmerston was re-elected.

Many of William's political stances, such as his discomfort with British imperialism, were highly principled. (His defense of slavery in the West Indies, in contrast, seems so much to do with protecting his family's interests that it makes us wince.) Some of his other activities seemed questionable both during and after his lifetime. For example, he took great personal interest in some prostitutes. This always ended badly, or, at the least, got him bad publicity. His diaries have revealed another odd sexual peccadillo, self-flagellation, which has also damaged his reputation. His religiosity struck many as extreme. An example of this was his final action with respect to Helen. She defied him and converted to Roman Catholicism. He never was able to accept this. At the time of her death, he insisted, with no evidence, that she had returned to the Church of England and arranged for her burial in a Church of England cemetery.

He was not as extreme when it came to laudanum. William, despite his observations of the harm laudanum did to his sister, was himself a laudanum user. He often drank laudanum in coffee before some of his orations in Parliament. For him, the combination of opium, alcohol, and caffeine was not harmful. Perhaps he was taking Wilberforce as an example. Wilberforce used laudanum every day for the last 45 years of his life because of problems with his bowels.

Notes

1. Olaudah Equiano, *The Interesting Narrative and Other Writings*, ed. Vincent Carretta. (New York: Penguin, 1995), 105.

2. S. G. Checkland, *The Gladstones: A Family Biography, 1764–1851* (London: Cambridge University Press, 1971), 353.

3. Philip Magnus, *Gladstone: A Biography* (New York: Dutton, 1964), 83.

4. Ibid.

5. Checkland, *Gladstones*, 377.

6. Julia Lovell, *The Opium War: Drugs, Dreams and the Making of China* (London: Picador, 2011), 107.

7. Magnus, *Gladstone*, 52.

19

Opium Smoking, the Opium Wars, and Emigration from China

Introduction

Some military conflicts are named after years, such as the War of 1812; other wars are named after flowers, such as the War of the Roses, or after cartographic features, such as the Battle of the Bulge. Not many conflicts are named after agricultural substances or beverages. The Whiskey Rebellion of 1791 in western Pennsylvania is one example. The Tea Party in Boston has become famous. Another example of an agricultural substance lending its name to a conflict is the nineteenth-century Opium Wars between Britain and China.

The background to this conflict consists of seeking profit while balancing trade. The English were addicted to drinking tea and the Chinese to smoking opium. The English wanted to trade one for the other. The Chinese government opposed this tea-for-opium switch and at one point confiscated and destroyed 20,000 chests of opium that the English wanted to sell to the Chinese. This and other incidents led to the Opium Wars. The result of these wars was a huge influx of opium, trade, and Christianity into China. Shanghai boomed, and Hong Kong changed from a barren island to a center of world commerce. The Chinese distrust of foreigners, particularly the English, increased. Opium is not smoked much in China these days, but heroin is injected, with more lethal consequences. The English still drink tea.

History of Opium in China

Poppies were grown in China for centuries, and the opium was used as an expensive medicine or tonic. Opium became more popular in China for a surprising reason: the introduction of tobacco. In the 1500s, tobacco was carried throughout world trading routes, and Portuguese colonizers began to cultivate tobacco in Brazil. The Portuguese introduced Brazilian tobacco to China in exchange for silk in the 1600s, and then the Dutch brought madak, a mixture of tobacco and opium, into China. In the late eighteenth century, the Chinese began to smoke pure opium in expensive pipes. An opium pipe was sometimes one to two feet long, engraved and bejeweled, and a sign of wealth. The wealthy smoked opium for recreation.[1,2] The preparation of the opium pipe took time and skill.[3]

Smoking opium became a more widespread habit when it became cheaper. The price dropped when the British began to sell Indian opium in large amounts to China, under the auspices of the British East India Company. To understand this odd commerce, we will review (briefly) the imperial exploits of the British.

The British East India Company dates back to Elizabeth I, who profited from the exploits of Francis Drake and wanted to continue international "trade." In 1600 she granted a royal charter to a small band of adventurers to develop trade in India. In other words, they were granted a monopoly over trade between England and Asia. These traders became so wealthy and influential that they came to be known simply as the Company.

The Company worked hand in hand with the British government to form the British Empire. Queen Victoria, three centuries after Elizabeth I granted the charter for the Company, considered the subcontinent of India, the huge expanse of Canada from the Maritimes to the Pacific, some of the savannas and jungles of Africa, and other parts of the world to be hers. Her soldiers brought *Pax Britannica*, railroads, the English language, democracy (after a fashion), and a disregard for the customs or culture of others to these regions. Although the British Empire never included China, that did not stop the English from making huge profits from that country. This profit making depended on English control of parts of India.

The connection between India, China, and English profit making began in 1750 when the Company gained control of the opium-growing districts of India. Poppies were grown in the fertile alluvial Gangetic plains and farther west in the province of Malwa. At the direction of the

Company, more agricultural lands were turned over to poppies. Indian peasants became sharecroppers, forced to agree to produce a certain amount of opium. As is always the case with such agreements, the sharecroppers did badly. Sharecroppers quickly became indebted to the Indian middle class of landowners and moneylenders. Indian farmers who grew opium became poor.

The Company had its own soldiers to protect what it saw as its rights. The Company's army was helped by internal conflicts among their enemies. Many Indians in Bengal resented the despotic Mughals who then ruled over this area, the richest province in India. The Company, with the help of Indians unhappy with their own rulers, engaged in a series of battles, most of them successful, against the French and unfriendly Indian forces. (The French had established the French East India Company and ruled a number of cities in India, including Pondicherry.)

The decisive battle took place in 1757 at Plassey against Siraj-ud-daullah, the last independent nawab, or Mughal, or Muslim prince of Bengal. Following this victory, the Company looted the Bengal treasury of 100 boatloads of gold and silver.[4]

Over the next 100 years, Company men became administrators and governors of large parts of present-day India. One of their main tasks, at which they were superb, was to collect taxes, which allowed the Company to maintain an army. They did a less efficient job of governing. Bengal had occasionally suffered from episodic droughts and food shortages, but the number of famines in Bengal increased once the Company was in power.

A major source of money for the Company continued to be opium. The cities of Ghazipur and Patna in the east of India employed many workers to process opium in opium factories, as Figure 19.1 shows. (The word *factory* was often used in those days when we might use the word *warehouse*.) Opium is still processed in Ghazipur, where the largest legal opium factory in the world is located.

Indian opium was of high quality, valued by the Chinese people, and illegal in China. Officially, England and the Company were responsive to China's concerns and did not allow importation of opium into China. But unofficially, and by crafting complicated arrangements with Indian merchants and country traders, the Company carried on a large and profitable opium trade. Country traders were English businessmen, ship owners, or merchants who traded within Asia and were the important middlemen. Opium grown in Bengal was sold in Calcutta (present-day Kolkata) to these private concerns that then sold it in China.

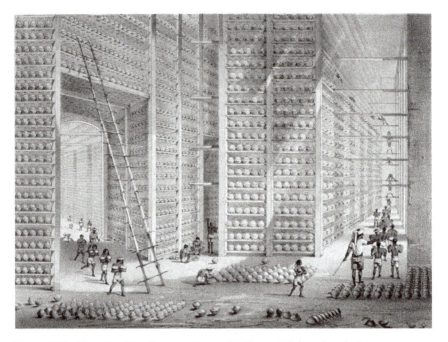

Figure 19.1   **Busy Stacking Room at Patna. (Wellcome Library, London)**

The country traders and the Company itself became wealthy by buying and trading many of the products of India. From the point of view of the Indians, the trades were not always done in a fair manner. Mir Kassim, a nawab of Bengal, described what he perceived to be the typical activity of the young men of the Company:

> ... Setting up the colours and showing the passes of the Company, they use their utmost endeavours to oppress the peasants, merchants and other people of the country ... In every village and every factory they buy and sell salt, betel-nut, rice, straw, bamboos, fish, gunnies, ginger, sugar, tobacco, opium and many other things ... They forcibly take away the goods of the peasant, merchants etc. for a fourth part of their value, and by ways of violence and oppressions they oblige the peasants to give five rupees for goods which are worth by one rupee, and for the sale of five rupees they bind and disgrace a man who pays a hundred rupees in land-tax ...[5]

As well as illustrating the arrogance of these young men, this passage shows that they bought opium as though it was just another product like rice or fish. This was true of their superiors as well. In 1772, Warren Hastings, the Company-appointed governor of Bengal, was openly involved in the opium trade.[6] Opium trading was part of what made so many Englishmen connected with India wealthy.

It was not just the British who profited from the opium trade. Opium leaving the west coast of India contributed to the wealth of a number of Indians as well. By the 1820s, a large number of wealthy Indian merchants and bankers of several ethnicities and religions—including Parsis, Marwaris, and Muslims—were involved in the opium trade at Bombay (present-day Mumbai). Opium from Malwa traveled to China through this city. Of the 42 foreign firms operating in China at the end of the 1830s, nearly half were owned by Parsis. One important Parsi was Jamsetjee Jeejeebhoy, who became a partner of the English country traders Jardine-Matheson. Jeejeebhoy owned ships and commercial clearing-houses, and was one of the six directors of the Bank of Bombay. He later became a knight, and then a baronet, and is much honored in Mumbai.

On the east coast, the Brahmin Tagore family in Calcutta developed great wealth by working for the Company. Dwarkanath Tagore was an officer in the Company's salt and opium department, a director of the Union Bank, and owner of indigo factories. His son continued the family's financial success and reforming zeal, but his grandson is the member of the family best known to Westerners. Rabindranath Tagore won a Nobel Prize in literature in 1913 and, as we shall see later in this chapter, was opposed to opium smoking.

England Imports Tea from China and Looks for Something to Export

England was intent on selling Indian opium to China because she wanted Chinese products such as ceramics, rhubarb, raw silk, and tea. The English mercantilists did not want to import manufactured products into England, and they certainly did not want silver leaving their shores. But they did want Chinese products, and one way of getting around this would have been to trade English products to China.

But China did not want English products. China thought of the Western cultures as chaotic, barbaric, and incapable of producing beautiful objects. The Chinese referred to their own country as the Celestial Empire or the Middle Kingdom. The term *Middle Kingdom* comes from the belief that China was the center of the world. They had little respect for other countries and referred to foreigners as barbarians, red bristle, or just the devil.

The Chinese had reason to believe that they were superior to others. Their government was based (theoretically) on sophisticated Confucian principles of benevolence, order, and self-control. The task of the emperor was to be virtuous, which would lead to safety and prosperity for his subjects. The Chinese possessed mechanical and artistic genius. For example, they developed gunpowder, wheelbarrows, paper, and printing far ahead of the rest of the world. They admired artistic and scholarly pursuits. Poets, painters, and calligraphers took precedence over peasants and soldiers. Calligraphy was an important and revered art form, in which beautiful brushwork added meaning to the Chinese characters. Commerce and war were not highly valued, and merchants occupied the lowest occupational order.

At this time, China was not actually ruled by Chinese. The Manchu had pushed over the Great Wall to conquer China in 1644 to establish the Qing Empire (1644–1911), and they assumed many of the values of the ethnic Chinese. Confucian values of respect for parents and ancestors persisted. Lack of interest in other cultures did not change. Chinese and Manchu alike saw China as the epitome of civilization.

In 1793, George III sent presents to the emperor of China to try to convince him of the value of English goods. He sent him a gold box studded with diamonds and the beautiful earthenware pottery of Josiah Wedgwood, England's famed potter. The emperor sent this clear reply:

> Our ways have no resemblance to yours, and even were your envoy competent to acquire some rudiments of them, he could not transplant them to your barbarous land ... Strange and costly objects do not interest me. As your Ambassador can see for himself, we possess all things. I set no value on strange objects and ingenious, and have no use for your country's manufactures.[7]

Chinese ceramics at that time were more sophisticated than equivalent English products. Potters in China, influenced by Persian artisans, had been making beautiful objects since the fourteenth century. Chinese ceramics were so thin and delicate that they were almost transparent. Their glazed surfaces were lustrous, and the colors were vivid. In comparison, Wedgwood's objects were dull and lifeless.

The use of the word *china* to describe porcelain is an ongoing tribute to the art of the Chinese ceramicists. Wedgwood learned to make the "bone china" that competed with Chinese products in fineness and translucency. English china became one of England's most respected products, but not until the early 1800s.

The most important export from China was tea. Tea drinking had been common in China for many centuries, and it spread to the rest of the world in the eighteenth century. Tea became a particularly popular drink in England and over time, it has become a symbol of the English way of life. The appetite for tea grew quickly in England and daily tea drinking replaced daily beer drinking.[8]

China had beautiful porcelain and tea. The English only had woolens, spices, and metals, and they were not able to sell enough of these to the Chinese to achieve a tolerable balance of trade. Without opium, and with no other product that was attractive to the Chinese, England would have had to pay for tea and other Chinese goods with silver. She was unwilling to do this.[9]

Trade at Canton: Admonish and Soothe

England and other European countries persisted in their attempts to trade, and China slowly began to have some contact with the "barbarians." Canton (present-day Guangzhou) at the mouth of the Pearl River, the only Chinese port open to Westerners, became the English entryway to China. The traders were allowed to live only in a small area, downriver from Canton, and their stay was restricted to the winter months, when tea was exported. Wives were not allowed. The Company established its factories in the trading quarters and carried out its transactions through the Chinese Hong merchants. Officially, the British traded textiles and woolen cloth, metals, pepper, and spices in exchange for tea, rhubarb, raw silk, china, porcelain, and objets d'art from China. Unofficially, they traded opium.

The emperor of China tried to control the Canton trade. He forbade opium smuggling and allowed other trade only if it was conducted in a circuitous way, with many restrictions on the English. According to the Confucian way of seeing things, the emperor was paternal and tender. His duty was to "admonish and soothe."[10] He sent encouraging messages to the Hoppo, a Manchu relative of the emperor who was the director of the Canton merchants and the customs men. For example, he suggested that the Hoppo should encourage the Hong merchants to *educate* the English. This is a typical message that the Hoppo sent to the Hong merchants of Canton:

> It is very difficult for the Barbarians to understand the proprieties of the Celestial Empire. Hence Hong merchants have been appointed to control commercial transactions. It is the duty of these merchants continually to instruct the Barbarians; to repress their natural pride and profligacy, and

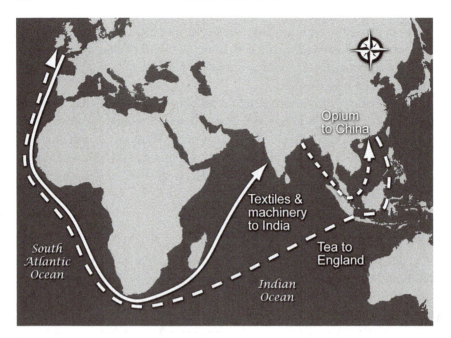

Figure 19.2   **Opium Trade Triangle.** (© 2013 Joan M.K. Tycko)

to insist on their turning their hearts to propriety, that all parties enjoy glad repose and gain, with each person in his place and minding his own business. Since the Hong merchants are men of property and good family, it becomes them to have a tender regard for their face, nor to cheat but trade justly, and so win devil confidence.[11]

This stern language glossed over the fact that the Hoppo and the Hong merchants were happy to be bribed by the contemptible Europeans.

East Indiamen and Clippers

A complex set of trade routes crisscrossed the oceans between India, China, and England in another trade triangle (see Figure 19.2). Textiles went from England to India, opium from India to China, and tea and porcelain from China to England. At first, the tea and opium were carried in lumbering ships known as East Indiamen. These boats sailed down the coast of Africa, sometimes stopping off at Madeira or St. Helena; rounded the Cape of Good Hope; stopped off at Madras or Calcutta to trade textiles for opium; threaded their way through Malaysia; and then sailed up to Canton. They retraced their route laden down with tea and porcelain. The round trip took up to two years.

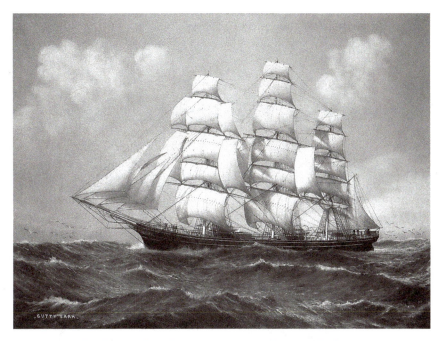

Figure 19.3   **The Clipper Ship *Cutty Sark*.** (© **Louis Papaluca/Corbis**)

Later, the trade was carried out by the famous "clippers" such as the *Cutty Sark*, the *Sylph*, and the *Sea Witch* (see Figure 19.3). The clippers were first built in the United States in the early to mid-1800s. They had narrow hulls and were rigged with many sails to take advantage of the winds. The vessels with diaphanous, white sails shining in the sun, sparkling in the salt spray, and skimming along the oceans of the world, seemed unearthly and romantic. The reality was quite different. The clippers were fast so that they could make three profitable trips a year between Calcutta and Canton. Because the English and Americans had become more sophisticated in their taste for tea, the freshest teas commanded premium prices. Speedy clippers also allowed vessels carrying chests of opium to evade Chinese officials. These beautiful ships were well armed in case they were unable to escape from Chinese or Malay pirates. Sometimes, clippers took the same routes as the East Indiamen; sometimes, they sailed the other way and traveled round Cape Horn.

The clippers, like all things of beauty, had a brief life. They were replaced by less elegant steamships when the Suez Canal, connecting the Mediterranean with the Red Sea, opened in 1869. The canal allowed steamers to refuel and eased the passage through the Middle East. The laborious and dangerous passage around the Capes of Africa or South

America and through the pirate-friendly Malacca Straits was no longer necessary. Never again would opium be associated with such elegance.

Chinese Opposition to the Opium Trade

Importation of opium into China had been forbidden since 1729. According to one historian, the Chinese government was opposed to opium smoking because it distracted people from their "duties and occupations" and loosened the "sense of restraint that holds convention together."[12] Another problem was more straightforward: the inflow of opium meant the outflow of silver that was needed to pay for public work projects and military salaries.[13] China had few silver mines of her own, and though she could have obtained silver from her neighbor Japan, she did not like to trade with that country. Much of the Chinese silver had come from Potosí via trade with the Spanish in Manila. Chinese silk was traded for Potosí silver.[14] (The Potosí silver, as we saw, was mined by Native Americans fortified by chewing coca.)

The focus on opium was also a useful way of diverting attention from problems within China itself—"economic stagnation, environmental exhaustion, overpopulation, decline of the army and general standards of public order."[15] In other words, officials blamed opium—or, as it was known in China, "foreign mud"—for the country's problems.

China was run by an organized bureaucracy consisting of a highly educated class of civil servants centered in Peking. These officials railed against opium. In this large empire, with local officials far from their superiors in Peking, communication could take weeks or months, so sometimes orders from Peking lost their urgency or relevance. As well, Chinese civil servants were paid little and were expected to support themselves by various methods of bribes and kickbacks.[16] Directions coming from Peking were often ineffectual.

Why was there such a market for opium in China? Although the Chinese Empire officially revered Confucian virtues, the country's rulers were often corrupt and inefficient. As a result, chaos and confusion marked many Chinese reigns. There was always fighting on the borders with Burma, Laos, Vietnam, and Tibet.

Chinese peasants welcomed opium because most were illiterate and did not benefit from the official resplendence of the empire. Most worked at jobs involving heavy labor. (The labor-saving invention of the steam-powered engine was late to come to China.) Famines were common.

Smoking opium brought some relief from tedium, physical pain, and the pangs of hunger.

Why not drink alcohol? Alcohol has never been very widely used in China, perhaps because many Chinese have an inefficient form of the enzyme aldehyde dehydrogenase, which means that high levels of acetaldehyde build up and lead to unpleasant flushes after consuming alcohol.

The opium trade grew throughout the late eighteenth century. In 1834, the Company lost its monopoly on Indian opium, and other companies, such as some of the country traders, developed their business and thrived. The most successful of the country traders came from Scotland.

William Jardine, born on a small Scottish farm, became a surgeon and worked for the Company. He left the Company to set up his own business and worked with Parsis, including Jeejeebhoy. In Bombay, he met James Matheson, son of a Scottish baronet. They combined forces in 1828 to become country traders, known as Jardine-Matheson. They were despised by many Englishmen, who found their straightforward enterprise unbecoming. Benjamin Disraeli, future prime minister of England wrote in his novel *Sybil* a description of a character based on Jardine (and also demonstrated the limitless range of prejudice):

> Oh! a dreadful man! A Scotchman, richer than Croesus, one McDruggy, fresh from Canton, with a million of opium in each pocket, denouncing corruption, and bellowing free trade.[17]

The opium trade was not purely a British enterprise. By the early 1800s, American traders—such as Charles Cabot and John Cushing of Boston as well as John Jacob Astor of New York—were also involved in this lucrative activity. Russell & Company was another prominent American firm. Poppies were grown in Turkey as well as in India, and the Americans sold Turkish opium to China.

In 1823, a 24-year-old American, Warren Delano, sailed to Canton and within seven years was a senior partner in Russell & Company. Delano returned to America as a wealthy man. His daughter Sara married James Roosevelt. They had one child, Franklin. He was given the name of his maternal grandfather as his middle name. So was named the thirty-second American president, Franklin Delano Roosevelt.

The trade needed interpreters. One small group of people who spoke both Chinese and English was the missionaries. Robert Morrison, for example, had learned Chinese by studying a New Testament translated into Chinese by a Jesuit who had lived in Peking. He served as an interpreter for the Company but also worked as a missionary. Another missionary was a multilingual Prussian, Karl Gutzlaff. He worked for the opium smugglers as they distributed opium up and down the Chinese coast. He distributed religious tracts from these ships, and his wife ran a mission school for blind Chinese girls. Many missionaries, including Gutzlaff, also distributed patent medicines. The distribution of tracts, charity, patent medicines, and opium was odd, but efficient.

Trade at Canton: "A Special Edict!"

As smoking opium became more widespread, the central Chinese government became increasingly concerned about opium smoking interfering with productivity and the drain on silver. The emperor once again ordered the opium smuggling to stop, but these orders continued to be ineffective. The Chinese Hong merchants continued to be friendly with the English and cooperative with the opium smugglers. They were bribed by all of the different parties involved in this trade and became rich. The Chinese navy, consisting of picturesque wooden junks, was neither able nor willing to stop the clippers.

In 1838, Lin Ze-Xu, an honest civil servant who did believe in the traditional Confucian virtues, was appointed commissioner of the Canton area. He broke with custom and did not accept bribes. He increased pressure on the English to stop the smuggling.

The English government officials were advised by—of all people—the opium smugglers Jardine and Matheson, who encouraged a hard line against the Chinese. They represented many other English merchants who found the soothing admonishments insulting. Jardine and Matheson had no faith in ongoing discussions with the emperor's representatives. They wanted to do whatever was necessary—including waging war—to increase trade opportunities with China.

Their job became easier when Lin decided to act to stop the trade by seizing the opium. He addressed the barbarians:

> I, Lin, Imperial High Commissioner of the Court of Heaven, President of the Board of War and Viceroy of Hu-Kuang, issue these my commands to the Barbarians of every nation. ... Let the Barbarians deliver to me every particle of opium on board their store-ships. There must not be the smallest atom concealed or withheld. And at the same time let the said Barbarians enter into a bond never hereafter to bring opium in their ships

and to submit, should any be brought, to the extreme penalty of the law against the parties involved ... Do not indulge in idle expectations, or seek to postpone matters, deferring to repent until its lateness renders it ineffectual. A special Edict![18]

The English chief superintendent, Charles Elliot, instructed the opium smugglers to comply, writing to London that the opium smuggling was "discreditable to the character of the Christian nations, under whose flag it is carried on ..."[19] Lin confiscated 20,000 chests of smuggled opium in 1839. Each chest of opium weighed about 140 pounds. He considered sending the opium to Peking but realized that the long journey would be too risky. Instead, in a move that foreshadows similar actions in the United States, he created a show in which the opium was destroyed while invited guests watched. He built special trenches; dissolved the opium in water, salt, and lime; and then dumped it all into the ocean.

Elliot, who had approved of the confiscation, was at the same time appalled by the destruction of the opium and saw this as interference with English commercial activities. (Actually, it was helpful for the opium smugglers because the price of opium immediately increased.) Elliot described it in a letter to the British foreign secretary, Lord Palmerston, as "the most shameless violence which one nation has ever yet dared to perpetrate against another."[20]

This language was driven by commercial concerns. The opium smuggling was a part of the web of English trade. Textile manufacturers in Manchester and other manufacturers in Leeds and London needed markets for their products. The port of Liverpool needed business. The opium smugglers may have been "discreditable" in their law breaking, but support of English industry trumped laws (especially another country's laws).

Lin was pleased with his progress. After the destruction of the opium, he had time for his calligraphy and poetry. He also wrote two letters to Queen Victoria pointing out the hypocrisy of her government. They probably never reached her.

The incorruptible and honest Lin did not understand the strong English feelings for their commerce. The English government detested the opium trade, but this paled in contrast to their hatred of foreign interference with English trade. Jardine traveled to London and consulted with Palmerston. They pored over maps of the Chinese coast and discussed the intricacies of trade between England and China. Jardine also helped to gather and coordinate protest from the English businessmen. Palmerston organized military action. He did not bother to run this decision by the House of Commons, which was distracted by an ongoing conflict in Afghanistan. Skirmishes between the English and Chinese developed into the First Opium War.

The First Opium War

The Chinese had invented gunpowder, had cannons surrounding the Canton harbor, and possessed an obvious home advantage. But the quality of the gunpowder was poor, the cannons were fixed in place, and their navy—such as it was—was weak. The years of the great Chinese navies were long past. The junks were wooden and no match for the English warships coming over from India.

The English navy was the finest in the world at the time. One of its proudest vessels was the world's first iron sail and steam ship, the *Nemesis*. The flat bottom of the ship allowed her to navigate the shallow river mouths at Canton. She carried guns on pivots and a rocket launcher. She sailed up river easily and bombarded the Chinese defenses mercilessly.

The war, consisting of many small battles, lasted from 1839 to 1842 and ended in defeat for the Chinese. The Chinese paid $6 million in silver in compensation for the destroyed opium and another $12 million to cover the British war expenses. In the Treaty of Nanking, five open treaty ports (Canton, Shanghai, Foochow, Ningpo, and Amoy) were established, and Hong Kong was ceded to the British. The five ports were open to American merchants also. Opium remained illegal in China, but the trading continued. This was the first of what are known to the Chinese as the "unequal treaties."[21]

Opium smuggling and opium smoking spread up the coast of China and along the navigable rivers. The opium trade more than doubled in the three decades following the Treaty of Nanking. Opium became the principal export of India in the 1800s and the largest single item of international commerce.[22] British critics of the trade became more vocal. Many British were embarrassed by the drug cartel–like activity of their government. In 1843, Anthony Ashley-Cooper, the future seventh earl of Shaftesbury and a philanthropist, deplored his country's involvement: "I am fully convinced that for this country to encourage this nefarious traffic is bad, perhaps worse than encouraging the slave trade." Dr Thomas Arnold of Rugby, the famous educator, described the opium trade as "a national sin of the greatest possible magnitude."[23]

The Second Opium War

Conflicts around the opium trade continued in China and came to a head in 1856 in a series of battles. The English steamed up the Yangtze River into the heart of China. At the same time, civil war and ethnic and border conflicts raged within China. The English looted the famous summer palace in Peking (present-day Beijing). The war again ended with defeat for the Chinese. Under the Treaty of Tientsin (1858) and the Peking Convention (1860), the Chinese opened new ports to trading and allowed foreigners and merchants to travel in the interior of China. Opium became legal in China, which meant that Peking could tax it, and missionaries were allowed to propagate Christianity throughout China.

The British (and American) traders profited greatly from this trade. Opium smoking became far more common, particularly in the western provinces of China. Shanghai became the main point of entry for opium into China. More companies and families became involved. Opium was transported on the ships of the Peninsular and Oriental Steamship Company. The Sassoons, a Jewish family from Bombay and Baghdad, created an international trading empire that was based in part on trade in cotton and opium between Canton, Shanghai, and Bombay. The family also became known for its philanthropy. The Chinese government reported that in 1906, more than a fourth of adult Chinese males smoked opium.[24] For the Chinese, a "century of humiliation" in which their wishes and their borders were ignored, and their people addicted to opium, had begun.

Chinese Women and Opium Smoking

Most of the literature about opium use in China is about men. This cannot be due to women not wanting to smoke it. Foot binding, common in China until the twentieth century, crippled women and consigned them to years of agony. But these women would have found it difficult to get access to pain-relieving opium unless the men in their family approved of it. From other countries, we know that opiates, at least in the form of laudanum, appeal to women just as much as to men. A few women in China did have access to opium. Prostitutes smoked opium, as did some wealthy women, sometimes while drinking tea and playing lengthy games of mah-jongg.[25]

Chinese Emigration, Smoking Opium, and Opium Dens

In 1736, the Chinese emperor forbade his subjects from leaving the country. This edict (often ignored) was repealed in 1868. The peak period of Chinese emigration to the west coast of the United States was during and shortly after the Opium Wars, from about 1852 to 1882. Many emigrants came from impoverished southeastern China, an area that was plagued by feudal warfare and famines. Chinese also emigrated to Southeast Asia and to Europe.

Some Chinese immigrants came to the United States when they heard about the discovery of gold in California in 1848. By 1852, there were 25,000 Chinese immigrants in California, where they were the largest ethnic minority. Eventually, the rich surface claims of gold became exhausted. The gold seekers who had flocked to California hoping to make their fortunes were bitterly disappointed. The Americans turned against the immigrants, and anti-Chinese sentiment grew. Caucasian Californians blamed the Chinese immigrants for working for lower wages and thus lowering their own wages

This situation changed with the establishment of the new transcontinental railroad system. The Central Pacific Company was in charge of laying railroad track eastward from Sacramento to Promontory, Utah. In 1865, the company brought over thousands of men from China to carve a passage through the Sierra Nevada Mountains, the granite mountain range just east of Sacramento. The work was dangerous, and many workers died in accidents, avalanches, and explosions.

After the railroad was completed, many immigrants moved to San Francisco, where they encountered prejudice, some fostered by the new trade union movement. Chinese immigrants, at various times subject to discriminatory laws or even riots, moved from San Francisco throughout the rest of the United States. Many moved north to Portland and Seattle, and then to Vancouver and Victoria in British Columbia, Canada.

Much of the emphasis on opium dens and the alleged connections with prostitution and white slavery resulted from bigotry and prejudice or—to put it another way—from those concerned with high wages and full employment for their own kind.

In the popular mind, the Chinese immigrants, most of whom were men, were associated with vices not uncommon to single men far from home, such as gambling and prostitution. Because the Chinese men also smoked opium, this habit acquired a dissolute reputation, and it became connected with the idea of criminal activity. The idea of opium dens populated with emaciated and depraved Chinese men with queues (braids of hair hanging down from the back of the head) infiltrated the popular literature. Charles Dickens described London opium dens and made them seem unsavory indeed. He describes an opium den in *The Mystery of Edwin Drood*, visited by John Jasper, a seemingly respectable choirmaster:

[Jasper] is in the meanest and closest of small rooms. Through the ragged window-curtain, the light of early day steals in from a miserable court. He lies, dressed, across a large unseemly bed, upon a bedstead that has indeed given way under the weight of it. Lying, also dressed and also across the bed, not longwise, are a Chinaman, a Lascar, and a haggard woman. The two first are in a sleep or stupor; the last is blowing at a kind of pipe, to kindle it ...

...

"Here's another [pipe] ready for ye, deary. Ye'll remember like a good soul, won't ye, that the market price is dreffle high just now? More nor three shillings and sixpence for a thimbleful! And ye'll remember that nobody but me (and Jack Chinaman t'other side the court; but he can't do it as well as me) has the true secret of mixing it? Ye'll pay up according, deary, won't ye? ... Ah, my poor nerves! I got Heavens-hard drunk for sixteen year afore I took to this; but this don't hurt me, not to speak of. And it takes away the hunger as well as wittles, deary."[26]

This unpleasant passage does make the interesting suggestion that alcohol is more harmful than opium. Dickens also notes that the woman boasts of her skill in preparing an opium pipe. This preparation, in which the opium is manipulated into a ball of the right size and consistency, and heated at the right temperature for the right amount of time, is sometimes known as "cooking" or "cheffing," and takes some practice.

Opium smoking was popular briefly in some of the artistic or Bohemian parts of Europe, where it became associated with a louche lifestyle. Opium smoking became a common feature of lurid books. The English author Sax Rohmer created the villain Fu-Manchu, who was connected with opium dens, attempts at international domination, and white slavery. Opium smoking developed a criminal and eroticized mystique.

The opium den has often been portrayed as a den of squalor and misery. The opium smoker and the absinthe drinker are both irresistible to the melodramatic artist. Photographs of the dens are a little different, as is shown in Figure 19.4.

Only men are present; they are neatly dressed and well groomed. They are smoking opium in pipes with a long stem and a small bowl that is held over a flame so that the opium can be vaporized. The length of the pipe

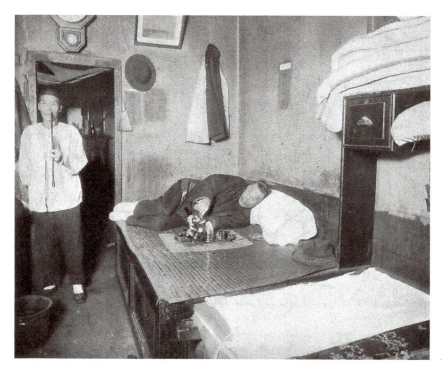

Figure 19.4   Opium Den in San Francisco. (Wellcome Library, London)

ensured that the heat from the opium would not burn the smoker's mouth. The scene is perhaps exotic but quite calm.

Somerset Maugham, in his 1922 dyspeptic book about China, criticizes everyone and everything in China, particularly his English fellow countrymen who lived there. One exception is the opium den. He visited one, expecting to see a dimly lit, squalid scene with stupefied victims at the mercy of villainous men. Instead, he found:

> ... a neat enough room, brightly lit, divided into cubicles the raised floor of which, covered with clean matting, formed a convenient couch. In one an elderly gentleman ... was quietly reading a newspaper, with his long pipe by his side. In another two coolies were lying, with a pipe between them, which they alternately prepared and smoked. They were young men, of a hearty appearance ... It was a cheerful spot, comfortable, home-like, and cosy. It reminded me somewhat of the little intimate beer-houses of Berlin where the tired working man could go in the evening and spend a peaceful hour ...[27]

Many historians support the view of Maugham and not those of Dickens and Sax Rohmer. Most of the Chinese opium smokers in

California were recreational smokers and not criminals at all. They smoked opium to relax in the evenings, but it had no obvious deleterious effect on their health. Few Chinese immigrants who came to the United States and smoked opium were addicted to it, and little harm can be documented from the occasional use of smoked opium.[28] The American and European perception of opium smoking as vice-ridden may have had more to do with its newness and fear of competition for jobs than it did with reality.

The Rise and Fall of Opium Smoking in China

At the beginning of the twentieth century, the opium trade began to decline for several reasons. Tea was being grown in large quantities in India and in Ceylon, so the English were no longer so dependent on Chinese tea. In 1909, the United States convened the first international meeting, the Shanghai Opium Commission, to regulate international opium traffic. One of the aims of this commission was to stop the importation of Indian opium into China. The United States, in part, wanted to placate China, a valuable commercial partner. The United States passed the Smoking Opium Exclusion Act in 1909, partly to prove to China that it was opposed to smoking opium.

Poppies continued to be grown in India but in smaller quantities. Indian farmers and processors had become addicted to opium, and there was increasing awareness of this as a problem. In the 1920s, Mahatma Gandhi and Rabindranath Tagore organized protests against opium. Within a decade, Indian poppy cultivation had decreased considerably.[29] The England-India-China opium trade ended.

At the same time, the Chinese domestic production of opium was increasing. By the late 1800s, China was exporting opium to other countries.[30] Chinese officials deliberately encouraged the growth of poppies in China. This had the advantage of keeping silver in China and weakening Western smugglers, who brought in Christianity along with the opium. The intention was to drive out the Westerners, smugglers, and missionaries by producing cheaper and legal Chinese opium. Then once there were no other sources of opium, they would close down the poppy fields.

One consequence of this was yet another increase in the number of opium smokers in China. The amount of money involved in the opium business also increased, and Chinese warlords and politicians, from Sun Yat Sen to Chiang Kai-Shek, were intimately involved in producing and selling opium to finance their armies. Japan occupied territories in some

Chinese cities and sold opium, and later morphine and heroin, to China for much of the first part of the twentieth century to finance her expansion and wars.

Not surprisingly, the addiction to poppies and their revenue and taxes was difficult to break. Corrupt enforcers and inconsistent policy through the first half of the twentieth century ensured that opium smoking in China would continue.

Profits were also made, as usual, by people selling opium addiction cures. In early twentieth-century China, the opium addict was offered a number of options, including some that seem similar to what is available in early twenty-first century America: tai-chi, hypnotism, confinement, and religion. Other treatments were more surprising—pomegranate skin and the combination of camphor and arsenic. Some treatments were the all-too-familiar tricks of hucksterism—morphine or heroin.[31]

Opium smoking in China finally ended in 1949, when the Communist victors of the Chinese Civil War (1927-1950) burned opium stores and ploughed under poppy fields. Opium taking was described as a capitalist activity and was linked with the Opium Wars, their "unequal treaties," the Japanese invasions, and the presence of Americans in Korea.

The Communists organized a multipronged three-year program involving antidrug propaganda meetings at mass rallies. The campaign was helped by the well-organized police, the Communist Youth League, and urban residents committees. Traffickers were executed at public trials. The numbers were small, but the effect was large. Opium addicts were offered treatment, but if their use continued, they were threatened with shooting or jail. Opium smoking ended. (Or, at least, it went underground.) Mao Zedong was more powerful than the earlier Qing emperors.

Opium smoking was a large part of the history of China and international trade yet now has almost disappeared. Tea drinking in contrast spread quickly, as did other minor addictions such as coffee, and these habits have persisted. Alcohol is worldwide, as is Coca-Cola. Opium smoking is not common now, perhaps because it is not a very efficient or easy way of consuming opiates. Smoking vaporized opium is a less potent way of using opium than taking it in by mouth or by injecting it. Cheffing, or preparing the opium and the pipe, is a painstaking procedure that takes time, skill, and patience. More potent drugs such as heroin and synthetic drugs (e.g., crystal methamphetamine), are now available. As noted earlier, tobacco smoking is common in China. It is possible that the tobacco smoking and use of other drugs are more harmful than was opium smoking.

Opium smoking persisted for many years in areas of Southeast Asia, such as Laos. It is now illegal there, and intravenous heroin use has become more common.[32] In a similar way, the decline in opium smoking in the United States following the Smoking Opium Exclusion Act was followed by an increase in heroin use. Some of those addicted to smoking opium were unable to give it up, and they and new opiate users began to use heroin.[33]

Notes

1. Timothy Brook, *Vermeer's Hat: The Seventeenth Century and the Dawn of the Global World* (New York: Bloomsbury, 2008), 147.

2. Timothy Brook and Bob Tadashi Wakabayashi, eds., *Opium Regimes: China, Britain, and Japan, 1839–1952.* (Berkeley: University of California Press, 2000), 5–8.

3. Peter Lee, *Opium Culture: The Art and Ritual of the Chinese Tradition* (Rochester VT: Park Street Press, 2006), 11.

4. Nick Robins, *The Corporation That Changed the World: How the East India Company Shaped the Modern Multinational* (London: Pluto Press, 2006), 3.

5. Geoffrey Moorhouse, *Calcutta* (London: Phoenix, 1998), 39.

6. Ibid., 49–50.

7. Jack Beeching, *The Chinese Opium Wars* (San Diego: Harcourt Brace Jovanovich, 1975), 17.

8. We rarely worry about tea being an addictive substance, since regular tea drinking does not lead to any clear harm to the body, intoxication, or interference with daily life. People do not seem to suffer withdrawal symptoms if they are not able to have it. Indeed, tea aficionados claim that tea is safe, mild, and invigorating. Some tea lovers claim that with the aid of tea, England changed from a nation of beer-addled rowdies to even-tempered gentlemen and ladies sipping tea from Wedgwood bone china. The tea drinkers, once they sobered up from their beer drinking, did not just savor tea and the English countryside. They began the Industrial Revolution and established the robust English Empire.

9. Tea drinking was also linked with slavery. Unlike the Chinese, the English tend to drink their tea with milk and sugar. Some of the sugar harvested by African slaves in the Americas was used to sweeten tea and thus ensure the booming market for tea from China. British abolitionists eschewed sugar-sweetened tea because of its provenance.

10. Maurice Corliss, *Foreign Mud: Being an Account of the Opium Imbroglio at Canton in the 1830s and the Anglo-Chinese War That Followed* (New York: New Directions Classic, 1946), 66.

11. Ibid., 65.

12. Julia Lovell, *The Opium War: Drugs, Dreams and the Making of China* (London: Picador, 2011), 35–36.

13. Ibid., 36.

14. William Bernstein, *A Splendid Exchange: How Trade Shaped the World* (New York: Grove/Atlantic, 2008), 203.

15. Lovell, *Opium War*, 37.

16. Martin Booth, *Opium: A History* (New York: St Martin's Griffin, 1996), 128.

17. Benjamin Disraeli, *Sybil, or the Two Nations*, 1845, reprinted with introduction and notes by Sheila Smith (Oxford: Oxford University Press, 1981), 46.

18. Corliss, *Foreign Mud*, 213–14.

19. Ibid., 241.

20. Ibid.

21. The English government was disconcerted by its unexpected capture of Hong Kong, an unpromising rocky island in the harbor. Eighty percent of the land was too mountainous for farming. The climate is awful: hot, humid, and stormy. A few rice farmers and fishermen eked out a poor living. The Japanese in World War II occupied Hong Kong and profited from an active opium trade. In 1949 when the Communists took control of China, Hong Kong remained a British protectorate. The island became a productive and refugee-rich city as well as a center of heroin smuggling, international finance, and manufacture. It was returned to China in 1997.

22. Jan Morris, *Hong Kong* (New York: Vintage, 1985), 22.

23. Booth, *Opium*, 136.

24. Alfred W. McCoy, *The Politics of Heroin: CIA Complicity in the Global Drug Trade*, 2nd rev. ed. (Chicago: Lawrence Hill, 2003), 88.

25. Lee, *Opium Culture*, 12–34.

26. Charles Dickens, *The Mystery of Edwin Drood*, 1870, ed. Arthur J. Cox, intro. Angus Wilson (New York: Penguin, 1985), 37–38.

27. William Somerset Maugham, *On a Chinese Screen*, 1922 (New York: Paragon House, 1990), 60–61.

28. E. Leong Way, "History of Opiate Use in the Orient and the United States," *Annals of the New York Academy of Sciences* 398, no. 1 (1982): 12–23.

29. Booth, *Opium*, 186–87.

30. McCoy, *Politics of Heroin*, 89

31. Lovell, *Opium War*, 304.

32. Joseph Westermeyer, *Poppies, Pipes, and People: Opium and Its Use in Laos* (Berkeley: University of California Press, 1982), 272–82.

33. David Courtwright, *Dark Paradise: A History of Opiate Addiction in America* (Cambridge, MA: Harvard University Press, 2001), 81–84.

20

The Brain

Introduction

This chapter reviews the structure of the brain and how the four substances of this book interact with it. Because of the complexity of the brain, this chapter will be best appreciated by those who already have a background in psychology, medicine, or biology.

Until recently, the brain has been *terra incognita*, and the complex details of what allows thought and perception were unknown. We are beginning to understand some of the mechanisms, but our minds still struggle to understand our brains.

Other parts of the body are more easily understood than the brain because we see what they do and can compare them to other devices. For example, we liken the work of our muscles, heart, and kidney to levers, pumps, or filters, but there are no obvious physical comparisons to brain activity. In the past, the brain was compared to hydraulics, looms, or telephone networks. The brain is now compared to computers, and the different parts of the brain are described in terms of electrical circuits. In the future, the brain will be compared to new technology, the nature of which today is unimaginable. Currently, it is difficult to see a link between form and function in the brain.

The names of different brain parts are odd. One example is the hippocampus. A Venetian anatomist in the 1700s gave this structure its odd name because it looked to him or her like a seahorse; others have compared it to a ram's horn. Its function of forming memories has nothing to do with its curving shape or with its fanciful name.

In the past, the brain was not always regarded as a part of the human world that even merited exploration. The Egyptians treated the dead body (if it was a royal one) with respect, but this did not extend to the brain. During the process of mummification, the brain was scooped out of the skull and tossed away. The Egyptians considered the *heart* to be the most important organ, and it was the only organ kept inside the dead body. Aristotle, the Greek philosopher and polymath, taught that the heart was the center of thinking and that the purpose of the brain was to cool the heart.

The Greco-Roman physician Claudius Galen was familiar with the human body from his work as surgeon to the gladiators. He also performed many dissections on Barbary apes, dogs, pigs, goats, and stags, as dissection of the human body was not allowed in ancient Rome. He extrapolated from his encounters with the wounded bodies of the gladiators and animal dissections, and he wrote prolific descriptions of anatomy and physiology. His work was medical dogma for 15 centuries.

Galen recognized the importance of the brain in controlling muscles but was mystified by its structure. He believed that "spirits," produced in the liver, were transported to the left ventricle of the heart and then to the ventricles in the brain, where they were stored.

Andreas Vesalius, the great European anatomist of the Renaissance, did carry out dissections of human corpses. He corrected many of Galen's mistaken extrapolations and described the human brain in exquisite detail. But despite his close scrutiny, the brain yielded few of its secrets. Looking at the brain was not enough.

The technology to explore the brain developed slowly. The scientists who discovered some of the secrets of the brain worked with single-celled fungi and an astonishing variety of animals. They used electric fish and sea squid from rivers and oceans, as well as more common laboratory animals such as frogs, rats, and monkeys. Advances were made when technology improved. For example, the invention of voltage clamps allowed scientists to examine sea squid axons. Weak stains were important, as we shall see. Development and improvement of microscopes were essential. Galen and Vesalius did not have the necessary tools to help them begin to understand the brain.

The brain is the target organ of alcohol, cocaine, nicotine, and opiates. In the text to follow, we will describe some of the discoveries of the past that have clarified the workings of the brain. We will begin with a description of the building blocks of the brain, from neurons to systems. Then we will discuss the neurotransmitters, the molecules that allow the brain to transmit information both within itself and to the rest of the body. How can plant-derived molecules affect the brain so strongly? It turns out that alcohol, cocaine, nicotine, and opiates affect and/or mimic the brain's neurotransmitters.

The Structure of the Brain

Neurons

The cell is the fundamental working unit of all living organisms, from single-celled microbes, such as yeast, to multicellular plants and animals. Each cell has a membrane around it that controls exchange of substances between the interior and exterior of the cell. Each cell (except the red blood cell) has a nucleus within it. Within the nucleus is the chromosome that contains the genes that direct each cell in its specific job or function.

Anatomists were not always certain that there were cells in the brain. The structure and composition of the brain were difficult to comprehend. It has a soft, gelatinous appearance quite different from other organs. Until the late nineteenth century, it was thought that the brain consisted not of individual cells, but of a continuous network or mesh. According to this theory, the entire body—with the exception of the brain—was made up of cells. Not until 1873 did it become possible to see brain matter clearly. In that year, Camillo Golgi, an Italian neuropathologist, developed a new technique. He sliced the brain, immersed the slices in potassium dichromate, and then reimmersed them into a weak solution of silver nitrate. The reaction between the potassium dichromate and silver nitrate resulted in silver becoming attached to some of the neurons. The structure of the brain emerged.

Stains were not new. They had been used 300 years earlier by Anton von Leeuwenhoek, the draper who first saw microorganisms. Stains distinguish between objects of interest and the background. Golgi's stain colored only about 3 percent of the neurons—and therein was its value. If all the neurons were stained, it would have been impossible to see an individual neuron. But this inefficient stain led to just a few neurons becoming encrusted with silver. When Golgi examined the stained neurons with his compound microscope, he was not convinced that the neurons were distinct from one another. Golgi believed that his new stain supported the idea that the brain was a network with no individual cells.

Golgi's stain was used by others, and most effectively by Santiago Ramón y Cajal, a Spanish neuroscientist. As a child, Cajal had wanted to be an artist. He retained an interest in drawing throughout his life as a scientist. He was enchanted by Golgi's silver nitrate stain and further refined the staining procedure. Cajal drew beautiful pictures of neurons and used these pictures to support a different conception of the brain—the neuron doctrine. According to this doctrine, the brain, like the rest of the body, is indeed composed of cells. These cells, neurons, are separate from one another. Cajal concluded that information travelled from neuron to neuron in one direction. He also thought that the little lumps on the neuron's dendrites, which he called spines, were not artifacts of staining, as others thought, but important parts of the dendrites.

Golgi and Cajal were fierce in their defense of their theories. The Nobel Prize committee was not sure who was right but, captivated by Golgi's staining and Cajal's drawings, awarded both scientists the Nobel Prize in Physiology or Medicine in 1906.

The dispute was settled by the development of the electron microscope in the 1950s. An electron beam, instead of light, forms an image with greater magnification and resolution. This improvement was another jump forward in the ability to see small objects and led to revelations just as Leeuwenhoek's simple microscope did several hundred years earlier. The electron microscope was powerful enough to show that Cajal had been correct. The neurons were separate cells.

The electron microscopist could see gaps between most neurons. Vesicles, or small bags, of neurotransmitters inside the neurons are on one side of the gap only, indicating that information flows in one direction. Neurons are independent and unidirectional units. Scientists also found that an increase in the number of spines is connected with learning and memory, as suggested by Cajal. His adversary and co–Nobel Prize winner, Golgi, could also feel vindicated. In the early twenty-first century, many discuss the brain once again in terms of networks.

We now know that the brain is composed of neurons and their support cells, the glial cells. The junction between two neurons is known as a synapse. The neuron consists of a cell body, dendrites, and an axon. The cell body contains the nucleus and machinery for making other cell structures. A presynaptic neuron's dendrites—or branches—studded with spines collect information from other neurons and send it to the cell body, and then the neuron's long axon sends the information to a postsynaptic neuron. Each neuron has up to 50,000 synapses. The brain is composed of about 100 billion neurons and 100 to 500 trillion synapses (see Figure 20.1). The functions of the glial cells, which outnumber neurons, are not well understood.

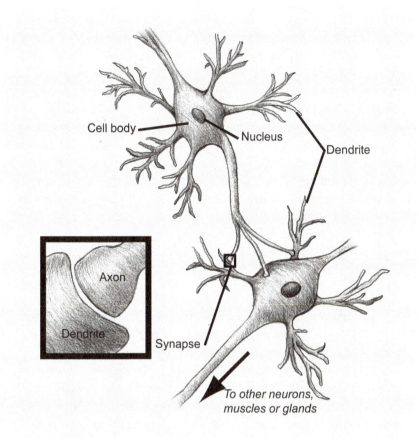

Figure 20.1   **Neuron and Synapse.** (© 2013 Joan M.K. Tycko)

The axons of the neurons are sometimes covered with myelin, a pale, fatty, insulating substance that allows for faster electric activity. Masses of nonmyelinated neurons appear gray, while masses of myelinated neurons appear white. This is the basis for the distinction between the gray and white matter of the brain.

The neurons are grouped together in different areas of the brain. Each group of neurons, sometimes known as a nucleus, is responsible for certain tasks or brain activities. (This is different from the nucleus in the cell body.)

Bundles of neuronal axons in the peripheral nervous system, that is, the nervous system *outside* of the brain and spinal cord, are known as *nerves*. There is, however, one set of important nerves arising within the brain, or cranium—the 12 pairs of cranial nerves. The first cranial nerve, the olfactory nerve, runs from the nasal mucosa to the olfactory bulb, which is part of the cerebrum, and allows us to smell. The second cranial nerve is the optic nerve, more accurately a tract, and runs from the eyes directly to the thalamus. It is the nerve of vision. The next 10 pairs of cranial nerves travel from the brain stem to the periphery, or the rest of the body. These nerves direct the muscles that move our eyes and allow us to chew and swallow. The nerves also carry sensation from our face and allow us to hear and taste. The vagus, or tenth cranial nerve, also affects many other parts of the body. We will return to the vagus nerve when we discuss an experiment with a frog. The larger nerves are thick and difficult to distinguish from blood vessels or tendons. Galen thought that nerves, similar to blood vessels, were hollow to allow for the passage of "animal spirits" from the brain's ventricles to the muscles.

Cerebrum, Cerebellum, and Brain Stem

Cerebrum

The cerebrum is the largest part of the brain and is divided into right and left hemispheres. Each hemisphere is divided into *frontal, parietal, occipital,* and *temporal* lobes, as Figure 20.2 shows.

The frontal and temporal lobes are affected by alcohol, cocaine, nicotine, and opiates. The frontal lobe is where we think, and the temporal lobe is concerned with hearing, emotions, and memory. Also contained in the cerebrum is the limbic system and most of the basal ganglia.

Cerebral Cortex   The cortex, or superficial part of the brain, is a gray, wrinkled covering of the cerebrum. The crumpling and crinkling increase the surface area. The word *cortex* comes from the Latin word for rind, which makes it sound like a covering for the more important "inside" parts of the brain. Vesalius drew the ventricles carefully but the cortex in a more impressionistic manner.

Thomas Willis, a British anatomist, was one of the first to appreciate the importance of the cortex. He believed that memory and will were localized here. He also described the ring of arteries supplying the base of the brain that is now known as the "circle of Willis." Willis collaborated with the multitalented Christopher Wren, who developed one of the first syringes. Wren was also an expert microscopist and artist who prepared the engravings for Willis's masterpiece, *The Anatomy of the Brain and Nerves*, first published in 1664.

The frontal lobe, or cortex, distinguishes us from other animals. It takes up more than a quarter of the cortex—a far higher proportion than is

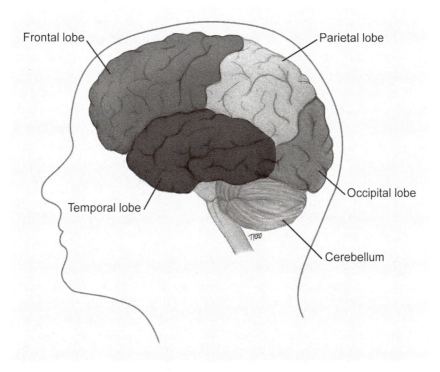

Figure 20.2 **Lobes of the Brain.** (© 2013 Joan M.K. Tycko)

found in any other animal. At the front of the brain, just behind the forehead, is the prefrontal cortex, where we plan, organize, and solve problems. Neuropsychologists describe these activities as "executive functioning." This phrase may evoke images of businessmen in three-piece suits running corporations. The prefrontal cortex allows us to do this and more. Unlike other mammals without a prefrontal cortex, we think about such abstract concepts as past, present, and future. Humans possess self-consciousness. Our prefrontal cortex allows us to face our own mortality.

The prefrontal cortex grows and becomes more effective as we move through adolescence and early adulthood. The brain's reward center (discussed later in this chapter), in comparison, seems to be more active during adolescence than during adulthood. This difference in rates of maturation explains, in part, the turmoil sometimes associated with this stage of life.

The prefrontal cortex is affected in many psychiatric illnesses, such as attention deficit hyperactivity disorder, schizophrenia, and some types of substance abuse and addiction. Impulsivity and difficulty sustaining attention are problems for people with these psychiatric disorders. Executive functioning is challenging to assess, since these abilities vary from person to person and change with the task or the person's attitude and energy. But a loss of executive functioning is devastating.

Excessive use of three of these substances—alcohol, cocaine, and opiates—can directly interfere with executive functioning. As well, people with addictions use much of their planning and organizing abilities to arrange ongoing use of these substances at the expense of other activities.

Some people welcome the loss of selected aspects of executive functioning. For example, our perception of the passage of time and our own mortality is not always welcome. Heroin, in particular, can take away the sting of this painful realization. Ann Marlowe, a memoirist and journalist who used heroin for some years, wrote:

> Heroin re-inserts you in a harsh chronology based, like the old, outmoded one, on the body, but this time on the waxing and waning of heroin in your bloodstream. "Here" is defined by where in the dosage schedule you are ... By incorporating a drug regularly into your body, you identify with a stable and predictable outside entity. Time, concretized as a powder, becomes fungible, and thus harmless. The past is heroin that has been consumed, and the future is heroin that you have yet to buy. There is nothing unique about the past to mourn, and nothing unique about the future to fear.[1]

Limbic System   The limbic system is difficult to describe and understand. Thomas Willis described a border of cortex different from the cerebral cortex in that it was deep and appeared to encircle the brain stem. He named this the cerebri limbus. In Latin, limbus means "border" or "edge."

Two hundred years later, in 1878, Pierre Paul Broca, a French physician and anatomist, described a large arc of structures lying deep in the brain around the lower edge of the thalamus, a brain structure just above the brain stem. (Broca was a skilled neuroanatomist known for his discovery that one particular region of the left frontal lobe controls the muscles involved with speech. This is now known as *Broca's area*.) He named this arc the *grande lobe limbique*. Neither Willis nor Broca was able to establish the purpose of this part of the cortex, although Broca thought that it might be connected with the sense of smell because of its proximity to the olfactory systems of the brain.

James Papez, an American neuroanatomist, thought that these structures were involved with emotions. Paul MacLean, an American physician and neuroscientist, further elaborated its importance by calling it the limbic *system* or "visceral brain" and noting that it exists in all mammals. He emphasized the importance of the limbic system in motivation, emotion, and the reproductive and parental behavior displayed by mammals. MacLean suggested that nurturing and social behaviors, found more consistently in mammals than reptiles, derive from the limbic system.

The exact functions of the limbic area are difficult to pin down, and not all neuroscientists accept the usefulness of the term. Among those who use the term, there is some discrepancy about the exact membership. Brain structures often assigned to the limbic system are the *amygdala, anterior cingulate cortex, hippocampus, hypothalamus*, and *nucleus accumbens*. The amygdala and nucleus accumbens are also sometimes assigned to the basal ganglia. The insula, a part of the cortex hidden deep within the brain, is also sometimes considered part of this system.

The amygdala is concerned with emotional responses and memory. The anterior cingulate cortex is part of the cingulate cortex that forms a collar around the corpus callosum, the part of the brain connecting the white part of the two hemispheres of the brain. The name cingulate comes from the Latin word for girdle or belt. The part of the cingulate cortex closest to the front of the head is known as the anterior cingulate cortex and is where we process many emotions, including our unpleasant responses to physical pain. We describe separation from those we love or depend on as "painful," and this feeling may also be processed in this part of the brain. The anterior cingulate cortex is rich in dopamine and opiate receptors.

The hippocampus is located in the temporal lobe and is where memories are formed. We process hunger, thirst, sleep, and sexual response in the hypothalamus. This small part of the brain regulates body temperature, blood pressure, and secretion of some hormones, including those from the pituitary gland. The pituitary gland secretes hormones that control or regulate sexual development, bone and muscle growth, and responses to stress.

The nucleus accumbens is part of the reward system. It has a role in tagging some behaviors as reinforcing so that we will do them again.

Strong reciprocal connections exist between the limbic system and prefrontal cortex. Without the limbic system, we would be colorless organizers and planners. Without the prefrontal cortex, we would be disorganized creatures bubbling with emotions. Together these systems form powerful brain experiences:

> *When to the sessions of sweet silent thought*
> *I summon up remembrance of things past,*
> *I sigh the lack of many a thing I sought,*
> *And with old woes new wail my dear time's waste:*
> *Then can I drown an eye, unused to flow,*

For precious friends hid in death's dateless night,
And weep afresh love's long since cancell'd woe,
And moan the expense of many a vanished sight:[2]

Shakespeare describes beautifully the bitter-sweet emotions brought forth by memory. Pain, grief, and remorse involve the limbic system, prefrontal cortex, and temporal lobe, and are sharpened—or, more often, blunted—by alcohol, cocaine, nicotine, and opiates. We described earlier how some people use heroin so that their brains are less apt to mourn the past.

Basal Ganglia   The basal ganglia are a group of nuclei that include the *nucleus accumbens, corpus striatum,* and *substantia nigra* in the base of the brain that modulates movements and certain aspects of motivation. These nuclei are tightly interconnected with the limbic system. The nucleus accumbens was discussed earlier in this chapter. The striatum has a role in forming memories of certain activities. For example, once we learn how to ride a bicycle, that memory is stored in the striatum. The substantia nigra, a "black substance," is part of the brain affected in Parkinson's disease. It contains a pigment, melanin, that makes it look black.

Cerebellum

This part of the brain is located at the base of the skull, tucked beneath the occipital lobes of the cerebral cortex and behind the brain stem (see Figure 20.2). Coordination of balance and muscular activity takes place here. Our ability to stand on one foot depends on the cerebellum. The cerebellum is sensitive to alcohol.

Brain Stem

The brain stem connects the cerebrum and cerebellum to the spinal cord. The brain stem includes, going from the bottom of the brain upward, the *medulla oblongata, pons,* and *midbrain.* The *locus coeruleus,* a nucleus that has a role in opiate withdrawal, is found in the pons. The substantia nigra, part of the basal ganglia, is located in the midbrain. Another structure in the midbrain is the *ventral tegmental area,* which is involved in the response to alcohol, cocaine, nicotine, and opiates. Most of the cranial nerves exit the brain through the brain stem. The brain stem controls breathing, digestion, heart rate, and blood pressure (see Figure 20.3).

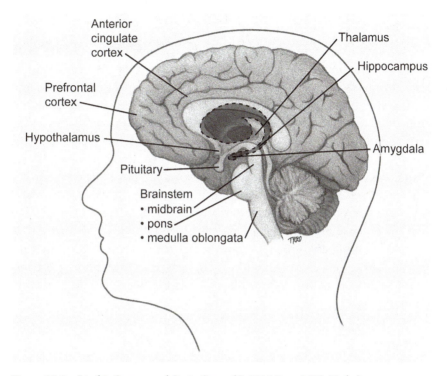

Figure 20.3   **Limbic System and Brain Stem.** (© 2013 Joan M.K. Tycko)

Interconnectivity and Systems

The white matter of the brain, which is the bulk of the deeper part of the brain, contains within it aggregates of gray matter such as the basal ganglia and parts of the limbic system. Connections between the various nuclei or cell clusters and other parts of the brain take up most of the matter of the brain and are just beginning to be studied. Most areas of the brain connect with one another. Some of these connections are known as pathways or systems.

The systems overlap and vary in evolutionary age and function. There is probably some redundancy in their functions. Some systems are defined by where they are and some by what they do. The nature of these systems or pathways is difficult to perceive, and their exact delineations and purposes are debated. The function of a system is not obviously related to its appearance. Some of these neural pathways are discussed in the following text. Extensive interconnectivity is an important principle in neuroscience and dauntingly difficult to study.

Plasticity

Plasticity usually means the ability to be physically molded. With respect to the brain, plasticity describes the ability of the brain to grow and change. The brain develops rapidly before birth, in infancy, and during childhood. Much of this growth is in the dendrites reaching out from maturing neurons. The number of neurons does not change much after birth, although new neurons do appear in the hippocampus. However, the number of synapses increases rapidly in babies. During childhood and adolescence, unused pathways are ruthlessly purged. For example, consider a child growing up in suburban America. The neural pathways that could make sense of Sanskrit disappear, and the pathways that make sense of video games are strengthened. This combination of synaptic pruning and growth is how we learn and adapt to the environment. A brain exposed to alcohol, cocaine, nicotine, and/or opiates changes, although not as dramatically as during normal childhood development.

Summary

The brain is made up of cells, just as is every other organ in the body. One of the unique features of the neuron is the great number of connections with other neurons. These neurons and synapses form multiple pathways and systems that transfer and synthesize information. Communication between the various parts of the brain is carried out by neurotransmitters. The neurotransmitter most often implicated in the use of alcohol, cocaine, nicotine, and opiates is dopamine. This molecule and other neurotransmitters are described in the next section.

Neurotransmitters and Receptors

Communication by Electricity or by "Chemical under His Fingernails"

The small space between the neurons that was so difficult for neuroanatomists to see and that caused such ill feeling between Golgi and Cajal was puzzling. In the early twentieth century, scientists thought that neurons must communicate with each other by electrical signals because communication is so rapid. That turns out to be true for only a small number of neurons. Most neurons communicate with each other using a surprising mechanism—the passage of small chemical substances known as neurotransmitters.

In London, chemist Henry Dale was working at the Wellcome pharmaceutical company with extracts from a one-celled organism, ergot that grows on rye plants. Ergot *(Claviceps purpurea)* is a fungus that makes a variety of substances that have plagued and benefited humanity for centuries. Bread made from rye infected with ergot led to epidemics of ergotism in the Middle Ages. Those infected acted strangely, hallucinated, developed gangrene of their limbs, and often died.[3] The cause of the clinical symptoms may have been the substance, ergotamine, which is a precursor to the hallucinogen lysergic acid diethylamide (LSD). Other ergot alkaloids have quite different effects. They increase uterine contractions and constrict blood vessels. Ergot was therefore used to speed birth and decrease postpartum bleeding for hundreds of years. Ergot compounds were also used to treat migraine and Parkinson's disease. The properties of this simple fungus were so varied, interesting, and powerful that Wellcome assigned Henry Dale to investigate this fungus for commercial uses.

By 1914, Dale had shown that one fungal extract, acetylcholine, could slow the beating of the heart. The next step was taken by Otto Loewi, an Austrian physician and pharmacologist.

Loewi wanted to prove that transmission of information was chemical and not electrical. He told this story of how he came to the proof. One night in the early spring of 1921, he dreamt of an experiment. He woke, wrote the details down, and went back to sleep. When he woke the next morning, he was unable to read his midnight scribbles. The next day was long and frustrating. That night he had the same dream. He woke and, this time, not trusting his ability to write legibly in the middle of the night, he got up and went straight to his laboratory, even though the weather was miserable, and performed the decisive experiment.

He removed the hearts from two frogs and placed the organs into two separate beakers. (Once again a frog was helpful, just as it was in the discovery of cocaine anesthesia.) He then electrically stimulated the vagus nerve that was attached to the first heart, causing the beating of the heart to slow. He took the solution surrounding the first heart and applied it to the second heart, which promptly slowed down. The important ingredient, which he named vagusstoff, turned out to be acetylcholine—the same substance that Dale had found in ergot.

Other scientists scoffed. The idea of molecules in solution changing the heart rate seemed ridiculous, and other scientists did not always get the same results. Even Loewi had difficulty replicating his experiment. It turned out that he had been lucky in his dream-inspired experiment.

The bad weather was fortuitous because enzymes that destroy acetylcholine are less active in cold weather. He chose the right animal. Not all species of amphibians, let alone all frogs, let alone all frogs of that particular variety, will behave as well. Finally, he had pipetted the correct amount of the solution from beaker to beaker.

Loewi continued his work, and after a decade, he convinced his skeptical colleagues. He had been fortunate in the circumstances of his first experiment, but this would not have been enough without a decade of persistence. He told a colleague that when repeating the experiment in front of others he

> had been obliged to stand at one end of the room and simply give instructions, so that the possibility of his secreting some chemical under his fingernails and dropping it on the preparation could be eliminated.[4]

Loewi had discovered that the vagus secretes a molecule that slows down the heart. The vagus is that large cranial nerve that travels from the medulla oblongata in the brain stem through the neck down to the gut. This journey is the source of the name—*vagus* is Latin for "wandering." Branches from this nerve control the muscles of the larynx, heart, lungs, esophagus, stomach, gallbladder, and small intestine. This nerve also affects gastrointestinal secretions. The vagus nerve is long, thick, and ideal for experimentation.

The vagus nerve is an important part of the frog and human autonomic nervous system. This is the part of the nervous system that controls many organs and muscles without our awareness or control. When the environment changes, the autonomic nervous system modifies its directions. This system is further divided into the oddly named sympathetic and parasympathetic systems. The sympathetic system of nerves was described and named by Galen, who thought that it represented "sympathy" between the various organs. The vagus is part of the parasympathetic system that balances or opposes the sympathetic system.

When the body encounters stress, the sympathetic nervous system goes into action. Blood pressure increases, and heart and breathing rate speed up. The pupils dilate, sweating increases, and activity in the gastrointestinal system slows down. Blood rushes to the muscles. The adrenal glands, located just above the kidneys, release epinephrine, a hormone that works in tandem with the sympathetic system. The person is aroused and ready to move.

At other times, the parasympathetic system is in charge. Blood pressure decreases, and heart and breathing rate slow down. The pupils contract, sweating stops, and activity in the gastrointestinal system resumes. Blood flow to the muscles slows. The adrenal glands stop releasing epinephrine. The body gathers itself together, calms down, and resumes its normal activities. In medical student shorthand, the sympathetic system is "fight or flight," and the parasympathetic system is "rest and digest."

We noted earlier that we are unaware of how our brain functions; most of the time, we are unaware even of the existence of the autonomic system that ensures a flexible response of our body to change. We will revisit the sympathetic system when we review the symptoms of opiate withdrawal.

Loewi had discovered, with the help of the frog vagus nerve, the first neurotransmitter. Dale and Loewi received the 1936 Nobel Prize in Physiology or Medicine for their work with neurotransmitters that confirmed the neuron doctrine.

How does the neuron work? The answer to this question was found in 1952 by Alan Lloyd Hodgkin and Andrew Huxley, two English neuroscientists working with the sea squid, a common marine invertebrate. They used the squid because it has the largest known nerve cell in the animal kingdom. The axon can be as large as a millimeter in diameter and almost a meter in length. The axon is about 1,000 times thicker than a human neuron and is large enough to be seen by the unaided eye. This makes for much easier manipulation by the neuroscientist.

Hodgkin and Huxley also used new technology, the voltage clamp, which they attached to the large axon. It was already known that each neuron, like all other cells, is polarized, meaning that the inside of the cell is negative with respect to the outside. Channels within the cell membrane allow positively and negatively charged ions in and out of the cell. Hodgkin and Huxley showed, with the help of voltage clamps and complicated mathematic equations, that during what is now known as an action potential, ion channels in part of the membrane of the neuron open, allowing positively charged ions in and negative ions out. That part of the neuron then becomes positively charged. This is depolarization, and it travels down the axon membrane like a wave. The squid showed us how the neuron works.

Hodgkin and Huxley, along with John Eccles (a neurophysiologist), received the 1963 Nobel Prize in Physiology or Medicine for this work. Hodgkin noted that perhaps the sea squid deserved the Nobel Prize too.[5]

After the neuron depolarizes and a signal reaches the end of an axon, neurotransmitters are released, and they move across the gap, or synapse, to the next neuron. The targets of the neurotransmitters are receptors, molecules that "recognize" the neurotransmitters and attach to them.

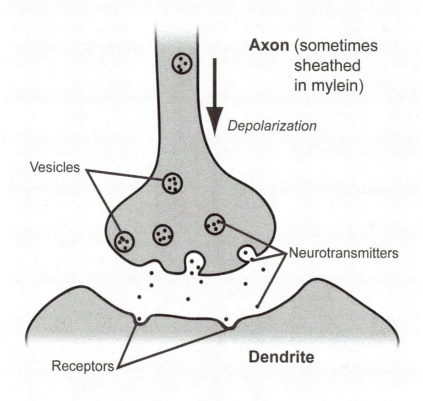

Figure 20.4   **Synapse in Action.** (© 2013 Joan M.K. Tycko)

Receptors usually are located in the cell membrane. This neuron in turn sends an electrical signal to the cell body and then down its axon to the next neuron. Some neurotransmitters facilitate depolarization, while others make it more difficult for neurons to depolarize. This is the basic component of information transfer (see Figure 20.4).

How does an action potential lead to the release of a neurotransmitter? How does a neurotransmitter latching onto a receptor lead to another electrical signal? These processes are known as signal transduction and are beyond the scope of this book.

In the early 1900s Dale and Loewi showed that acetylcholine, from ergot or the vagus, slowed the heart; then in the 1940s and 1950s, scientists discovered that dopamine, epinephrine, norepinephrine, and serotonin are also neurotransmitters. Each of these substances contains one amino group (NH_2) and is thus known as a monoamine neurotransmitter. Amino acids, including aspartate, gamma-aminobutyric acid

(GABA), glutamate, and glycine, which are found in abundance throughout the body, carry out many functions, including neurotransmission.
Other neurotransmitters include the gases, carbon monoxide and nitric
oxide, and neuropeptides. Among the neuropeptide neurotransmitters
are opioids, somatostatins, oxytocin, vasopressin, and secretins. Scientists
have now discovered about 100 neurotransmitters. The neurotransmitters
particularly affected by alcohol, cocaine, nicotine, and opiates are acetylcholine, the monoamine neurotransmitters, the amino acids GABA and
glutamate, and the opioid neuropeptides.

Acetylcholine (The Ubiquitous Neurotransmitter)

Acetylcholine is a neurotransmitter at multiple places in the body. As
we know from Otto Loewi's frogs, it is active in the parasympathetic nervous system. It also has a role in the sympathetic nervous system and is a
neurotransmitter at synapses between neuron and muscle. As we reviewed
in the story of the discovery of the opiate receptor, acetylcholine is the
neurotransmitter used in the electric organs of fish. Acetylcholine is also
a neurotransmitter throughout the brain.

There are two types of acetylcholine receptors, and they are named after
toxins that bind strongly and specifically to them. Muscarine, a toxin from
mushrooms, binds to one type of acetylcholine receptor. The other type of
receptor responds to another toxin—nicotine. Henry Dale worked out
some of these details. Neither muscarine nor nicotine is naturally found
in the human body, and both are poisonous at high doses. Both stimulate
acetylcholine receptors and so are known as cholinergic agonists.

Acetylcholine is metabolized by the enzyme acetylcholinesterase.
Acetylcholinesterase inhibitors are medications that block this enzyme and
therefore increase acetylcholine levels. They are used, with modest results,
in the treatment of Alzheimer's disease, the neurodegenerative illness of older
adults marked by loss of memory. The side effects of this treatment are what
would be expected from an increase in acetylcholine. Activity in the parasympathetic nervous system increases, leading to a slower heart rate and
increased gastrointestinal activity, which sometimes results in diarrhea.

Dopamine Pathways

Until the 1950s, dopamine was thought of only as a precursor to
norepinephrine, a hormone and neurotransmitter. In 1958, Arvid
Carlsson in Sweden discovered that the molecule is a neurotransmitter.

Carlsson's discovery was met with widespread disbelief. The theory of neurotransmitters had not been fully worked out, and many scientists, as noted earlier in this chapter, believed that neurons in the brain must communicate with one another through electrical, not chemical, impulses. Chemical impulses were thought to be too slow. Nevertheless, Carlsson was correct, and dopamine became—and remains—a molecule of great interest.

Carlsson also did much work with respect to the role of dopamine in diseases such as Parkinson's disease and schizophrenia and, along with Eric Kandel and Paul Greengard, received the 2000 Nobel Prize in Physiology or Medicine.

Dopamine is made by neurons and by the medulla, or inner part, of the adrenal gland. Within neurons, dopamine is packaged into the small sacs known as vesicles. The vesicles from a presynaptic neuron release the dopamine into the synaptic gap (see Figure 20.4). A receptor molecule on a postsynaptic neuron takes up the dopamine. The dopamine has delivered its message. The receptor then releases the dopamine, which is promptly taken back into the first neuron by the dopamine transporter and either broken down or repackaged.

There are different types of dopamine receptors and several dopamine pathways in the brain that can be defined both anatomically and functionally. The midbrain is a major starting point for dopamine pathways. Since the midbrain is also known as the mesencephalon, two of the dopamine pathways have *meso* in their name (see Figure 20.5).

Mesolimbic

Dopamine-producing neurons in the ventral tegmental area in the midbrain have axons reaching into the nucleus accumbens, amygdala, and hippocampus, and then up into the prefrontal cortex. (In Figure 20.5, for clarity, only the neurons from the ventral tegmental area to the nucleus accumbens are shown.) This is the reward system or pathway, so-called because it is associated with motivation and pleasure, and is thought to be the key pathway of substance use. In evolutionary terms, the reward system should be involved whenever the person is engaged in anything to do with successful reproduction. This includes sexual activity and whatever makes the person attractive to others and healthy enough to be able to reproduce and take care of offspring.

The reward system responds strongly to alcohol, cocaine, nicotine, and opiates. The rush, or high, that drugs produce is stronger than that

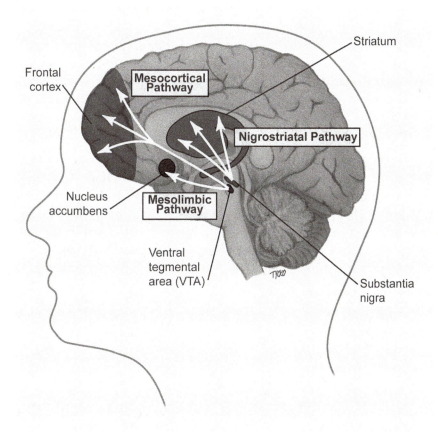

Figure 20.5   **Dopamine Pathways. (© 2013 Joan M.K. Tycko)**

produced by other activities and is not connected, in any obvious way, with reproduction or a long and healthy life. These substances trick the reward center. This system is influenced by another neurotransmitter, glutamate, which is discussed later in this chapter. The connection with the prefrontal cortex may explain some of the problems in executive functioning seen in addiction. This pathway is also involved with psychotic symptoms, such as hearing voices and having strange thoughts.

Nigrostriatal

Most of the brain's dopamine is located in this pathway in the basal ganglia. The pathway runs from the substantia nigra to the striatum. This pathway is involved with control of movements. The dopamine activity is balanced by acetylcholine activity.

Mesocortical

This pathway connects the ventral tegmentum in the midbrain to the frontal lobes of the cerebral cortex, including the prefrontal cortex and anterior cingulate cortex. This pathway involves motivation and emotion. If this pathway is underactive, the person will feel depressed and apathetic.

Tuberoinfundibular

This pathway runs between the hypothalamus and the anterior pituitary gland. Hypothalamic dopamine inhibits the secretion of prolactin from the anterior pituitary gland. (The pathway is not shown in Figure 20.5) Inhibition of dopamine release can increase blood levels of prolactin, and thus cause hyperprolactinemia, which is associated with sexual dysfunction, abnormal lactation, and, in women, menstrual changes.

Dopamine Disorders

Disturbances in dopamine-related areas are associated with the following three disorders.

Parkinson's Disease

Parkinson's disease is a good example of a neurotransmitter-related illness. In this common degenerative disease, dopamine-synthesizing cells in the substantia nigra die, and activity in the nigrostriatal pathway lessens. The person develops a tremor, becomes slowed down and stiff, and is sometimes depressed and apathetic. Treatment consists of dopamine replacement. This is difficult because dopamine itself does not cross the blood-brain barrier. Levodopa, a dopamine precursor molecule, does cross the blood-brain barrier and, once in the brain, is converted to dopamine. Levodopa is the gold standard for treatment of this illness. While patients with Parkinson's disease who are treated with dopamine medications rarely become addicted to these drugs, the treatment can be difficult. Some people treated with levodopa or similar medications develop disturbing psychotic symptoms such as visual hallucinations. This happens because the extra dopamine in the brain is active not only in the nigrostriatal pathway, but also in other areas, such as the mesolimbic pathways.

Schizophrenia

Schizophrenia is a poorly understood chronic psychiatric disorder in which the person has psychotic symptoms such as delusions and hallucinations. Perhaps more disruptive to their lives is the trouble that they have with executive functioning and interpersonal relationships.[6]

Chlorpromazine and other antipsychotic medications block the activity of dopamine at certain dopamine receptors. Carlsson in Sweden, Philip Seeman in Toronto, and Solomon Snyder in Baltimore suggested that overabundance of dopamine leads to schizophrenia. This was the first theory of schizophrenia that could be rigorously tested in the laboratory and clinic, and it led to some optimism that the illness could be understood and treated. But the illness is more complicated than just too much dopamine. While there may be too *much* mesolimbic activity, leading to hallucinations, at the same time there may be too *little* mesocortical activity, leading to apathy. Other neurotransmitters such as glutamate are involved.

Effective medications in schizophrenia remain those that target dopamine receptors. The medications affect other neurotransmitters, including acetylcholine, histamine, and serotonin.

Because dopamine blockade occurs throughout the brain, including at the nigrostriatal pathway, the person with schizophrenia who is treated with some dopamine antagonists may develop Parkinsonian symptoms, such as drooling and walking stiffly and slowly. Tobacco smoking is common in patients with schizophrenia, perhaps because nicotine leads to more rapid metabolism of the antipsychotic or antidopamine medications, thus to some extent relieving the lifeless feelings associated with Parkinsonism. Other substances of abuse may "replace" the dopamine activity that is quelled by medication.

People with schizophrenia who are medicated with some dopamine antagonists and people with Parkinson's disease have a disturbed dopamine-acetylcholine balance. One of the disabling results of this can be severe tremors. Anti-acetylcholine medications restore the dopamine-acetylcholine balance in the substantia nigra and thus dampen the tremor. Unfortunately, the person may develop side effects from these medications, including problems with memory, dry mouth, urinary retention, or constipation. This is a familiar story in medicine. Restoring one system often alters others. We are not as adept as our own autonomic system is in balancing opposing forces.

Attention Deficit Hyperactivity Disorder

Attention deficit hyperactivity disorder is a common childhood psychiatric disorder marked by inattentiveness, impulsivity, and difficulty paying attention. These problems in executive functioning persist into adult-hood. People with this disorder may be at higher risk of developing substance abuse and addiction than are others. Dopamine-enhancing or -increasing medication such as methylphenidate (Ritalin) is helpful in attention deficit hyperactivity disorder.

Norepinephrine (The Sympathetic System, Depression, and Opiate Withdrawal)

Norepinephrine is the other neurotransmitter (in addition to acetyl-choline) at peripheral nerves of the autonomic system and is the main transmitter of the sympathetic division of that system. It is synthesized within the neuron, stored inside the vesicles, and released into the synapse when an action potential travels down the axon. A major site of synthesis of norepinephrine within the brain is the locus coeruleus, a small blue nucleus in the pons in the brain stem. The locus coeruleus is blue because of the presence of melanin in the cells that make norepinephrine. This is the spot in the brain that generates panic. The locus coeruleus generates the fight or flight response when we are in danger. Norepinephrine is also synthesized in the adrenal medulla. When it is secreted into the bloodstream from this gland, it acts as a hormone and not as a neurotransmitter.

Norepinephrine plays an important role in understanding and treating depression. Depression is marked by low mood, disturbed sleep, poor appetite, low energy, and often a profoundly lowered self-esteem. In the 1950s, a theory that depression was due to a deficit in norepinephrine developed, and indeed, several classes of antidepressants seem to work by increasing brain norepinephrine. Monoamine oxidases are enzymes that break down monoamine neurotransmitters, including dopamine, sero-tonin, and norepinephrine. Monoamine oxidase inhibitors are medica-tions that prevent the enzyme from doing its work and therefore increase levels of these three neurotransmitters. Monoamine oxidase inhibitors were among the first drugs used to treat depression. Some antide-pressants such as desipramine are strong norepinephrine reuptake inhibitors. By blocking uptake, they increase the amount of norepinephrine in the syn-aptic gap. Other drugs known as "dual action" antidepressants lead to increases in both serotonin and norepinephrine.

Two other monoamine neurotransmitters are also involved with low mood. Serotonin will be discussed later in this chapter. Dopamine may also be involved. Bupropion is an antidepressant that increases dopamine levels. This drug is also used to help people stop smoking tobacco, as mentioned earlier.

Depression worsens all medical problems, including substance abuse. It works the other way around also—substance abuse and medical problems worsen depression. People are often tempted to treat their depression with substances. A cigarette or a drink may lift the person's spirits, but only for the moment. People who resort to heavy use of substances to treat their depression become more depressed. Suicide, the most serious outcome of depression, is more common when the person also has a problem with substance abuse. This relationship is clearest with alcohol, which can increase both depression and impulsivity.

The most effective treatment of depression is electroconvulsive therapy. The important element of this therapy is a seizure. Why this is effective is not known. Another treatment for depression involves the wandering nerve, the vagus, which was discussed earlier in this chapter. Stimulation of this nerve has been used successfully in treatment-resistant epilepsy. Because some people became less depressed after this treatment, vagus nerve stimulation is now sometimes used to treat depression.

Norepinephrine is also important in understanding the appeal of opiates and the misery of opiate withdrawal. Opiates decrease the activity of the locus coeruleus and eliminate any sense of danger. This feeling of safety makes opiates very appealing. But once opiates are withdrawn, the locus coeruleus springs back into action, and the sense of panic returns. The jitteriness, insomnia, tremors, high blood pressure, and rapid pulse of withdrawal are due to norepinephrine activity from an overactive locus coeruleus. The sympathetic system is activated, and the combination of panic and other opiate withdrawal effects makes opiate withdrawal intolerable for many. Medications that decrease norepinephrine activity, such as clonidine, are sometimes used in the medical treatment of opiate withdrawal.

Serotonin

Serotonin is made from the amino acid tryptophan. Most of the body's serotonin is in the gut and blood platelets. Serotonin cannot cross the blood-brain barrier, but tryptophan can. Dietary tryptophan travels into the brain and once there is converted into serotonin. Neurons using serotonin as a neurotransmitter are located primarily in a cluster of cells in the brain stem called the raphe nuclei and reach into almost all brain areas. The well-known antidepressant fluoxetine (Prozac) is a serotonin reuptake inhibitor, meaning that it increases serotonin levels at some synapses. This may be how it treats depression.

Serotonin also modulates some dopamine activity. Many antipsychotic drugs, particularly the newer ones, block some serotonin as well as dopamine receptors.

GABA (and Anxiety)

Gamma-aminobutyric acid (GABA), a common amino acid, is the chief inhibitory neurotransmitter in the brain and can be thought of as an "antianxiety" neurotransmitter. It slows down many neurons, including dopamine neurons. Alcohol increases GABA activity. Many other drugs that decrease anxiety, including benzodiazepines such as lorazepam and diazepam, also increase GABA activity. In contrast, caffeine, a well-known stimulant, inhibits release of GABA.

As well as decreasing anxiety, GABA is involved with decreasing electrical activity in the brain. If a person who is taking large quantities of lorazepam or alcohol suddenly stops this use, there will be a rebound decrease in GABA, and this (along with changes in the NMDA receptor, discussed later in this chapter) can lead to an increase in electrical activity and seizures. Alcohol withdrawal can be lethal because of this. This situation is further discussed later in this chapter and in the chapter about alcohol.

Glutamate

Glutamate, another amino acid, is the main excitatory neurotransmitter in the brain. There are several types of glutamate receptors. The N-Methyl-D-aspartate (NMDA) glutamate receptor is the most complicated of all of the neurotransmitter receptors. NMDA is a *synthetic* substance that binds to and activates this receptor and gave its name to the receptor. This is similar to the naming of the muscarinic and nicotinic acetylcholine receptors.

This receptor has at least five binding sites that regulate its activity. It recognizes glutamate, glycine, magnesium, zinc, and phencyclidine— as well as NMDA—and is involved in memory. A memory can be understood as a stronger connection between two neurons, or a stronger synapse, meaning that the presynaptic neuron is more likely to activate a postsynaptic neuron. NMDA receptors are found throughout the brain but are most densely concentrated in the cerebral cortex, as well as the hippocampus, amygdala, and basal ganglia.

Glutamate is an important neurotransmitter in the development of addictions. Glutamate pathways run from the prefrontal cortex to the ventral tegmental area and nucleus accumbens. These pathways go in the opposite direction of the dopamine pathways that are shown in Figure 20.5. Glutamate regulates the sensitivity of the dopaminergic reward pathway and is also involved with the memory of experiences with alcohol, cocaine, nicotine, or opiates. Thus, it may be part of craving, an important part of addiction.

Alcohol affects brain activity in part through its inhibition of NMDA receptor activity. Excessive glutamate activity is associated with withdrawal seizures, brain damage in Alzheimer's disease, epilepsy, strokes, and traumatic brain injury. NMDA receptor antagonists such as memantine are now also used to treat Alzheimer's disease, often in conjunction with the acetylcholinesterase inhibitors, but once again with only modest results.

Peptide Neurotransmitters

Peptides are short chains of amino acids with many functions in the body. Some peptides are neurotransmitters that bind to the same postsynaptic receptors that opium does. There are about 20 opioid peptides belonging to three separate classes—endorphins, enkephalins, and dynorphins.

Substances and the Brain

The skull protects the brain from physical blows, but the brain also needs protection from a different type of danger. The supply of necessary nutrients to the neurons of the brain by blood must be steady and uncontaminated. The blood vessels themselves form a defense known as the blood-brain barrier. This is not an inanimate wall, but rather an active series of gates and pumps formed by the capillaries. Tight junctions between the cells that line the capillaries prevent foreign or large molecules in the bloodstream from getting into the brain. Enzymes within the blood-brain barrier break down unwanted molecules or pump them out of the brain. Other molecules in the barrier do the reverse and carry some water-soluble molecules, such as glucose and some amino acids, across the barrier into the brain. The blood-brain barrier allows water, oxygen, carbon dioxide, and some small fat-soluble molecules, such as general anesthetic medications, easy access to the brain. The filmy blood-brain barrier allows the blood to provide the brain with desirable material while keeping out what is objectionable. When it is working well, the barrier ensures that the brain is unaffected by changes in blood composition. Each of the four substances of this book crosses the blood-brain barrier quickly. We will review how they breach the usually impermeable defenses of the blood-brain barrier and then what each substance does in the brain. Each substance leads to a marked increase in dopamine in the reward system but also has other effects.

Alcohol

Alcohol is fat soluble and slips through the blood-brain barrier easily. We do not understand the next steps very well. This is in part because alcohol is active throughout the brain and leads to changes in many interacting neurochemical pathways. These changes differ according to whether alcohol levels are increasing or decreasing. Some of the effects are the following. Alcohol promotes GABA activity and inhibits NMDA glutamate receptors. It leads to increased activity in the dopamine pathways running from the ventral tegmental area to the nucleus accumbens. Both alcohol and nicotine may also activate pathways in the brain used by the brain's endorphins and cannabis-like substances. It is challenging to put these many changes together in a way that describes the difference between grape juice and wine. The fermentation of carbohydrates into alcohol changes a pleasant but uninteresting fruit juice into a beverage that figures prominently in many of our ceremonies and celebrations. Yet how exactly alcohol manages to do this is far from understood.

Cocaine

Cocaine passes through the blood-brain barrier quite slowly if it is taken in by mouth. For example, if a Peruvian coquero drinks coca tea, there are no rapid effects. But if a Manhattan socialite "snorts" cocaine, it is absorbed into the brain within two or three minutes. If an inner-city youth or Hollywood movie producer smokes some crack cocaine, it gets into the brain within 10 seconds.

Cocaine temporarily disables the transporter protein that removes dopamine from the synapse. Excess dopamine remains to act on the postsynaptic neurons. This is how cocaine enhances some dopamine pathways, which leads to increased energy, motivation, and pleasure but also psychotic symptoms. Cocaine also blocks the norepinephrine and serotonin uptake transporter, thus increasing general monoamine neurotransmitter activity. In addition, cocaine activates the glutamate pathways that travel between the prefrontal cortex and nucleus accumbens. These pathways may be important in the disturbed executive functioning seen in people addicted to cocaine.

Nicotine

Nicotine is another simple molecule that has no trouble getting past the blood-brain barrier. Inhaled nicotine gets into the brain within seven to 10 seconds.

Nicotine is a molecule made by the tobacco plant and not found in humans, yet it acts as though it were a neurotransmitter that the brain "forgot" to make. Nicotinic acetylcholine receptors are found throughout the brain and in parts of the peripheral nervous system. Nicotine acting at these receptors activates pathways, including the important mesolimbic dopamine reward pathway.

Nicotine also increases the activity of other neurotransmitters, such as acetylcholine itself and glutamate. The release of acetylcholine within the brain may help to explain the improvement in concentration and memory that follows the administration of nicotine. The release of glutamate may also activate some dopamine pathways such as the mesocortical pathway, thus increasing concentration and motivation, as is seen with cocaine. Nicotine leads to the release of epinephrine that activates the fight or flight syndrome and suppresses the appetite. This explains, in part, the appeal of nicotine to people trying to control their appetite.

Other ingredients in tobacco smoke include molecules with monoamine oxidase inhibiting activity. By blocking the activity of the enzyme monoamine oxidase, the levels of a number of neurotransmitters are increased. Some monoamine oxidase inhibitors are used to treat depression, as noted earlier in this chapter, or Parkinson's disease. The monoamine oxidase inhibitors may also increase the energizing properties of tobacco smoke.

The increase of neurotransmitters due to nicotine has inevitably led some scientists to wonder if this effect could be used in a therapeutic manner. Perhaps nicotine administered in ways other than through tobacco could be helpful in the prevention or treatment of dopamine deficiency illnesses such as Parkinson's disease, or to prevent, treat, or alleviate diseases such as Alzheimer's disease in which there may be deficits of acetylcholine.

Opiates

Opiates are highly and artificially rewarding when they cross into the brain quickly and in large amounts. Heroin, not itself an active drug, crosses the blood-brain barrier very easily thanks to the two acetyl groups put on morphine by Bayer. Once in the brain, it is converted to morphine, an active drug.

Opiate-like substances are already in our brains in the form of endorphins, which are opioid neuropeptides. Endorphins do not lead to euphoria and addiction in quite the same way that opiates or opioid drugs from outside the body do, presumably because their release is slower and more modulated.

There are mu, delta, and kappa opiate receptors. The mu receptor, found throughout the central nervous system and the gut, is most relevant to addiction. Opiates activate mu receptors, which inhibit GABA interneurons, which in turn inhibit dopamine ventral tegmental area neurons. The result of this inhibition of inhibition is an increase in dopamine in the reward system. Opiates act directly at mu receptors in the nucleus accumbens independent of dopamine to cause euphoria and also at mu receptors at the locus coeruleus neurons to inhibit the sensation of panic.

Opiates are active at some parts of the parasympathetic system, which explains the pupillary constriction associated with opiate use. On the other hand, specific opiate receptors in the bowels lead to constipation that is not a parasympathetic response.

Opiate withdrawal leads to rebound anxiety that can be worse than the original distress. The locus coeruleus is activated, and the person becomes restless and fearful. Opiate withdrawal is often described as the worst of all of the withdrawals, although it is less life threatening than is alcohol withdrawal. Some people who are addicted to a variety of substances say that nicotine is more difficult to withdraw from than is heroin. But opiate withdrawal is associated with the most vivid descriptions.

Integration: Structure, Neurotransmitters, and Addiction

We have reviewed the effects that alcohol, cocaine, nicotine, and opiates have on neurotransmitters, and the role of the neurotransmitters in Alzheimer's disease, attention deficit hyperactivity disorder, depression,

Parkinson's disease, and schizophrenia. This is not the entire explanation of how the brain works or how disorders occur. Looking at the brain just in terms of neurotransmitters is to look at it as though it is a bowl of soup perched on our neck. If depressed, add a teaspoon of serotonin or dopamine; if Parkinsonian, add a dash of dopamine. If psychotic, skim off the dopamine. But the soup metaphor is, of course, misleadingly simple. The neurotransmitters act at many types of receptors and circuits within the brain, most of which interact with one another, develop, and change.

Moreover, disorders of the brain are more complex than simple problems in neurotransmitter quantities. Schizophrenia may begin at birth or even earlier and is a problem of brain development in which certain parts of the brain seem to develop in an aberrant way. Adjusting neurotransmitters by giving antipsychotic medications can relieve symptoms but cannot "fix" schizophrenia. Levodopa alleviates some of the symptoms of Parkinson's disease but does not cure it.

With respect to alcohol, cocaine, nicotine, and opiates, people can develop chronic problems with the prolonged use of these substances. Oscillations in dopamine and glutamate change the brain.

Consequences of High Dopamine in the Nucleus Accumbens

Alcohol, cocaine, nicotine, and opiates are distinct from each other in their effects. Yet all activate dopamine neurons projecting from the ventral tegmental area to the nucleus accumbens and the prefrontal cortex. This flood of the reward system with dopamine far exceeds what is associated with nondrug events. The euphoria is more intense than the usual good feelings caused by more "natural" behaviors such as eating or socializing. But this is temporary, and another response is about to occur.

Like much of the body, the brain regulates itself to keep the internal environment in a stable condition. This is known as homeostasis. If the person uses any of these four substances to excess, the brain adapts to these powerful increases in dopamine. It produces less dopamine and reduces the number of dopamine receptors in the reward circuit. The brain of the person who uses these substances in excess actually changes.

Why should the laws of homeostasis apply to the reward system? Why should we not always have high dopamine levels and be happy? Perhaps the answer is that the brain specifically "wants" to keep the activity in the reward center steady—and on the low side. The happy person who already has her reward center swimming in dopamine may not care to reproduce or hunt for food. The brain, therefore, will do what it needs to do to keep dopamine levels low enough so that the reward system will not be satisfied.

The way in which drug use leads to lower dopamine levels probably involves activity at the level of the genes. Chronic drug use activates proteins that regulate the expression of genes and thus protein production. Some proteins dampen or stifle the reward circuitry, meaning that the person is unrewarded, or depressed. Life is dreary without the drug. Other proteins lead to increased sensitivity to the drug. For the brain to return to its pre–drug abuse levels of these proteins can take months to years.

Conclusion

In this chapter, we have reviewed the brain and its interactions with alcohol, cocaine, nicotine, and opiates. The brain manages such complex phenomena as digestion, temperature regulation, and breathing. It also directs activities unique to humans such as speaking, writing, and worrying about the future. Four small molecules, derived from the fermentation of grape juice or barley, or from the coca bush, tobacco plant, or poppy, slip easily into the brain and can improve or disturb all of these activities.

These molecules have been used by humanity worldwide and for centuries. In moderation, they improve the functioning of our brains or at least make us feel that our brains are humming along productively and that we have nothing to worry about. They do this by firing up the reward system or pathway that runs from the ventral tegmental area to the nucleus accumbens to the prefrontal cortex. But sometimes they are used in such a way that we feel worse and, strangely, unable to stop consuming these molecules. Substance abuse and addiction are common and are discussed in the next chapter. Travel on the reward pathway can be treacherous.

Notes

1. Ann Marlowe, *How to Stop Time: Heroin from A to Z* (New York: Basic Books, 1999), 58–59.

2. William Shakespeare, "Sonnet 30," lines 1–8.

3. Some historians wonder if ergotism led to behavior that Europeans in the Middle Ages and then later the Puritans in seventeenth-century Massachusetts blamed on witchcraft.

4. Elliot S. Valenstein, *The War of the Soup and the Sparks: The Discovery of Neurotransmitters and the Dispute over How Nerves Communicate* (New York: Columbia University Press, 2005), 61.

5. Eric R. Kandel, *In Search of Memory: The Emergence of a New Science of Mind* (New York: W.W. Norton & Company, 2006), 88.

6. An important clue to the cause and treatment of schizophrenia was discovered by chance. In the early 1950s, a French surgeon-anesthetist looking for safer anesthetic agents discovered that chlorpromazine had tranquilizing properties. It was the first drug to lessen incessant and threatening auditory hallucinations. This discovery was the beginning of a glorious decade of discoveries in psychopharmacology described in Jean Thuillier, *Ten Years That Changed the Face of Mental Illness,* trans. Gordon Hickish (London: Martin Dunitz, 1999).

21

Addiction

Alcohol, cocaine, nicotine, and opiates cause pleasure, lessen anxiety and pain, and increase energy. Some people benefit from these drugs, using them with ease and flexibility, stopping and starting as they choose. For example, friends end a meal with brandy. Young professionals experiment with cocaine. Many have given up cigarettes. After a tooth extraction, someone takes two to three Percocet and throws away the rest of the pills. But in earlier chapters of this book, we have mentioned other properties of these substances, evident in the gin drinkers caricatured by Hogarth in *Gin Lane*, the crack cocaine smokers of the inner cities of America, the patients with obstructive lung disease who still smoke while on oxygen, and those with back pain who "doctor shop" for oxycontin.

These four molecules, derived from simple plants, can parasitize the reward pathway and subjugate the prefrontal cortex. In other words, they can lead to addiction, which is the continued use of drugs despite clear evidence of harm to the user. Addiction is antithetical to health and happiness. Experts in this area distinguish between addiction, abuse, and dependence, but these distinctions are of greater academic than general interest. Addiction involves tolerance, compulsion, craving, and dependence. *Tolerance* means that the person takes larger amounts of the drug with fewer effects. If the person feels that he must have the drug, then he has a *compulsion* to use. When not taking the drug, if the person thinks about it incessantly, then she has a *craving* for the substance. *Dependence* involves unpleasant psychological and physical symptoms when he stops using the drug. These last symptoms are known as withdrawal. After

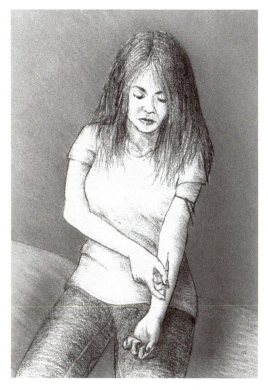

Figure 21.1 **Heroin Addict.** (© 2013 Joan
M.K. Tycko)

going through the agony of withdrawal, some never use drugs again. But
others stop their use, stay clean or sober for lengthy periods of time, resume
work and relationships, and then "pick up" again. People may start using
again because of a physical problem, stress at home, or no apparent reason.

The four substances of this book are different in many ways, but all are
active at dopamine pathways and other circuits in the brain. A person who
is addicted uses his prefrontal cortex or executive functions to hunt for
drugs; this takes precedence over other activities. The alcoholic loses her
job, and the heroin addict becomes emaciated. The addicted person notes
this but feels powerless to change course. Tobacco is the least harmful of
these substances to the brain in that it does not cause intoxication or damage the prefrontal cortex as severely as do the other drugs, but it more than
makes up for this by its devastating effects on general health. Even so, the
prefrontal cortex of the tobacco smoker does not work as well as it should.

A good example of the power of nicotine is the story of Rose Cipollone,
recounted in an earlier chapter. She was a respectable woman who loved

her family. Her husband told her repeatedly how harmful cigarettes were. She believed him, but she could not stop smoking. She smoked throughout her pregnancies as well as her labor and deliveries.[1] She looked through trash for butts.[2] Nicotine had taken control of her prefrontal cortex.

The rituals leading up to the drug use and the anticipation that accompanies them can be as pleasurable as the actual drug use and also play a part in addiction. For example, the author Caroline Knapp wrote about the powerful way alcohol muted her self-consciousness; this was so welcome that she also fell in love with the sounds that preceded the actual drinking:

> Yes: this is a love story. It's about passion, sensual pleasure, deep pulls, lust, fears, yearning hungers. It's about needs so strong they're crippling ... I loved the way drink made me feel, and I loved its special power of deflection, its ability to shift my focus away from my own awareness of self and onto something else, something less painful than my own feelings. I loved the sounds of drink: the slide of a cork as it eased out of a wine bottle, the distinct glug-glug of booze pouring into a glass, the clatter of ice cubes in a tumbler. I loved the rituals, the camaraderie of drinking with others, the warming, melting feelings of ease and courage it gave me.[3]

For those enslaved by these drugs, rituals may exacerbate the problem. Drugs sometimes are no longer enjoyable, but the search for and build up to using them are still craved. The addicted person can be "triggered" to use again when exposed to the ritual itself. Some heroin addicts will inject themselves, even knowing that there is no drug in the syringe. The ritual can sometimes work *against* the addiction, if it is too complicated. For example, it is difficult to prepare opium for smoking because the "cheffing," or cooking, requires some paraphernalia, expertise, and patience. The intricate preparation may add to the pleasurable anticipation, or it may seem tedious and too finicky to some people. Perhaps this is one of the reasons that opium smoking is less popular now than it was in the past.

We do not know why people who use drugs become addicted, although there is no shortage of theories. Much of the clinical literature and research generating the various theories come from experience with addicts who are in treatment. Clinical researchers tend to think that patients in a clinical setting represent all people with that condition. However, people who come to treatment are not the same as those who do not come for treatment. Clinicians see people with addictions who also have other illnesses. (The medical word for this is *co-morbidity.*) But this is not all, or even most, of the addicted population. Addicts who do not come for treatment have less co-morbidity and outnumber those who come to treatment.[4] Another related difficulty in understanding addictions is that people, out of a sense of shame, often hide their addictions from family members or physicians. Addictions suffered by the quietly ashamed are not always known about.

Nonetheless, theories abound, three of which are the following. Drug addiction might be a disease of the brain caused by the drug, or perhaps a way of lessening one's own unhappiness, or just a choice. The theories are not mutually exclusive or even consistent for one person. A person can develop or maintain an addiction for more than one reason. Someone can be addicted to several substances for different reasons. Sometimes reasons for addiction change over time. One person may have a constant drug of choice; another may change his drug or pattern of use as circumstances in his life change.

Some groups of people are well known for succumbing to addiction: antisocial people, adolescents, searchers, or artists. A person can belong to more than one group at the same time. These groups are all people who are in the public eye or have been available to researchers. They attract attention to themselves or are in institutions such as hospitals or prisons. The quiet person who is addicted but stays out of trouble is less often a subject for theorizing or describing.

For simplicity, each theory and each group of people will be discussed individually, but the distinctions between the theories and groups are somewhat artificial. There will be some back and forth in this chapter as the various theories and objections to them are reviewed.

Explanations of Addiction

A Disease of the Brain Caused by Drugs

This theory is based on the supposed ability of the four botanical molecules of this book to change the brain. In the previous chapter, the way in which these substances increased dopamine at the nucleus accumbens was described, but the impact on the person was not discussed.

It is difficult to ask a person what increased dopamine at the nucleus accumbens means or how it feels, because the nucleus accumbens is located in the limbic system, deep in the brain. Words are not the main currency of this system. We struggle to use our prefrontal cortex—the part of our brain where we reason—to understand our limbic system. To ask the addict why she smokes crack cocaine is as instructive as it is to ask someone else why he enjoys a hot bath. The person can describe their sensations but not in a way that is convincing to a person who has not had that experience.

One approach to understanding the effects of dopamine increase in the nucleus accumbens is to study the effects of drugs on the non-human brain. Since addiction begins below the cerebral cortex and since subcortical structures in humans are similar to those in other mammals, perhaps some generalizations can be made from studies of mammalian addiction. The animals most often used are rats and monkeys.

Scientists who study animal brains can control the environment and the animals in ways that they cannot for humans. Two experts in addiction, Eric Nestler and Robert Malenka, summarized much of this work in 2004:

> ... rats, mice and nonhuman primates will self-administer the same substances that humans abuse. In these experiments, the animals are connected to an intravenous line. They are then taught to press one lever to receive an infusion of drug through the IV, another lever to get a relatively uninteresting saline solution, and a third lever to request a food pellet. Within a few days, the animals are hooked: they readily self-administer cocaine, heroin, amphetamine and many other common habit-forming drugs.
>
> What is more, they eventually display assorted behaviors of addiction. Individual animals will take drugs at the expense of normal activities such as eating and sleeping—some even to the point that they die of exhaustion or malnutrition. For the most addictive substances, such as cocaine, animals will spend most of their waking hours working to obtain more, even if it means pressing a lever hundreds of times for a single hit. And just as human addicts experience intense cravings when they encounter drug paraphernalia or places where they have scored, the animals, too, come to prefer an environment that they associate with the drug—an area in the cage in which lever pressing always provides chemical compensation.[5]

In other words, some of the experiences of nonverbal mammals exposed to drugs are similar to those of people addicted to these same substances. Some animals choose cocaine over food and sleep.

Researchers do more than expose animals to drugs and describe their behavior; they also explore their brains. For example, they inject radiolabeled substances into the animals' brains and map the reward pathways. These and other studies show that the brain adapts to the drug-caused powerful surges in dopamine by sensing that there is "too much" neurotransmitter activity, producing less dopamine, and reducing the number of dopamine receptors in the reward circuit. Without more drug the reward pathway is depleted of dopamine and with fewer receptors the pathway is less responsive.

Similar reactions occur in humans who use drugs. Once the person stops using the drug, activity in the reward circuit slows down. The only immediate solution is to continue the drug. Each time the person uses the drug, there is an increasingly disappointing reaction as the number of dopamine receptors continues to decrease, and the person will need more drug to get a "rush." Euphoria is in the past. The reward circuit has slowed down so much that the addicted person feels flat and lifeless when not repeatedly consuming these dopamine-increasing molecules. Many addicts say that eventually they no longer enjoy their drugs and use them only to prevent withdrawal.

Scientists point to the animal experiments to agree with the temperance workers who referred to alcohol as demon rum, able to enslave anyone. These botanic molecules are dangerous. Avram Goldstein, who did much work related to the opiate receptor, wrote that animal work illuminated the ability of drugs to cause addiction:

> If a monkey is provided with a lever, which he can press to self-inject heroin, he establishes a regular pattern of heroin use—a true addiction—that takes priority over the normal activities of his life . . . Since this behavior is seen in several other animal species (primarily rats), I have to infer that if heroin were easily available to everyone, and if there were no social pressure of any kind to discourage heroin use, a very large number of people would become heroin addicts.[6]

Even before animal experiments, many in the past have thought that addiction to alcohol or drugs was a disease; the most famous person probably being Benjamin Rush.[7] The animal work allows some scientists to declare addiction to be an "official" illness in the United States. The clearest and most influential statement about this was made by Alan Leshner, then the director of the U.S. National Institute of Drug Abuse (NIDA). In 1977 in an article for *Nature*, he wrote:

> Scientific advances over the past 20 years have shown that drug addiction is a chronic, relapsing disease that results from the prolonged effects of drugs on the brain. As with many other brain diseases, addiction has embedded behavioral and social-context aspects that are important parts of the disorder itself. Therefore, the most effective treatment approaches will include

biological, behavioral, and social-context components. Recognizing addiction as a chronic, relapsing brain disorder characterized by compulsive drug seeking and use can impact society's overall health and social policy strategies and help diminish the health and social costs associated with drug abuse and addiction.[8]

Leshner was careful to say that the disease results *from* prolonged drug use. Initial drug use is voluntary, but continued drug use changes the brain so that it becomes diseased. This approach came from animal work as described previously and was also consistent with the medical approach taken at the Lexington Narcotic Farm.[9] Drug addiction at the Farm was considered to be a disease like asthma, osteoarthritis, or high blood pressure. All are chronic illnesses with frequent relapses, often with an unsatisfactory response to treatment.

The theories about addiction as brain disorder were supported by Vincent Dole and Marie Nyswander. In the 1960s, they gave methadone to heroin addicts and described extended periods of stability with no euphoria and reduced drug-seeking behavior. They concluded that heroin addiction responded to methadone much as diabetes responded to insulin. A drug had treated the brain disease.

This medical approach has been supported by evidence of changes in the brains of addicts. The belief that the brain, once past adolescence, could not develop, has been weakened by the development of new technology. "Neuroimaging" allows us to see the brain in detail. Using a variety of techniques such as structural magnetic resonance imaging (MRI), functional MRI, magnetic resonance spectroscopy (MRS), position emission tomography (PET), and single photon emission computed tomography (SPECT), neurotransmitter activity, blood flow, energy utilization, and drug distribution in the brain can be seen. Change can be quantified.

One of the best-known examples of the ability of the brain to change and of the usefulness of neuroimaging comes from the work of Eleanor Maguire, a professor of cognitive neuroscience who wondered why some people are better than others at remembering directions. She and her colleagues at University College London studied the brains of 16 London taxi drivers, each of whom had mastered the layout of the 25,000 streets of London. MRI showed that the taxi drivers had a larger posterior hippocampus than control subjects. The longer they had been on the job, the larger their posterior hippocampus, particularly on the right side, suggesting that this difference was acquired and that their hippocampi had changed over time.[10]

If the brain changes when learning the map of London, then it is not surprising that the brain changes when an addiction develops. Neuroimaging shows that people who are addicted to various substances do have brains that look different from others in a number of ways. For example, compared to those not using drugs, those who use large amounts of alcohol, cocaine, or heroin have smaller frontal or prefrontal lobes, suggesting the importance of this part of the brain in addiction.[11] These imaging findings may explain, in part, why it is so difficult for addicts to explain or understand why they continue to use drugs. A disordered or diseased limbic system drives the person to make a poor decision, that is, to use drugs, that his diminished prefrontal cortex can no longer challenge.

If addiction is a brain disease, common sense would suggest that there might be a hereditary component to it, since it is not unusual to see drug addictions "run" in families. It is, however, difficult to distinguish between genetic and environmental factors. Genetic factors have been studied most closely in alcoholism, and many experts believe that there is a genetic component to alcoholism, which is consistent with the concept of alcoholism being an illness with an inherited biological vulnerability.

The classic way of exploring genetic contributions to illnesses is by studying twins, which allows, to some extent, environmental and genetic influences to be separated. Work with identical twins suggests that perhaps as much as half of a person's risk of developing an addiction is genetic.[12] A number of different genes are probably involved in the inheritance of substance abuse or, more accurately, a predisposition to substance abuse. In this respect, addiction is similar to other diseases such as high blood pressure, in which there is a genetic predisposition but no one single gene.

Both addiction and high blood pressure are influenced by nongenetic factors. A person with a genetic predisposition to high blood pressure may never develop the problem, or at least control it better, if he follows a careful diet and exercise program; a person with a genetic predisposition to addiction may never develop that problem if she avoids alcohol and drugs.

The genetics of these two disorders are not straightforward and environmental factors are important. By likening drug addiction to illnesses such as diabetes or high blood pressure, the stigma of addiction is lessened. Being considered ill is unpleasant but less so than being called weak or immoral.

Not everyone is comfortable with the idea that addiction is an illness. Despite the neuroimaging findings (which are still produced only by researchers), the biological underpinnings of addiction remain elusive. There is no malignant cell transformation, infectious organism, inflammation, or degeneration as there are in so many other diseases. There are no physical values such as blood sugar or blood pressure to quantify. No diagnostic lab tests exist. Most importantly, there is no disease without the decision to take the substance. The elements of decision, choice, and desire present in addiction are unusual in medicine. No one wants to encounter the tuberculosis bacillus, but many people do want to use drugs. The person only has to avoid the substance and then there is no illness.

The botanical molecules, powerful as they are, do not convert all animals into addicts. In Nestler and Malenka's description of animal work, they refer to *individual* rats. The reasons for these differences between the rats are not known. It would be interesting to see if the brain of the addicted rat is different *before* the addiction begins. In a similar way, many people are exposed to drugs; not all become addicts. Perhaps the person who is to become an addict has different dopamine pathways than others. This is difficult to show, since there is no easy way of predicting future substance abuse.

With respect to humans, many theoreticians invoke other factors. Perhaps the reason some people exposed to a drug become addicted and others do not may lie in quite a different sphere—not in the brain but in the personal or social history of the person.

Self-Medication

Perhaps all pleasure is only relief.[13]

A different theory of addiction focuses on the unhappiness of the person and not on the strength of the drug. Unhappiness has many causes, ranging from the personal to the philosophical. Distress can be caused by a variety of intolerable emotions, such as fear, loneliness, or anger. Some people say that they use drugs to relieve agony caused by the knowledge of the briefness and fragility of life. Russell Brand, the British comedian and ex-addict, writes that "... the priority of any addict is to anaesthetise the pain of living to ease the passage of the day with some purchased relief."[14]

But the drugs do not solve the problem that leads to the emotion. They "ease the passage of the day" for only a brief moment. The relief is temporary, the "pain of living" continues, and the drug's effects lessen with repeated use. Therefore, the use of drugs tends to increase over time. Eventually, the person becomes addicted, and the original problem leading to the emotion is often worse. This is the self-medication hypothesis of addiction.

Recent discoveries about the limbic system support this theory. Many emotions that seem to be unendurable have to do with our relationships or attachments to others. Successful social attachment, beginning with our connection with our caregivers, leads to the release of endogenous opioids within the limbic system. Lucky children grow up being able to trust that their parents are predictably kind, caring, and present. These children have limbic systems well bathed in endorphins. Less fortunate children who have cruel or absent parents (or differently configured brains) may have limbic systems without such a good supply of endorphins.

One part of the limbic system with particular relevance to early childhood, relationships to others, pain, and substance abuse is the anterior cingulate cortex. Both physical pain and the experience of romantic or social rejection activate the anterior cingulate cortex.[15] Many people with the most difficult to quit addictions have had empty or traumatic childhoods; it is almost as though their anterior cingulate cortices were endorphin deprived, and once exposed to opiates or the like, they do not want to let go. Opiates and their derivatives ease pain, whether physical or otherwise. Drugs can relieve pain or help people control their distress.[16]

Some support for this way of understanding substance abuse comes again from animal work, beginning with experiments done by Marian Diamond in California with rats. Scientists had been uneasy about the common practice of housing laboratory rats in single cages because in the wild, rats are lively and social creatures. In the early 1960s, Diamond compared the brains of rats that were housed with other rats and toys to the brains of rats living with neither. The brains of the rats housed in the enriched settings had brains with neurons that had more and longer dendrites with more spines. In other words, environment affects the rat brain.[17]

This work was expanded upon and made relevant to substance abuse in an imaginative series of animal experiments in the late 1970s. Bruce Alexander, a psychologist at Simon Fraser University in British Columbia, built a large and more natural living space for his rats. This was a plywood enclosure about the size of 200 usual cages. The enclosure was painted with bright colors and pictures of trees. It was furnished with cedar shavings, boxes, and tin cans for play, hiding, and nesting. Sixteen to 20 rats of both genders lived together, and baby rats were born.

Following the construction of Rat Park, the experiments began. The researchers developed morphine addiction in their rats by giving them sweetened morphine-laced water for two months. (Rats love sweetened water.) Some rats were kept in single cages, and others were moved to Rat Park. The experimenters offered all the rats a typical morphine solution alongside their normal water, thus giving them the choice to use the morphine or not. The expectation was that all the rats would continue to choose the morphine solution to support their well-established "morphine habit." But this did not happen. The rats in Rat Park took about one-twentieth as much of the morphine as did those in single cages, showing that their morphine habit was affected by their living circumstances. In other words, rats are more likely to use opiate drugs when confined, bored, or lonely. The well-housed rat with playmates is less likely to have a morphine-sensitive limbic system.[18]

It is tempting to apply this finding to the human condition. If Alexander is correct, conclusions from experiments on animals that are caged in isolated and cramped circumstances apply most accurately to people who themselves are living in restricted and miserable circumstances with no meaningful occupation.

As always in science, it is important to replicate the experiment. Some researchers have repeated Alexander's work with variations and found similar results, but other researchers have not. Defending the theory that addiction is a brain disease, Goldstein dismissed Alexander's work:

> A rat addicted to heroin is not rebelling against society, is not a victim of socio-economic circumstances, is not a product of a dysfunctional family, and is not a criminal. The rat's behavior is simply controlled by the action of heroin (actually morphine, to which heroin is converted in the body) on its brain.[19]

Alexander argues, in turn, that history supports his Rat Park findings. He worked in British Columbia and so, from his point of view, he was witness to the effects of British colonialization on the lives of the aboriginal people in British Columbia, and suggests that at least some drug abuse is in reaction to the long lasting effects of this cultural dislocation.[20] Gabor Maté also describes tragic patterns in aboriginal people in this part of Canada who have trouble adjusting to the predominant culture. Children are abused by their own drug-abusing parents and grow up to treat their own children badly, all the time smoking and drinking heavily.[21]

Another example comes from the work of the anthropologist Philippe Bourgois. He lived in the *barrio* of Spanish Harlem in New York City for three-and-a-half years and wrote a gritty account of the use of heroin and crack cocaine there. He blamed the widespread addictions at least in part on the difficulties facing the Puerto Ricans who had moved to the city. He described the loss of job opportunities for the working class, the marginalization of the Puerto Rican population, and the difficulty of people migrating from an economy based on subsistence farming to one based on white-collar work.[22]

But of course morphine does not change the reality of life for the caged rat, nor does it solve the problems of people coping with traumatic childhoods or cultural upheaval. Some people find temporary relief from these problems in drugs, but this may develop into an addiction that will not address the initial problem and that will often compound the misery. The American novelist Stephen Crane described the appeal and the problems of substance abuse when, as a journalist, he wrote about denizens of the late nineteenth-century New York opium den:

> The problems of life no longer appear. Existence is peace ... The universe is readjusted. Wrong departs, injustice vanishes; there is nothing but a quiet, a soothing harmony of all things—until the next morning ... Opium holds out ... its lie, and they embrace it eagerly, expecting to find a definition of peace, but they awake to find the formidable labors of life grown more formidable. And if the pipe should happen to ruin their lives they cling the more closely to it because then it stands between them and thought.[23]

Not everyone agrees that addiction is just "purchased relief." Not all people with addictions have had obvious traumas or struggles with injustice, and not all people with terrible childhoods become addicted to substances. Vulnerability and its opposite, resilience, are not well understood. One person with abusive alcoholic parents becomes an alcoholic; another person makes a decision to never use alcohol. There seems to be an element of choice involved.

Choice

Some experts believe that drug addiction is not a disease or a way of coping with unhappiness, but simply a choice. Because this choice hurts themselves and others, addiction is disapproved of in a way that other illnesses such as asthma, high blood pressure, and diabetes are not.

This theory seems quite different from the two earlier theories, but even those who do see addiction as a disease, such as Benjamin Rush, sometimes simultaneously seem to see it as a bad choice and will use language indicating disapproval when referring to the behavior of people who are addicted. Rush wanted a drunkard to be "as infamous in society as a liar or a thief," and he constructed a "moral thermometer" comparing the ill effects of various beverages.

Another example of disapproval can be found in Alcoholics Anonymous (AA). AA, ambivalent about whether alcoholism is an illness, teaches that the use of alcohol is about loss of control of one's own behavior. The language of AA contains notes of censure. For example, the Twelve Steps of AA refer to "a searching and fearless moral inventory" and "defects of character." AA also mentions the wrongs done by the alcoholic to others. Health care providers urge people with some chronic illnesses to eat less salt, exercise more, or the like. But dietary indiscretions or refusal to exercise are not described as "defects of character," and health care providers do not exhort those with high blood pressure to continue to "take personal inventory."[24]

If drug use is a choice, a person should be able to choose to stop it. Leshner argued that the initial use may be voluntary, but then the person's brain changes and the person can no longer stop. However, some say that addicts *can* stop, once the consequences of their continued use are dire enough. If true, this makes addiction very different from other brain diseases such as Alzheimer's disease or Parkinson's disease.

Gene Heyman develops this argument at length in his book *Addiction Is a Choice*. He notes that addicted physicians and pilots have high rates of recovery. The professional associations make the choice clear for their members: stop the addiction or lose your job. The associations know that the choice is not easy, and so they monitor the former addict closely. An addicted physician stops her use of opiates if she knows that "dirty urine" found on random testing will mean that she loses her job. She chooses to use and she chooses to stop.

Another example that Heyman uses of people choosing to stop when the consequences worsen comes from mid-twentieth-century China. Mao Zedong declared opium addiction to be criminal and that trafficking would be punished by death. Addiction rates plummeted.

Heyman also argues that stopping substance abuse is common and is often preceded by concerns about health or finances, or is simply due to growing up. Large epidemiological surveys find that people quit drugs, may relapse again, but "by about age 30 most have quit for good."[25] Recovery from other chronic illnesses rarely follows this pattern. As a person with arthritis, diabetes, or high blood pressure ages, the illness usually worsens.

Even within populations where substance abuse is common, individual choice is important. In his description of life in East Harlem in the 1980s, Bourgois notes that most of the residents in El Barrio did not use drugs. Furthermore, those who used drugs often at some point chose to stop.

Those who believe that addiction is a choice argue that to call the persistent use of drugs a reaction to a difficult childhood or cultural problems, or a disease, is not only incorrect, but harmful because the person provided with either explanation will now have a "reason" to feel hopeless and to continue using the drug. To call addiction a brain disease discounts the autonomy of the addict.

If addiction is a choice and the choice to stop sometimes happens when the consequences are bad enough, that explains the common belief that the addict sometimes has to "hit bottom"—that is, sustain serious losses of job, family, housing, or health—before he chooses to stop using drugs. This also means that treatment may prolong the substance abuse by deferring the losses. Detoxification programs and treatment facilities sometimes "enable" the addict. And, indeed, treatment results in addiction programs are notoriously poor.

How does this theory that addiction is a choice, not a brain disease, fit in with the findings that the brains of the addicts are different? The answer to this question is that, as noted earlier, most of the imaging findings are from the brains of those who have already "chosen" to use drugs, and it is difficult to know if the brain of the person about to become an addict is significantly different from that of the non-addict.

As well, perhaps the brain changes that we see are not necessarily prolonging the addiction; perhaps they are just a result of other activities associated with addiction. It is not surprising that what goes on in the brain of an addict looking for heroin is different from what goes on in the brain of a sober person. But it is a leap to go from that to saying that the addict *has* to look for heroin. The crux of the matter, so the argument goes, is not the craving for the drug; it is the decision of the person to act on the craving, and that decision is too complex to be captured by neuroimaging. A person with little reward circuit activity can still choose whether to inject heroin. The assertion of NIDA that there is a compulsion in addiction is only that: an assertion. What is compulsion to one person is to another person weakness or a conscious decision to give in to an impulse. A hungry person who steals some food makes a bad choice. However, we would not be so quick to make that judgment if we knew the person had had no food for several days. Whether the addicted person is closer to the hungry or the starving person is difficult to determine.

This theory makes many uncomfortable, particularly those who have sympathy for people with unfortunate childhoods. Is it not true that bad childhoods can lead to bad choices? Those who say that drug abuse or addiction is a choice argue that it is mistaken to assume that a terrible childhood has anything to do with the decision to use drugs. We like our lives to be meaningful rather than a random series of incidents; we seek patterns. Something happens, and we look for a cause. We invent our own narratives. If we are addicts, we look back to our childhoods to find the reason. Those who see addiction as a choice, and not related to bad childhoods, can point to people with traumatic childhoods who do not develop addictions.

This theory is about choice, which itself is a complicated concept. Often we believe that we are "choosing," but actually we are responding to cues of which we are unaware. Sometimes we are merely copying others. French painters saw each other drinking absinthe and did the same. Wilkie Collins used laudanum, and so did his friend Samuel Coleridge. This tendency to copy others applies to drug use and to quitting drug use, and has been most clearly shown with respect to smoking cigarettes. Nicholas Christakis argues in his finely grained analysis of Massachusetts smokers that a person's decision to stop smoking reflects a group decision.[26] In colloquial language, he explains:

> A smoker may have as much control over quitting as a bird has to stop a flock from flying in a particular direction.[27]

A teenager begins to smoke because of all his friends are smoking. The friends of a heroin addict give up heroin, and she decides to stop using. In both cases, they think that they have made a choice, but they are—to use Christakis's analogy—just like geese flying south in the winter. The choice that the person does make is who she chooses to befriend. The importance of our friends and our tendency to be animals of the herd is reflected in the maxim heard at AA meetings: If you want to fly like the eagles, don't hang out with the turkeys.

Who Are the People Who Develop Addictions?

If none of these theories—addiction is a brain disease, self-medication, or choice—is able to satisfactorily explain drug abuse, can we at least *describe* the people who become drug addicts? The task is difficult because it involves looking backward at people before they started their addiction, and that can be misleading. Also, there may be different answers with respect to different substances, in different times, and in different cultures.

There are, however, some groups of people who develop addictions that lead to trouble or publicity and who are therefore well-described. These are the antisocial, young, searchers, or artists. The categories are not exclusive of one another, since one can belong to several groups at the same time. The number of people who develop addictions who do not fit into any of these categories is not known.

The Antisocial Person

Personality disorders are a group of psychiatric conditions marked by pervasive patterns of maladaptive thoughts or behavior. One of the best defined is antisocial personality disorder, which is marked by a persistent disregard for the rights or welfare of others. There is an overlap between antisocial personality disorder and substance abuse or addiction.[28] People who break laws are not afraid of negative consequences, and they value immediate gratification. Routine is irksome; thrills and novelty beckon. They are comfortable with behavior that violates the rules of society. Abuse of alcohol, cocaine, and opiates is consistent with all of these qualities. These addictions interfere with education, steady work, and/or good health. People who use these drugs to excess choose pleasure over responsibility. Criminality and a disrespect for society are consistent with substance abuse and addiction.

The connection is strongest with respect to addiction to opiates. Evidence can be found in Lee Robins's work, described in the opiates chapter, in which earlier antisocial behavior predicts heroin use. Robins inquired about the lives of soldiers before they went to Vietnam, looking into what might have predicted or led to heroin use. In medical or epidemiological terms, she was looking for "risk factors." The risk factors she found were "deviant behaviors" such as fighting, arrests, drunkenness, school expulsion, and drug use.[29]

In other words, those soldiers who had used heroin were more likely to have had behavioral problems as youngsters than were the soldiers who had not used this drug. (Her work also supports the idea that a clear consequence—in this case, the threat of not being able to leave Vietnam—stops the heroin use.)

Other experts agree. In a study of Lexington Farm heroin addicts, about half had been antisocial *before* they began to use heroin. Few had stable work records.[30] James Inciardi, a leading researcher into the relationship between criminality and drug abuse, writes:

> ... while drug use tends to intensify and perpetuate criminal behavior, it usually does not initiate criminal careers. ... among the majority of street drug users who are involved in crime, their criminal careers were well established prior to the onset or either narcotics or cocaine use.[31]

Under the influence of drugs, people often do things that hurt others or put them at risk. They drive recklessly while using alcohol and steal from their friends and family. People go through cycles of drug abuse and sobriety, and often choose to use again, knowing yet ignoring how dangerous this can be to others.

Those who do see antisocial behavior leading to addiction think of treatment as problematic, since there is no accepted treatment for antisocial personality disorder. Treatment, since it implies that an illness is present, can give antisocial people an excuse for their bad behavior and may also foster the addiction. Some people, for example, choose to enter a facility for a detoxification program, not for help in giving up an addiction, but to prolong or nurture it. They enter a hospital for a few days to get some decent food and rest, or for what is known as "three hots and a cot." Having been refreshed, they leave and are able to resume their addiction. They now have lowered their tolerance so that their drug habit has become cheaper.

The difficulty of treating addiction was evident at the Lexington Narcotic Farm in Kentucky, where many of the patients had, at the least, antisocial traits. The high relapse rate was partly responsible for the pessimism with which many came to regard heroin addiction. Some people came to the Farm for a brief detoxification, with no intention of stopping their drug abuse. Also, some patients were able to go to the Farm and receive free opiates in return for participating in experiments. These patients had little interest in staying away from drugs.

Many experts argue that the association between substance abuse and antisocial behavior goes the *opposite* way. They suggest that it is the illegality of substance abuse that causes antisocial behavior. The addicted person is unable to work at a regular job because she has no easy or socially accepted way of buying drugs and must use much of her time to find them. The addict needs a rapid supply of money, and since he is already acquainted with lawbreakers who supply him with the drug, it is a small step to activities such as prostitution, pimping, gambling, or selling drugs so that he can support his addiction.

Illegality of substances is a boon to criminal enterprise, as was well demonstrated during Prohibition. During those years, people who formerly bought alcohol from legal stores supported the underworld by buying it from bootleggers. Many bootleggers were also involved in other illegal activities such as gambling and prostitution. Other consequences involved violence. Disputes between gangs could not be settled in courts and sometimes were settled by bribery or murder. One of the reasons for the repeal of Prohibition was the fear that it was fostering widespread disrespect of the law.

Dole and Nyswander were articulate proponents of this point of view. They also thought that some people have a physiological need for opiates. Combining both of these opinions—that illegality of drugs was part of the problem, as was a metabolic need for opiates—they criticized the suggestion that there was any connection between antisocial personality disorder and addiction:

> ... addicts are self-centered and indifferent to the needs of others. To the family and community the addict is irresponsible, a thief, and a liar ... The rapid disappearance of theft and antisocial behavior in the patients on the methadone program strongly supports the hypothesis that crimes that they had previously committed as addicts were a consequence of drug hunger, not the expression of some more basic psychopathology. The so-called sociopathic personality is no longer evident ...[32]

Methadone allows opiate addicts to satisfy their "drug hunger" legally. As noted earlier and in the opiates chapter, Dole and Nyswander were successful. Their methadone-treated patients stopped stealing and became productive law-abiding members of society. The connection with antisocial personality disorder was broken.

Fifty years later, this eloquent argument and Dole and Nyswander's excellent results have lost their luster. Methadone clinics, still successful, nonetheless are associated with many problems, including abuse of other substances, such as alcohol and cocaine, diversion, and deaths due to methadone overdoses.[33]

A final complication of the possible connection between antisocial personality and addiction is the question of money. Rich antisocial people drink champagne; poor antisocial people drink gin or malt liquor. Rich people snort cocaine powder; poor people smoke crack cocaine. The rich have skilled attorneys to help them evade the consequences of their misdeeds; the poor do not. This is not a new phenomenon. In 1686, Increase Mather, father of Cotton Mather, said:

It is an unhappy thing that in later years a Kind of Drink called Rum has been common among us. They that are poor, and wicked too, can for a penny or two-pence make themselves drunk.[34]

This was the same complaint made by eighteenth-century Londoners— that gin was so cheap anyone could drink it. If drugs are cheap, then the "poor and wicked" have easy access to them. The message is clear: poor people have no business breaking the law, getting drunk, or using drugs; rich people who are wicked are given more latitude.

The Adolescent

Adolescence is a time of exploration and experimentation. Our reward system reacts to thrill seeking, as well as to drugs, and develops earlier than does our prefrontal cortex. Young people lead lives unhindered by their prefrontal cortices. The perils of various activities are not as apparent to them as they are to older people. They make a reckless decision to use drugs, and the substances further impair their executive functioning. They can develop addictions and become entangled in a life of perilous excitement.

Addiction also appeals to some adolescents because it provides challenge and structure. Heroin addiction, for example, is not easy. Addicts have to hunt for heroin. For some adolescents with no job, education, or clear goals, the life of searching for heroin can be fulfilling.[35] For other adolescents, the appeal of drugs is different. These young people chafe against the confinements of home, school, or job and can be seduced, sometimes by their musical heroes, into believing that drugs lead to freedom, creativity, and a way out of their dull lives.

Adolescence is also a phase of life when many feel anxious and uncertain. Tobacco companies thought about these issues a great deal and, of course, did what they could to recruit new smokers by exploiting the adolescent's sense of awkwardness as he approaches adulthood as well as his adventurousness. A research agency working for a tobacco company offered this cold-blooded advice on how to make cigarette smoking appealing to adolescents:

An attempt to reach young smokers, starters, should be based . . . on the following major parameters: Present the cigarette as one of a few initiations into the adult world. Present the cigarette as part of the illicit pleasure category of products and activities. In your ads create a situation taken from the day-to-day life of the young smoker but in an elegant manner have this situation touch on the basic symbols of the growing-up, maturity process. To the best of your ability (considering some legal restraints), relate the cigarette to "pot," wine, beer, sex, etc.[36]

As the person grows up and becomes interested in her own family or in becoming productive, she stops using drugs. The person's prefrontal cortex catches up to his reward system, and enthrallment with danger diminishes. The prefrontal cortex asserts its primacy in adulthood.

Charles Winick, a New York psychologist and colleague of Nyswander, saw that heroin addicts gave up their addiction as they reached their forties and described this as "maturing out." He thought that this process was not to do with the life cycle, but rather the number of years of the actual addiction process.[37] Whichever explanation one favors, many adolescents do—eventually—stop using drugs or alcohol in an addictive manner.

The Searcher

It is not only the adolescent who has trouble finding her place in the world and who agonizes over the purpose of life. A person of any age may use drugs as a way of "finding" her true self or deciphering the mysteries of the universe. Some people cannot accept the mundane facts of their lives and search for more. Are birth, disillusionment, and illness all there is to life? Drugs can "anesthetize" us to the realization of the futility of life or lead us to an intimation of a greater or more reassuring truth. Often the drug chosen for this quest is a psychedelic drug, which is not the subject of this book. However, each of the four drugs of this book has, on occasion, been used for this purpose.

Alcohol and cocaine can convince the person that she understands herself and her place in the world. Tobacco in very high doses leads to visions and was used for this purpose by shamans in the Americas. Opiates usually alleviate pain or anxiety but have been associated with hallucinations. Samuel Taylor Coleridge might have written the poem *Kubla Khan* under the influence of opium and may be referring to opium in the last lines of this poem:

Weave a circle round him thrice,
And close your eyes with holy dread,
For he on honey-dew hath fed,
And drunk the milk of Paradise[38]

The searcher sometimes adopts a "junkie" lifestyle as a way of asserting himself as an individual and not just another unthinking cog in a society with its plethora of oppressive rules and expectations. Taking drugs can seem to be an act of authenticity.

William S. Burroughs, discussed in the opiate chapter, was the scion of a successful Midwestern family. From childhood, he was unsettled. He graduated from Harvard and then began a (long) life as a drug taker and drifter. His best seller *Junky* is a semiautobiographical description of his life as an opiate addict. He is not complimentary of other addicts, but he is fascinated by them:

> Waves of hostility and suspicion flowed out from his large brown eyes like some sort of television broadcast … The man was small and very thin, his neck loose in the collar of his shirt. His complexion was fading from brown to a mottled yellow, and pancake make-up had been heavily applied in an attempt to conceal a skin eruption. His mouth was drawn down at the corners in a grimace of petulant annoyance.[39]

His narrator later descends into the world of another addict:

> The apartment was dark and musty. Clothes, books, newspapers, dirty plates and glasses were scattered around on chairs and tables and on the dirty floor. I pushed a stack of magazines off a ratty-looking couch.
> "Sit down," I said. "You got the stuff on you?"
> "Yeah, I got it planted." He opened his fly and extracted a rectangular paper packet—the junkie fold, with one end fitting into another … He placed the papers on the table … His mouth, toothless and tightly closed, gave the impression of being sewed together …[40]

The squalor of these scenes does not deter Burroughs from using drugs. The frankness of these descriptions appeals to some, while to others, the book is a litany of criminal activities, irresponsibility, and illness. The perception of drug abuse as a rebellion against the stifling mores of mainstream culture is common among adolescents and those who cannot tolerate the humdrum routines of normal life.

The romanticization of addicts had a supporter in Nyswander. She thought that some of her patients were free:

> In one sense, some of those I know up here strike me as among the few comparatively free people I meet during the day. Of course, they have a compulsion; but their compulsion is to drugs, not to smiling when you

don't mean it and entertaining the boss for what you're going to get from him. Except when he's scrounging for drugs, the addict's relationships are usually honest and direct. He's not "refined" in the way that striving for upward mobility necessitates . . .

She went on to compare some of them to mystics:

In India and throughout the East they've had their lotus eaters—their drug addicts—for centuries. They grow up with them, they feed them, and they consider the addict part of the whole community as a balance against the materialistic proclivities of their society. In some cultures, moreover, religious mystics are forbidden to involve themselves in the tensions and desires of ordinary life. They're supposed to just sit and think. But there's no room for a mystic here . . .

Here the addict is forced into the abyss. He is forced to look at something in himself that every man has in him but that few men have fully faced—the fear of basic, total failure. . . . Hasn't nearly every great religious leader and artist and writer gone through horror, agony, torture, and temptation . . . an addict confronting his reality existentially is different from the man who commutes on the train, drinks too much, sleeps with call girls at conventions or with his neighbor's wife. I wonder which of those two kinds of experience is more apt to lead a man to discover the truth about himself . . .[41]

Nyswander suggests that much of our day-to-day life depends on routine and politeness, or, in her words, "smiling when you don't mean it." Is this an admirable way of spending our few years on earth? The lotus eaters described by Nyswander and the addicts described by Burroughs refuse to be enslaved to the "materialistic proclivities" of society. Drugs let a person escape to a world without conformity or perceived hypocrisy.

Most would not think that the answer to the search for the meaning of life can be found through drugs or a life of addiction. Nevertheless, health care professionals working with people with addictions do sometimes note that their patients or clients can have a variety of emotions and experiences denied to the more restrained or buttoned-up professional.

The Artistic or Creative Person

We usually accept what is around us in an unquestioning way, but the creative person sees the world from his own perspective and fashions new things. This gift allows the person to see the world with freshness and to experience the thrill of creation. Yet this gift does not make the creative person immune from substance abuse. Whether creativity and substance abuse are connected is difficult to determine, but there are so many dramatic descriptions of artists abusing and celebrating substances that the association is difficult to ignore.

Creative persons use alcohol or other substances to spur on their flight from convention, spark insights, or release their inhibitions. They drink to court Dionysus. There are other reasons for the creative person to use drugs. The work of an artist is personal, and judgment of others on one's expressions of individuality stings. Success comes with expectations of even better work to come, and that is terrifying. If the work is condemned, mocked, or—worst of all—ignored, then the artist has to cope with rage and self-doubt. Alcohol and/or drugs briefly quell these feelings. The person may be swept away by the drugs into intoxication or oblivion, which, for brief periods, is a world where there are no critics or adoring crowds demanding more.

Writers

Addiction is a natural subject for storytelling. The narrative begins with pleasure and intoxication accompanied by a glorious sense of revelation and adventure. This is followed by dependence, pain, and chaos. Sometimes there is recovery and redemption. As previously discussed, opiates were popular among eighteenth- and nineteenth-century writers. Some writers draw on personal experiences to write about addiction. For example, Eugene O'Neill wrote about his mother's physician-caused morphine addiction in *Long Day's Journey into Night*.

A well-known writer-addict was the English poet Samuel Coleridge. Coleridge wanted to stop his use of opium and so decided to live with a London surgeon, Dr. James Gillman. The plan was that the good doctor would gradually wean Coleridge off the drug. Coleridge lived with Gillman for 18 years, and Gillman did succeed in lowering his dose. But Coleridge was ambivalent. Unbeknownst to Gillman, Coleridge visited a "chemist's assistant" who surreptitiously supplied him with "a 12-ounce pint of laudanum every five days."[42] This kind of deception is surely familiar to those with a personal knowledge of addiction. The addicted person, no matter how brilliant and accomplished, has wavering resolve.

Absinthe and Creativity

One type of alcoholic beverage, absinthe, was associated with a remarkable outpouring of literature and art. It was a liberating but destructive drug for many in nineteenth-century Europe. Absinthe was reported to have caused hallucinations and, in part because of this, was highly valued. The writers who drank absinthe, and were often addicted to it, included Guillaume Apollinaire, Charles Baudelaire, Burroughs, Ernest Dowson, Alfred Jarry, Arthur Rimbaud, Paul Verlaine, and Oscar Wilde. Ernest Hemingway is reported to have written *For Whom the Bell Tolls* under the influence of absinthe.

Absinthe was a favorite subject in many paintings of the time, most notably in posters by Henri de Toulouse-Lautrec. The artist kept absinthe in the cane that he used to help him walk. Honoré Daumier, Edgar Degas, Viktor Oliva, Pablo Picasso, Vincent van Gogh, and others also painted pictures in which absinthe and its drinkers can be seen. These pictures exude Belle Époque decadence and cynicism—deeply alluring to many.

Rituals were pleasing to painters of absinthe drinkers. The clear green absinthe was poured into a glass, and then water from a pitcher or siphon was added through a lump of sugar held over the glass in a special slotted spoon called an absinthe spoon. As the sweetened water was poured in, the absinthe turned a milky, pale yellow-green. This green gave rise to absinthe being called *la fée verte* and the afternoon hours, when absinthe was often drunk, *l'heure verte*. The ceremonies of absinthe drinking and the green drink can be seen clearly in the portrait of Henri Boileau that was painted by Toulouse Lautrec (see Figure 21.2).

In 1901, Pablo Picasso painted *Woman Drinking Absinthe* with quite a different feeling to it. This is a picture that might belong to a book written by Burroughs (see Figure 21.3).

An historian of absinthe described Picasso's subject in this way:

> The long arms and sinewy hands enfold her meager body while her eyes glow with what may be carnal contemplation. Before her sits the absinthe. In the mirror behind, the images of the outside world flatten and change form.[43]

Absinthe was identified with a culture of abandon and recklessness and with the celebration of death. The French poet, Paul Verlaine, when intoxicated on absinthe, shot his lover, the poet Arthur Rimbaud, in the arm and was jailed for two years. Picasso, although fascinated by absinthe, was not himself particularly fond of it. He had a longer and more productive life than other artists who did drink absinthe.

Musicians

Addiction plagues musicians. John Coltrane, Miles Davis, Billie Holliday, and Charlie Parker, all jazz musicians, were addicted to heroin.

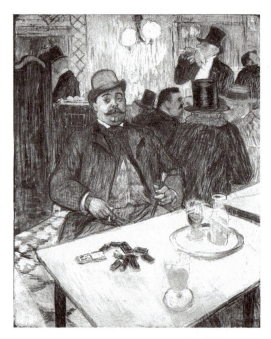

Figure 21.2   **Monsieur Boileau at the Café, 1893.**
(Henri de Toulouse-Lautrec [French, 1864–1901].
Gouache, 80 × 65 cm. Cleveland Museum of Art,
Hinman B. Hurlbut Collection 394.1925.
Photograph © The Cleveland Museum of Art)

There is a sad list of musicians who have died in their twenties due
to overdoses of alcohol and or drugs: Kurt Cobain, Jimi Hendrix,
Janis Joplin, Brian Jones, Jim Morrison, Gram Parsons, and Amy
Winehouse. The lack of a steady income or, on the other hand, sudden
success with wealth, high expectations, and relentless public scrutiny do
not make the lives of artists easy. Musicians and artists often espouse a
hard-living and hard-partying lifestyle in which they disavow any connection with the sober establishment.

Is There a Connection?

These lists do seem to support the theory that artists have a disproportionate share of addictions. However, we may be misled by what we read,
since articles, news reports, and biographies are not often written about
people with normal or happy lives. If Dylan Thomas, the Welsh poet
who died at the age of 39 from alcoholism, had not been such a rowdy
drinker, his life would be less interesting to read about. The artists
themselves may be more given to self-disclosure than the rest of us.

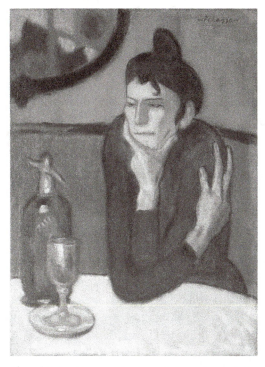

Figure 21.3 *Woman Drinking Absinthe*, 1901, Pablo
Picasso. (State Hermitage Museum, St. Petersburg.
Photograph © The State Hermitage Museum/photo
by Vladimir Terebenin, Leonard Kheiferts, Yuri
Molodkovets)

The brilliance of their descriptions of substance abuse and its miseries
creates an impression that artists are more prone to addictions than others.
Some have tried to determine the existence of such an association in a
quantitative way. For example, Felix Post reviewed the biographies of
291 world-famous men and found a higher incidence of depression and
alcoholism in artists and writers than in scientists or politicians.[44] Joseph
Schildkraut looked at American abstract expressionists, a New York painting movement of the mid-1940s, and found that at least five and possibly
seven of the 15 were alcoholics. Of these seven, one committed suicide,
and two died in single car accidents that might have been suicides.[45]
These and other studies are far from conclusive but do suggest that the
creative process may indeed be linked with depression, substance abuse,
and addiction. Or at the very least, the studies suggest that alcoholism
does not stop the creative person from being productive; nor does
creativity keep a person safe from depression or alcoholism.

Conclusion

This debate over the nature of addiction will not soon be resolved. We know something about addicts who come to treatment or go to jail but less about those who keep quiet about their problems. None of the explanations or descriptions is adequate. Not everyone with a terrible childhood or with two biological parents with alcoholism becomes an addict, and some people who have no genetic loading for the problem and benign childhoods do become addicted.

People who are able to drink wine in moderation look down on the homeless Listerine drinker: "I can control my drinking; why can't she? All she needs is some will power." But it is impossible to judge the strength of the compulsions that afflict others. The question of what is will power is unanswerable.

The dispute may be of more theoretical than practical importance. If addiction is a brain disease, it is still influenced by stress, life circumstances, and choices. If addiction is a choice, it is still affected by the wiring of the individual brain. No matter what the causes, some people have great difficulty in controlling their use of alcohol, cocaine, nicotine, and opiates despite serious and health-damaging consequences. Education, careers, health, and families fall prey to addictions.

The choice of whether to use drugs, how and when to use them, and which drug to use is always affected by culture and circumstance, as well as by the architecture and molecular makeup of the particular person's brain circuitry. Our *milieu intérieur* determines how we feel, but it is affected by a myriad of events in the *milieu extérieur*. Whether substances are legal, cheap, or approved of by society at large will affect how the drugs are used. Legalizing a drug makes it safer and weakens the connection with criminality but makes it more widely used and increases addiction.

Notes

1. Richard Kluger, *Ashes to Ashes: America's Hundred-Year Cigarette War, the Public Health, and the Unabashed Triumph of Philip Morris* (New York: Vintage, 1997), 646.

2. Allan M. Brandt, *The Cigarette Century: The Rise, Fall, and Deadly Persistence of the Product That Defined America* (New York: Basic Books, 2007), 335.

3. Caroline Knapp, *Drinking: A Love Story* (New York: Dell, 2006), 5–6.

4. Gene Heyman, *Addiction: A Disorder of Choice* (Cambridge, MA: Harvard University Press, 2009), 82–85.

5. Eric Nestler and Robert Malenka, "The Addicted Brain," *Scientific American*, March 2004, 80.

6. Avram Goldstein, "Heroin Maintenance: A Medical View; A Conversation between a Physician and a Politician," *Journal of Drug Issues* 9 (1979): 342.

7. William L. White, *Slaying the Dragon: The History of Addiction Treatment and Recovery in America* (Normal, IL: Chestnut Health Systems/Lighthouse Institute, 1998), 2.

8. Alan Leshner, "Addiction Is a Brain Disease, and It Matters," *Science* 278, no. 5335 (1997): 45.

9. Nancy Campbell, J. P. Olsen, and Luke Walden, *The Narcotic Farm: The Rise and Fall of America's First Prison for Drug Addicts* (New York: Abrams, 2008), 190.

10. Eleanore Maguire et al., "Navigation-Related Structural Change in the Hippocampi of Taxi Drivers," *Proceedings of the National Academy of Sciences USA* 97, no. 8 (2000): 4398–4403.

11. Rita Z. Goldstein and Nora D. Volkow, "Drug Addiction and Its Underlying Neurobiological Basis: Neuroimaging Evidence for the Involvement of the Frontal Cortex," *American Journal of Psychiatry* 159, no. 10 (2002): 1642–52.

12. NIDA, "Genetics of Addiction: A Research Update from the National Institute on Drug Abuse, April 2008," http://www.drugabuse.gov/publications/topics-in-brief/genetics-addiction (accessed August 18, 2013)

13. William S. Burroughs, *Junky* (New York: Penguin, 2003), xxxix.

14. Russell Brand, "Comments on the Death of Amy Winehouse," *Guardian.com*, July 24, 2011, http://www.theguardian.com/music/2011/jul/24/russell-brand-amy-winehouse-woman (accessed August 18, 2013). His comments were in response to the overdose death of the musician Amy Winehouse.

15. Naomi I. Eisenberger and Matthew D. Lieberman, "Why Rejection Hurts: A Common Neural Alarm System for Physical and Social Pain," *Trends in Cognitive Science* 8, no. 7 (2004): 294–300.

16. Edward J. Khantzian, "The Self-Medication Hypothesis of Substance Use Disorders: A Reconsideration and Recent Applications," *Harvard Review of Psychiatry* 4, no. 5 (1997): 231–44.

17. Marian C. Diamond, David Krech, and Mark R. Rosenzweig, "The Effects of an Enriched Environment on the Rat Cerebral Cortex," *Journal of Comparative Neurology* 123 (1964): 111–19.

18. Bruce K. Alexander et al., "Effect of Early and Later Colony Housing on Oral Ingestion of Morphine in Rats," *Pharmacology, Biochemistry, and Behavior* 15 (1981): 571–76.

19. Avram Goldstein, "Neurobiology of Heroin Addiction and of Methadone Treatment," American Association for the Treatment of Opioid Dependence, plenary speech 1997, reprinted by the American Association for the Treatment

of Opiate Dependence, April, 2013 http://www.aatod.org (accessed August 18, 2013).

20. Bruce K. Alexander, *The Globalisation of Addiction: A Study in Poverty of the Spirit* (Oxford: Oxford University Press, 2008), 131–36.

21. Gabor Maté, *In the Realm of Hungry Ghosts: Close Encounters with Addiction* (Berkeley, CA: North Atlantic Books, 2008), 263–80.

22. Philippe Bourgois, *In Search of Respect: Selling Crack in El Barrio* (New York: Cambridge University Press, 1996), 319.

23. Stephen Crane, "Opium's Varied Dreams," *New York Sun*, 1896, in ed. Phillip Lopate, *Writing New York: Literary Anthology* (New York: Literary Classics of the United States, 1998), 313.

24. AA quotes come from "The Twelve Steps" of AA, found in *Alcoholics Anonymous*, 4th ed. (New York: A.A. World Services, 2001), 59.

25. Heyman, *Addiction*, 77.

26. Nicholas A. Christakis and James H. Fowler, "Quitting in Droves: Collective Dynamics of Smoking Behavior in a Large Social Network," *New England Journal of Medicine* 358, no.21 (2008): 2249–58.

27. Nicholas A. Christakis and James H. Fowler, *Connected: The Surprising Power of Our Social Networks and How They Shape Our Lives* (New York: Little, Brown, 2009), 116.

28. Deborah S. Hasin et al., "Personality Disorders and the 3-Year Course of Alcohol, Drug, and Nicotine Disorders," *Archives of General Psychiatry* 68, no. 11 (2011): 1158–67.

29. Lee N. Robins et al., "Vietnam Veterans Three Years after Vietnam: How Our Study Changed Our View of Heroin," *American Journal on Addictions* 19 (May–June 2010): 203–11.

30. George E. Vaillant, "What Can Long-Term Follow-Up Teach Us about Relapse and Prevention of Relapse in Addiction?" *British Journal of Addiction* 83 (1988): 1147–57.

31. James Inciardi, *Legalize It? Debating American Drug Policy* (Washington, DC: American University Press, 1993), 204.

32. Vincent P. Dole and Marie Nyswander, "Heroin Addiction: A Metabolic Disease," *Archives of Internal Medicine* 120 (July 1967): 21.

33. Theodore Dalrymple, *Romancing Opiates: Pharmacological Lies and the Addiction Bureaucracy* (New York: Encounter Books, 2006), 44–56.

34. Alice Morse Earle, *Customs and Fashions in New England*, 1893 (repr., Williamstown, MA: Corner House, 1974), 175.

35. Ann Marlowe, *How to Stop Time: Heroin from A to Z* (New York: Basic Books, 1999), 57–58.

36. Quoted in Simon Chapman, *Great Expectorations: Advertising and the Tobacco Industry* (London: Comedia, 1986), 32.

37. Charles Winick, "Maturing Out of Narcotic Addiction," *U.N. Bulletin on Narcotics* 14, no. 1 (1962): 1–7.

38. Samuel Coleridge, *Kubla Khan*, lines 51–54.

39. William S. Burroughs, *Junky*, 4.

40. Ibid., 118.

41. Nat Hentoff, *A Doctor among the Addicts* (New York: Rand McNally, 1968), 22–24.

42. Alethea Hayter, *Opium and the Romantic Imagination* (London: Faber, 1968), 194.

43. Barnaby Conrad III, *Absinthe* (San Francisco: Chronicle, 1988), 79.

44. Felix Post, "Creativity and Psychopathology. A study of 291 world-famous men," *British Journal of Psychiatry* 165 (1994), 22–34.

45. Joseph Schildkraut, Alissa Hirshfeld, and Jane Murphy, "Mind and mood in modern art, II: Depressive disorders, spirituality, and early deaths in the abstract expressionist artists of the New York School," *American Journal of Psychiatry* 151, no. 4 (1994), 482–88.

Glossary

acetyl: An organic group used by the Bayer Company in chemical transformations to make aspirin and **heroin.** The chemical formula is $COCH_3$.

acetylcholine: The chemical compound that was the first **neurotransmitter** to be discovered. It is active at **synapses** in the brain, in the **parasympathetic system,** and also at **synapses** between **nerves** and muscles.

acetylcholine receptor: The **receptor** that recognizes **acetylcholine;** one type recognizes **nicotine,** and one type recognizes muscarine.

acid: In chemistry, refers to a structure that can donate protons or accept electrons, the opposite of a **base.** In water, acids produce H^+ ions. **Base** and acid together form **salts.**

action potential: A brief electrical signal running down the **axon** to the terminal of the **neuron** terminal that triggers release of **neurotransmitters.**

addiction: Compulsive use of a **substance,** such as **alcohol, cocaine, nicotine,** or **opiates,** despite adverse consequences. Involves craving, **dependence, tolerance,** and **withdrawal.**

adrenal gland: Small **gland** located just above the kidney. The inner part of the **gland,** or medulla, produces the **hormones norepinephrine** and **epinephrine.**

agonist: A **drug** that is active at a **receptor.** It acts like a **neurotransmitter** at the **synapse.** *See also* **antagonist.**

alcohol:

1. In this book, alcohol usually refers to **ethanol,** or ethyl alcohol, a molecule composed of two carbon atoms, six hydrogen atoms, and one oxygen atom. At room temperature, it is a clear and colorless liquid. It boils at 78.5 degrees Celsius. It has multiple effects on **neurotransmitters** and **cell membranes.** Alcohol is a solvent (see also **laudanum**). The chemical formula is C_2H_5OH or CH_3CH_2OH.

2. Class of chemical compounds where there is an –OH or hydroxyl group, containing **ethanol** and **methanol.**

3. Sometimes used as shorthand for an alcoholic beverage.

ale: Type of beer made with top fermenting yeast, associated with the English. *See also* **lager.**

alewife: Woman in medieval England who **brewed** beer at home. *See also* **brewster**.

alkaloid: A naturally occurring chemical compound, often found in plants, containing nitrogen, usually with a bitter taste. Some examples are caffeine, **cocaine, morphine, nicotine**.

alveolus: The small pocket of lung tissue surrounded by **capillaries**, where the gases oxygen and carbon dioxide are exchanged. There are about 300 million alveoli in each human lung.

Alzheimer's disease: A common degenerative illness in older adults, marked by memory loss and disturbances in **executive functioning**.

amine: An organic compound derived from ammonia, containing nitrogen, a **base.**

amino acid: An organic compound containing an amine, carboxylic acid, and a side-chain. Twenty different types of **amino acids** are the building blocks of **proteins**. Some amino acids (**GABA** and **glutamate**) also serve as **neurotransmitters**.

amygdala: The almond-shaped region of the brain in the **limbic system,** sometimes considered part of the **basal ganglia**, concerned with emotions, especially fear. The name comes from the Latin word for almond.

analgesia: The relief of pain or the inability to feel bodily sensations, especially pain.

anesthesia: Deliberately caused unconsciousness for the purpose of a surgical operation.

antagonist: Drug that binds to a **receptor** but does not activate it. It interferes with the action of a **neurotransmitter**. *See also* **agonist.**

anterior cingulate cortex: The part of the cingulate **cortex** that forms a collar around the corpus callosum, a bundle of fibers between the two hemispheres. Belongs to the **limbic system** and is involved in emotional responses to pain, empathy, decision making, conflict, and reward anticipation. Rich in **dopamine** neurons and **opiate** receptors.

attention deficit hyperactivity disorder (ADHD): Common childhood psychiatric disorder that may persist into adulthood, marked by impulsivity and inattentiveness, or problems in **executive function**. May be associated with **substance abuse** and **addiction.**

autonomic nervous system: A part of the **peripheral nervous system** that controls many organs and activities, such as digestion, heart rate, and blood flow, without our awareness or control. Made up of the **sympathetic** and **parasympathetic** systems.

axon: Long thin projection of a **neuron** carrying messages from the **neuron cell** body to another **neuron** (or muscle cell or **gland**). Each **neuron** has one axon that may branch.

barley: A grass in the genus *Hordeum*, native to temperate regions, having flowers in dense spikes. The word also refers to the **grain** used to feed livestock and to produce **malt** and **cereal.**

basal ganglia: A group of **nuclei** in the base of the brain, involved with the control of movements and some aspects of thinking and **addiction.** Includes the **nucleus accumbens, corpus striatum, substantia nigra** (and some neuroanatomists place the **amygdala** here).

base: In chemistry, refers to a structure that can donate electrons or accept protons, the opposite of an **acid.** In water, bases produce OH⁻ ions. Base and **acid** together form a **salt.**

benzopyrene: A **polycyclic aromatic hydrocarbon** found in coal **tar** and **tobacco smoke**; causes cancer. The chemical formula is $C_{20}H_{12}$.

blood-brain barrier: The **capillaries** that supply blood to the brain are lined with **cells** that are tightly joined. **Enzymes** in the barrier break down unwanted molecules or transport wanted molecules into the brain.

bootleg: The *noun* refers to illegal **liquor**; the *verb* refers to selling illegal **liquor.**

bootlegger: Seller of illegal **liquor.**

brain stem: Central core of brain structures between the spinal cord and the **cerebrum.** Contains the **medulla oblongata, pons**, and **midbrain.** It controls essential survival functions such as breathing and arousal.

brew: To steep a **substance** in water so that the water becomes infused with the flavor of this material. This is how beer, coffee, and tea are prepared. The brewing of beer is a multistep process.

brewer: Man who **brews** beer.

brewster: Woman who **brews** beer.

bronchitis: Infection or **inflammation** of bronchi, the passages in the lungs that transport air to and from the **alveoli.** The person with bronchitis coughs and is short of breath. **Tobacco smoking** can lead to chronic bronchitis, in which excessive **mucus** is produced, **inflammation** worsens, and **chronic obstructive pulmonary disease** may result.

buprenorphine: A semisynthetic **opioid.** Partial **mu opiate agonist** that binds tightly to **mu opiate receptors** without activating them fully; used to treat **opiate addiction.**

burn:

1. At high temperatures, a **substance** exposed to flame and oxygen rapidly changes its chemical nature and produces **smoke.** When **tobacco** is burned and then **smoked, nicotine** is drawn deeply into the lungs. **Nicotine** is not changed during the burning of **tobacco.** Hundreds of **substances** are formed when

tobacco is burned, many of which can cause cancer and/or harm the lungs and
cardiovascular system.

2. A gentle flameless process whereby the body gets its energy. **Cells** burn **carbohydrates** with oxygen. The results are water, carbon dioxide, and energy.
The chemical formula is:**carbohydrate** (CH_2O) + oxygen $(O_2) \rightarrow$ water
(H_2O) + carbon dioxide (CO_2) + energy. **Cells** can also burn **proteins** or
fats for energy.

capillary: A small blood vessel.

carbohydrate: A large group of compounds that includes **sugars** and **starches,**
produced by photosynthetic plants and used as energy source and building
material by animals. Contains carbon, hydrogen, and oxygen in a ratio of
roughly 1:2:1. The chemical formula is CH_2O or $C_6H_{12}O_6$.

cartel: An organization of businesspeople that fixes production, marketing, and
prices; to do with a **commodity.**

cell: The smallest structural unit of all living things. Some microorganisms,
such as **yeast,** consist of only one cell. Humans consist of about 100 trillion
cells.

cell membrane: Membrane separating the inside from the outside of the **cell;**
where most **receptors** are located. The membrane is made up of fats and **proteins** and allows fat-soluble **substances,** such as **alcohol** or **heroin,** into the
cell more easily than other molecules. There are also "ion channels" passing
through membranes; **local anesthetics** block these.

central nervous system: The brain and spinal cord, made up of **neurons** and
glial or supporting **cells.**

cereal: Annual grasses such as **barley,** corn, oats, rye, and wheat that produce edible **grains. Fermentation** of some of these grains leads to **alcohol.** Also refers
to **grain** itself and to breakfast food made from these **grains.**

cerebellum: The "little brain" located beneath and behind the **cerebrum.**
Coordinates muscular activity; needed for fine motor movements and balance.
The cerebellum is sensitive to **alcohol,** so a common sign of excessive **alcohol**
intake is clumsiness, uncoordinated movements, or inability to maintain balance. Long-term, heavy **alcohol** use damages the cerebellum.

cerebral cortex: The gray outermost part, or surface, of the brain where we
"think," about 1.5 to 4 mm thick, covering the **cerebrum,** folded into wrinkles
known as gyri and sulci, increasing the surface area of the brain.

cerebrum: The upper, large, and main part of the brain; large, round structure
divided into the right and left hemispheres, each of which is divided into the
frontal, parietal, occipital, and temporal lobes. It also contains the **limbic
system** and **basal ganglia.**

chromosome: A thread-like linear strand of **DNA** wrapped around **proteins** in
the **cell nucleus;** composed of **genes** and other less well understood material.

chronic obstructive pulmonary disease (COPD): Chronic lung disease that worsens over time. Can be **bronchitis** or **emphysema** and is usually caused by **tobacco smoking.**

coca: A **shrub** that grows in the Andes, *Erythroxylon* (or *Eryrthroxylum*) *coca.* Also refers to the dried leaf.

cocaine: An **alkaloid** produced by the leaves of the **coca shrub.**

cocaine hydrochloride: A **salt** of **cocaine,** a white crystalline powder, soluble in water, breaks down above 197 degrees Celsius. Injected or **snorted cocaine** has **psychoactive** properties and is **addictive.**

coca paste: An intermediate product between **coca** and **cocaine hydrochloride;** can be **smoked.**

cocktail: A beverage containing **distilled alcohol** and another ingredient, such as fruit juice, honey, milk, or soda. The cocktail became popular during **Prohibition**, perhaps to disguise the poor quality of much of the **bootlegged liquor.**

commodity: A good for which there is a demand. One way of understanding the history of the **drugs** discussed in this book is to see each as a commodity that is bought and sold for profit.

corpus striatum. Part of the **basal ganglia,** involved with muscular memories.

cortex: The outermost layer of an organ, such as the brain or **adrenal gland**. The name comes from the Latin for bark or rind.

crack cocaine: A form of **free base cocaine** that is prepared with baking soda or sodium bicarbonate. Crack cocaine **vaporizes** at 89 degrees Celsius and does not lose its **psychoactive** properties. **Smoked** crack cocaine can get into the brain within 10 seconds.

cure: With respect to **tobacco**, to age and to preserve by drying. After the **tobacco** leaf is harvested, it is dried either by air, exposure to fire, heat, or sun, and flavors develop.

denatured alcohol: Alcohol that is undrinkable because of the addition of poisonous **substances** such as **methyl alcohol**.

dendrite: A branch of a **neuron** carrying messages toward the **cell** body. Each **neuron** has thousands of dendrites studded with spines.

dependence: A state in which the person adapts to **alcohol, cocaine, nicotine,** or **opiates** and undergoes a **withdrawal** syndrome when no longer using the **substance**, particularly in the setting of **addiction.**

desensitization: A decrease in number and sensitivity of **receptors** that causes **tolerance.**

distillation: A method of purifying a **substance** based on difference in boiling points. If a liquid containing **alcohol** is heated, the **alcohol evaporates** at a lower temperature than the water. The **vapor** can be captured and condensed, and it becomes a liquid, known as **liquor,** containing more **alcohol** than the original liquid.

DNA: Deoxyribonucleic **acid**, makes up **genes**, in the form of a double stranded helix.

dopamine: A **neurotransmitter** that acts at dopamine **receptors**. It also is a **hormone;** it inhibits the release of prolactin from the **pituitary gland.** It is a precursor to **epinephrine** and **norepinephrine.** A rapid increase in dopamine in the **nucleus accumbens** or **reward system** is important in **addiction.** In **Parkinson's disease,** there is too little dopamine. Many medications used to treat **schizophrenia** are dopamine **antagonists.**

drug: A **substance** from outside the body that changes or restores the **homeostasis** of the body. It can be medication prescribed by a health care provider or an illegal **substance.**

drunkenness: Behavioral changes due to **intoxication** with **alcohol.** Influenced by social expectation.

emphysema: A type of **chronic obstructive pulmonary disease,** usually caused by **tobacco smoking,** in which the small airways and **alveoli** of the lung are damaged. **Alveolar** walls are destroyed and/or become less elastic.

endorphin: A **peptide neurotransmitter** with **opiate** like activity, produced in the brain. Shortened form of the phrase, "endogenous **morphine.**" Composed of five to forty **amino acids.** Leads to **analgesia** when binds to endorphin **receptors.**

enzyme: A **protein** that increases the rate of chemical reactions, made up of **amino acids.**

epinephrine: A **hormone** produced by the **adrenal gland.** Epinephrine means "on top of the kidney." In countries other than the United States, it is often referred to as adrenaline.

ethanol: Grain alcohol, or ethyl **alcohol,** a beverage. The chemical formula is C_2H_5OH. *See also* **alcohol;** *compare to* **methanol.**

evaporate: To change into a **vapor.**

excise: A tax on consumption of luxury or nonessential products, such as **alcohol** or **tobacco.** Often included in the price of the product. *Compare to* **tariff.**

executive functioning: A set of brain activities carried out in the **prefrontal cortex,** including inhibiting impulses, initiating tasks, planning, and self-monitoring. Working memory and cognitive flexibility are also part of executive functioning. It is impaired in **addiction, Alzheimer's disease, attention deficit hyperactivity disorder,** some brain injuries, and **schizophrenia.**

factory: In the past, a warehouse or establishment for merchants, often in a foreign country. There were large **opium** factories in Canton, China; in North American factories, furs were traded for **alcohol.**

fermentation: The transformation of **glucose** or fructose to **alcohol** and carbon dioxide, usually catalyzed by the **enzyme** zymase, which is found in **yeast.** The chemical formula is:**glucose** $(C_6H_{12}O_6) \rightarrow$ **ethanol** $(2C_2H_5OH)$ + carbon dioxide $(2CO_2)$ + energy

Fertile Crescent: A region in Asia, considered by some to be the cradle of civilization. Includes land within present-day Iran, Iraq, Israel, Jordan, Lebanon, Syria, and Turkey.

free base: The basic form of an **amine**, usually an alkaloid. When a proton is removed, the molecule becomes neutral and is thus "freed" from the anion to which it was previously bound. The free base form of some **drugs** is absorbed quickly. Free base **cocaine** is prepared by adding ammonia to the **salt, cocaine hydrochloride.** Free base **cocaine** is **smoked. Crack cocaine** is a form of **free base cocaine.** Free base **nicotine** is also usually prepared by adding ammonia to **nicotine salts.**

fruit: The soft, fleshy seed-associated structures of flowering plants that are sweet and edible in the raw state.

GABA (gamma-aminobutyric **acid**): an **amino acid** that is also the chief inhibitory **neurotransmitter** in the **brain.**

gene: A sequence of **DNA**, the basic unit of heredity that carries information to direct the activities of the **cell,** found on **chromosomes.**

gland: An organ that produces **hormones,** for example, the **pituitary.**

glucose: A **sugar** or **carbohydrate** used by **cells** as a source of energy and building other molecules, such as cellulose and **starch.** The chemical formula is $C_6H_{12}O_6$.

glutamate: An **amino acid** that is also the principal excitatory **neurotransmitter** in the brain. There are several glutamate **receptors,** one of which is the **NMDA receptor.**

grain: A small, hard, edible **fruit** or seed of **cereal** grasses, such as **barley,** corn, oats, rye, wheat. Grains differ from **fruit** in their hardness and the need to be germinated or cooked before they can be eaten. **Cereal** grains are the main source of food energy worldwide. **Fermentation** of some of these grains leads to **alcohol.**

gut: The stomach and small and large intestine.

heroin: Morphine with two **acetyl** groups added to it. It is highly lipid- or fat-soluble and passes easily through the **blood-brain barrier.** Once in the brain, it is metabolized into the active drug **morphine.** It can be injected, **smoked, snorted**, or taken in by mouth.

hippocampus: A large seahorse-shaped structure in the **limbic system** where memories are first formed. Sensitive to **alcohol.** The name comes from the Greek words for horse and sea monster.

homeostasis: Constancy of environment or of **cell** activity, or maintenance of equilibrium.

hormone: A molecule produced by **glands** that is secreted into the bloodstream to act on other organs.

hypothalamus: A small structure in the brain, below the **thalamus,** that controls the **pituitary gland;** regulates the body's **hormones,** temperature, fat **metabolism,** thirst, and hunger.

Inca: A group of Quechuan peoples, who ruled a large part of Andean South America from 1200 to 1600 CE. Also refers to the emperor of this group.

inebriation: Drunkenness.

inflammation: The process by which the body defends itself against infection or other injuries. White blood **cells** release **substances** that lead to heat, pain, redness, and swelling; sometimes caused by **tobacco smoke**; a risk factor for cancer.

intoxication: A condition of unstable emotions, lack of coordination, slurred speech, impaired judgment, sedation, or excitement; caused by **alcohol, cocaine,** and **opiates**.

lager: A type of beer made with bottom fermenting **yeast**, associated with the Germans. *See also* **ale.**

laudanum: Opium dissolved in **alcohol.** Classic example of the combination of **addictive drugs**. The name comes from the Latin word for praise.

limbic system: Found in mammals, a ring of interconnected structures deep in the brain involved in emotion, memory, and motivation. Includes the **amygdala, anterior cingulate cortex, hippocampus, hypothalamus, nucleus accumbens, prefrontal cortex,** and septal nuclei. The name comes from the Latin word for border.

liquor: A **distilled** beverage with high **alcohol** content.

local anesthesia: Analgesia in one area of the body, with no loss of consciousness. **Cocaine** was the first local anesthetic.

locus coeruleus: A blue **nucleus** in the **pons** in the **brain stem;** one of the places where **norepinephrine** is synthesized. **Opiates** depress activity in this part of the brain. The symptoms of **opiate** withdrawal are partly due to overactivity in this area and are experienced as anxiety. The name comes from the Latin words for place and blue.

madak: Mixture of **opium** and **tobacco, smoked** in seventeenth- and eighteenth-century China.

malt: Grains (usually **barley**) that have begun to germinate. They are then dried so that the germination stops. Used to make beer.

malt liquor: A **lager** of high **alcohol** content; too **alcoholic** to be sold as beer.

maltose: A double **glucose,** found in grains, especially **barley**, formed from **starch** by the **enzyme** diastase, which is active in germinating **barley.**

mash: Produced after **malt** is steeped in water and the **starch** is converted to **sugar** by **enzymes** within the **grains.**

Master Settlement Agreement: A 1998 agreement between the large **tobacco** companies and attorneys general of 48 states.

medulla oblongata: The lowest part of the **brain stem**, just above the spinal cord. The **vagus** originates here.

mercantilism: A European economic theory of the sixteenth to eighteenth centuries that suggested that governments should keep wages low, encourage exports, discourage imports, and use **tariffs** and subsidies to protect domestic industry, and that the role of colonies was to produce and export raw material to the mother country, where manufacture and industry were located. *See also* **triangular trade.**

mesencephalon: Midbrain. The name comes from the Greek words for middle and brain.

mesocortical pathway: A **dopamine** pathway reaching from the **midbrain** to the **cortex.**

mesolimbic pathway: A **dopamine** pathway reaching from the **midbrain** to the **nucleus accumbens, amygdala, hippocampus,** and **prefrontal cortex.** *See also* **reward system.**

metabolism: Chemical reactions in the body that break down food, **drugs,** or other **substances** to maintain the body's processes and help the body grow and reproduce. Most metabolism takes place in the liver, but some takes place in the **gut.**

methadone: Synthetic **opioid.** Full **agonist** at the **mu opiate receptor.** Used to treat pain and **opiate addiction.**

methanol: Wood **alcohol,** also known as methyl **alcohol.** In the past, often made as a by-product of **burning** of wood. Poisonous. The chemical formula is CH_3OH. *Compare to* **ethanol.**

midbrain: The top of the **brain stem,** also known as the **mesencephalon,** containing the **substantia nigra** and **ventral tegmental area.**

moonshine: What is smuggled at night by the light of the friendly moon. Often refers to whiskey produced illegally in the Appalachians.

morphine: The active ingredient of **opium;** it is an **analgesic** and **addicting alkaloid.**

mu opiate receptor: The **opiate receptor** subtype important in **opiate addiction.**

mucous membrane: The linings of body passages that come into contact with air or the outside environment, such as the nose and the **gut;** protected by **mucus.**

mucus: A thick, protective liquid produced by some **mucous membranes.** Mucus-producing **cells** in the lungs multiply and produce more mucus in response to irritants such as **tobacco smoke.**

NMDA: N-methyl-D-aspartate, a synthetic derivative of the **amino acid** aspartate.

NMDA receptor: A **glutamate receptor,** usually inactive, closed by magnesium. **Alcohol** inhibits NMDA receptor activity. Increased NMDA receptor activity, as in **alcohol** withdrawal, causes seizures and **cell** death. Part of memory formation. Also involved in **Alzheimer's disease, nicotine addiction,** and **schizophrenia.**

narcotic: a confusing word with related but separate meanings.

1. An **opiate.**
2. The Harrison Narcotics Act of 1914 used the word in this sense: any **addictive drug,** including **opiates** and **cocaine.**

3. Any **drug** that that reduces pain and induces sleep or stupor.

nerve: A bundle of **axons** found in the **peripheral nervous system.**

nervous system: The brain, spinal cord, and **peripheral nervous system.**

neuron: A specialized kind of **cell,** also known as **nerve cell,** that processes information. Neurons receive messages or information at their **dendrites** and send information along an **axon** to other neurons, muscle tissue, or **glands.** Sensory neurons transmit information to the brain. Motor neurons transmit information from the spinal cord or brain to muscles and **glands.**

neurotransmitter: One of about 100 types of chemicals that carry information across **synapses;** molecules bind to **receptors.**

nicotine: An **alkaloid** produced by the leaves of the **tobacco** plant, *Nicotinia,* perhaps acting as a natural insecticide. Nicotine mimics **acetylcholine** at **presynaptic acetylcholinergic nicotinic receptors,** exciting **dopaminergic neurons** in the brain's **reward system.** It is **addictive,** whether consumed by **smoking,** chewing, or **snorting.**

nicotinic acetylcholine receptors: A type of **acetylcholine receptor** that responds to **nicotine.**

norepinephrine: Also known as noradrenaline. Norepinephrine is **epinephrine** without a radical group—hence the "no r" in the front of the word. **Hormone** and also a **neurotransmitter** in the **central** and **sympathetic nervous system.**

nucleus:

1. The center of every **cell** containing **genetic** material.
2. A group of **cell** bodies of **neurons** in the **central nervous system.** An example is the **nucleus accumbens.**

nucleus accumbens: A **nucleus** in the **limbic system;** part of the **basal ganglia.** It receives **dopamine** input from the **ventral tegmental area.** Most **neurons** in this area produce **GABA.** Part of the **reward system** and therefore important in **addiction.**

opiate: Related to **opium.** Strictly speaking, refers only to natural **substances** that come from **opium.** Sometimes used interchangeably with **opioid.**

opiate receptors: There are three subtypes—**mu,** delta, and kappa—to which **opiates** bind.

opioid: A substance that acts on the **opiate receptor.** Sometimes used interchangeably with **opiate.** Some opioids, such as **methadone,** are synthetic, that is, made in a laboratory. Some, such as **buprenorphine,** are semisynthetic in that they are based on an **opiate.**

opioid peptide: A **neurotransmitter** produced by the human body involved in mood, brain **reward systems,** and **pituitary gland hormone** release.

opium: Natural substance produced by the unripe seed capsule of the opium poppy, *Papaver somniferum.*

parasympathetic system: Part of the **autonomic system** that acts in opposition to the **sympathetic system** and calms the body. The main **neurotransmitter** is **acetylcholine.** This system leads to "rest and digest." Blood pressure goes down, pupils constrict, and activity in the **gut** increases.

Parkinson's disease: A degenerative disease caused by loss of **dopamine** in the **substantia nigra;** leads to slow movements, tremors, rigidity, and loss of motivation.

pasteurization: Heating a beverage, such as milk or beer, to kill microorganisms that could cause disease, spoilage, or undesired **fermentation.**

peptide: A short sequence of **amino acids.**

peripheral nervous system: All parts of the **nervous system** outside of the brain and spinal cord; consists of the **somatic** and **autonomic nervous systems.**

pituitary gland: Pea-sized "master **gland**" that releases **hormones** that regulate body activities or stimulate other **glands** to release **hormones.**

polycyclic aromatic hydrocarbons: Group of chemicals made up of carbon and hydrogen atoms connected in ring-like forms; often formed during burning of coal, oil, **tobacco,** or other **substances.** Some may lead to cancer.

pons: The middle of the **brain stem;** where the **locus coeruleus** is located.

postsynaptic neuron: A **neuron** that receives a message from a **presynaptic neuron.**

postsynaptic receptor: A **receptor** located on a **postsynaptic neuron.**

prefrontal cortex: The most anterior or forward part of the **cerebral cortex.** The part of the brain where we organize, plan, or carry out **"executive functioning."** Thought to be impaired in **addiction, attention deficit hyperactivity disorder,** and **schizophrenia.**

presynaptic neuron: A **neuron** that sends a message to a **postsynaptic neuron.**

prohibition: Banning of goods or services; sometimes decreases consumption and almost always a boon to criminals. When capitalized (Prohibition), refers to the ban placed on sale, manufacture, and transportation of **alcohol** in the United States from 1919 to 1933.

protein: A molecule made up of **amino acids;** serves as a building block or an **enzyme;** can be **burned** for energy.

psychoactive: Affecting the mind.

receptors:

1. **Protein** molecules that "recognize" other molecules and attach to them, sometimes compared to a key opening a lock, usually located in the **cell membrane** of a **gland, a** muscle cell, or **neuron.** In the **nervous system,** they recognize **neurotransmitters** (released from the **axon** of another **neuron**), bind them, and then act on the message.

2. Part of a sensory **neuron** that responds to stimuli such as light, movement, sound, or pain.

reticular activating system: An area of **neurons** in the **brain stem** that controls arousal or wakefulness; sensitive to **opiates.**

reuptake: Neurotransmitters are sometimes taken back from the **synapse** into the **axon** of the **neuron** from which they came. **Cocaine** prevents **dopamine reuptake,** and this prolongs the action of the **dopamine** in the **synapse.**

reward system: A theoretical system, pathway, or circuit reaching from the **ventral tegmental area** in the **midbrain** to the **nucleus accumbens** to the **prefrontal cortex.** Rapidly increasing **dopamine** levels in the reward system are thought to be important in **addiction.**

salt: In chemistry, a compound that is formed from the reaction of an **acid** and **base. Cocaine hydrochloride** is a salt.

schizophrenia: A poorly understood chronic psychiatric disorder in which the person may hear voices, have strange thoughts, and have difficulty with **executive functioning** and interpersonal relationships. People with schizophrenia have high rates of **substance abuse,** possibly as a way of treating their symptoms.

sensitization: Increase in number and sensitivity of **receptors.**

serotonin: A **neurotransmitter** primarily found in the **gut**; also involved in the action of platelets. Many antidepressants are serotonin **reuptake** inhibitors. Also involved in the activity of psychedelic drugs.

smoke: *noun*, the gaseous products of **burning**, such as **burning tobacco**; *verb*, to inhale smoke or **vaporized substances,** such as **crack cocaine** or **opium.**

snort: Common method of using powdered **cocaine, heroin,** or **tobacco.** The powder is sniffed and is absorbed through the **mucous membranes** lining the **turbinates** of the nose.

snuff: Ground up **tobacco** leaves, sniffed or **snorted.**

somatic nervous system: Part of the **peripheral nervous system** to do with sensation and control of our muscles. The **neurotransmitter** is **acetylcholine.**

speedball: Mixture of **heroin** and **cocaine.**

starch: Carbohydrate found in plants, often white and tasteless, used as an energy source, made up of **glucose** units joined together.

stimulus: A change in environment that leads to a response.

substance: In this book, usually refers to **alcohol, cocaine, nicotine,** or **opiates.** Also refers to matter.

substance abuse: Harmful use of a **substance.**

substantia nigra: Part of the **midbrain,** deeply pigmented with melanin so that it appears black. Affected in **Parkinson's disease.** The name comes from the Latin word for black.

sucrose: Table **sugar.** Formed of fructose and **glucose.** A white crystalline **carbohydrate.** The chemical formula is $C_{12}H_{22}O_{11}$.

sugar: Dextrose, **glucose**, or **sucrose**. Sugars are sweet and crystalline.

sympathetic system: Part of the **autonomic system** that acts in opposition to the **parasympathetic system** and gets the body ready for action. This system leads to "fight or flight." Blood pressure goes up, pupils dilate, and activity in the **gut** stops. This system is active in **opiate withdrawal.**

synapse: A junction between two **neurons**, **neuron** and muscle, or **neuron** and **gland.** Most of these junctions are chemical; some are electrical. There are 100 to 500 trillion synapses in the human brain.

synaptic cleft or gap: A space measuring about a millionth of an inch between two **neurons,** or between **neuron** and muscle or **gland.**

synaptic plasticity: A change in number of **synapses** involved in learning and memory.

tar: Thick, black, sticky matter released from the decomposition of a complex **substance,** such as wood or coal, by heating it in the absence of air. It also forms when **tobacco burns.**

tariff: A government tax on imports or exports; used to help the country's own manufacturers. *Compare to* **excise.**

temperance: Moderation or avoidance of excess. Also the social/political/moral movement against **alcohol.** Many have commented on this movement's lack of moderation at times.

teratogen: A **substance** that causes malformation of an unborn baby. An example is **alcohol.**

thalamus: The relay center of the brain, located just above the **brain stem.** All incoming (sensory) and outgoing (motor) signals pass through this brain structure.

tobacco:

1. Plant in the genus *Nicotinia.*
2. Product of the leaf of the plant. When **cured,** it can be **burned** and **smoked,** leading to the inhalation of several thousand chemicals, including **nicotine, tars,** and many other **substances,** some of which are still unknown. It can also be chewed or **snorted** as **snuff.**

tolerance: Exposure to a **drug** causes a smaller response over time, particularly in the setting of **addiction.** This may lead to an increase in the dose of the **drug.** It is one of the ways in which the **central nervous system** maintains **homeostasis,** is the opposite of **sensitization,** and is sometimes referred to as desensitization.

triangular trade: Trade between three regions; usually depends on complicated trade agreements and the exportation of raw materials from underdeveloped to developed countries. *See also* **mercantilism.**

turbinates: The bones covered with **mucous membrane** in the nose. Inspired air is heated, filtered, and humidified as it passes over the turbinates on its way to the **alveoli.**

vagus nerve: The long thick tenth cranial **nerve** descending from the **medulla oblongata** to heart, lungs, and **gut**. It is part of the **parasympathetic** branch of the **autonomic nervous system.** The name comes from the Latin word for wandering.

vapor, vaporization: The heating of a **substance** so that it evaporates, that is, changes into a vapor, its gaseous state. This is in contrast to **burning,** in which many different by-products are formed. When people **smoke crack cocaine, free base cocaine,** or **opium,** they are **smoking** a vapor.

ventral tegmental area: A part of the **midbrain;** sends messages, using **dopamine**, to the **nucleus accumbens** and **prefrontal cortex;** involved in the **reward system** and **addiction.**

vesicles: Sacs storing **neurotransmitters** at the end or terminal of **axons.**

vitalism: The theory that there is something different or vital to living things, separate from physics or chemistry.

withdrawal: Physical and/or psychological distress when a **substance** is withdrawn, particularly in the setting of **addiction.** The best known examples are **alcohol** withdrawal in which increased **NMDA** activity leads to seizures and **opiate** withdrawal, which is due in part to increased **norepinephrine** in the **locus coeruleus** and often characterized as "cold turkey"—goose flesh, diarrhea, nose running, and malaise. Usually withdrawal symptoms are the opposite of those produced by the **substance.**

yeast: Single-**celled** microorganisms belonging to the kingdom of fungi. Despite their small size and simplicity, these microorganisms have a large number of **enzymes.** Important in **fermentation** and the formation of **alcohol.**

Index

About the Author

FRANCES R. FRANKENBURG, MD, is Professor of Psychiatry at the Boston University School of Medicine, lecturer in psychiatry at Harvard Medical School, and adjunct Clinical Professor at Massachusetts College of Pharmacy and Health Sciences. She is chief of inpatient and consultation-liaison psychiatry at the Edith Nourse Rogers Memorial Veterans Administration Medical Center in Bedford, Massachusetts, where she is also responsible for medical student education. She has published widely in the field of psychiatry and has published a book about the discovery of vitamins.

DATE DUE

PRINTED IN U.S.A.